Neurocircuitry of the Retina
A Cajal Memorial

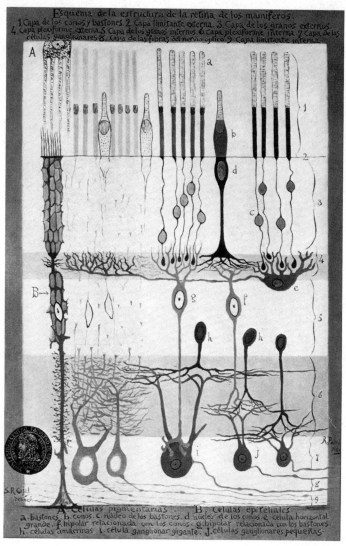

Esquema de la estructura de la retina de los mamíferos.
1 Capa de los conos y bastones. 2. Capa limitante externa. 3. Capa de los granos externos.
4. Capa plexiforme externa. 5 Capa de los granos internos. 6. capa plexiforme interna. 7 Capa de las células ganglionares 8. Capa de las fibras del nervio óptico. 9 Capa limitante interna.

S.R Cajal
delineó

A. Células pigmentarias. B. Células epiteliales.
a. bastones. b. conos. c. núcleo de los bastones. d núcleo de los conos. e. célula horizontal grande. f. bipolar relacionada con los conos. g. bipolar relacionada con los bastones. h. células amacrinas. i. célula ganglionar gigante. J. células ganglionares pequeñas.

La retina fue uno de los órganos en los que Cajal profundizó más en sus investigaciones, haciendo descubrimientos definitivos. Sus estudios de histología comparada de la retina son clásicos e indispensables para el que quiera penetrar en el conocimiento de este apasionante tema. Sus descubrimientos en este órgano, como decimos, son numerosos (sobre las bipolares, sobre las amacrinas, etc.). Además debemos a Cajal la sistematización de la retina, que en vertebrados superiores se estratifica en diez clásicas capas descritas por él. Sus interpretaciones sobre el significado del entrecruzamiento de las fibras del quiasma (total o parcial según la especie zoológica) han quedado como un ejemplo de descubrimiento científico genial.

LUIS ZAMORANO
Catedrático de Histología y Embriología
Universidad Complutense, Madrid

Neurocircuitry of the Retina
A Cajal Memorial

Edited by

Antonio Gallego, M.D.

Universidad Complutense
Instituto de Investigaciones Oftalmologicas
Facultad de Medicina
Madrid, Spain

and

Peter Gouras, M.D.

Columbia University
Department of Ophthalmology
College of Physicians and Surgeons
New York, New York

Elsevier
New York • Amsterdam • Oxford

This book has been registered with the Copyright Clearance Center, Inc.
For further information, please contact the Copyright Clearance Center,
Salem, Massachusetts.

Published by:

Elsevier Science Publishing Co., Inc.
52 Vanderbilt Avenue, New York, New York 10017

Sole distributors outside the United States and Canada:
Elsevier Science Publishers B.V.
P.O. Box 211, 1000 AE Amsterdam, the Netherlands

Library of Congress Cataloging in Publication Data

Main entry under title:

Neurocircuitry of the retina.

Proceedings of a symposium held Oct. 5, 1984, in Alicante, Spain, in conjunction with
the 6th International Congress of Eye Research; held in commemoration of Santiago
Ramón y Cajal.
Includes index.
1. Retina — Congresses. 2. Neural circuitry — Congresses. 3. Neural transmission —
Congresses. 4. Ramón y Cajal, Santiago, 1852-1934 — Congresses. I. Gallego, Antonio. II.
Gouras, P. III. Ramón y Cajal, Santiago, 1852-1934. IV. International Congress of Eye
Research (6th: 1984: Alicante, Spain) [DNLM: 1. Retina — cytology — congresses.
WW270N494 1984
QP479.N48 1985   596'.01823   85-16306
ISBN 0-444-00999-X

English translation of frontispiece quotation from Luis Zamorano:

The retina is one of the organs which Cajal studied intensively and in which he
made many important discoveries. His studies of the comparative histology of the
retina are classic and indispensable to anyone who wishes to understand this
fascinating field. His retinal discoveries are numerous (about the bipolar cells, the
amacrine cells, etc). We are also indebted to Cajal for the classification of the retinas
of vertebrates into ten well defined layers. His interpretation of the significance of
the crossing of the optic nerve fibers in the optic chiasm (either total or partial
according to zoological species) has remained as an example of the scientific
discovery of a genius.

Manufactured in the United States of America

CONTENTS

FRONTISPIECE... ii

FOREWORD... vii

PARTICIPANTS... ix

J.E. Dowling, E.M. Lasater and L.H.Y. Young, Some New
Approaches and Directions in Retinal Research...........................1

R.A. Normann, I. Perlman and H. Kolb, Chromatic Interactions
Between Cones of Differing Spectral Classes: Anatomical and
Electrophysiological Studies in Turtle..................................19

G. Falk, The Transmission of Rod Signals to Horizontal
and Bipolar Cells..34

M. Slaughter and R.F. Miller, The Role of Glutamate Receptors
in Information Processing in the Distal Retina.........................51

M. Piccolino, P. Witkovsky, J. Neyton, H. M. Gerschenfeld and
C. Trimarchi, Modulation of Gap Junction Permeability by
Dopamine and GABA in the Network of Horizontal Cells of the
Turtle Retina..66

K. Negishi, T. Teranishi and S. Kato, Dopaminergic Interplexiform Cells and Their Regulatory Function for Spatial
Properties of Horizontal Cells in the Fish Retina.....................77

A. Kaneko and M. Tachibana and T. Ohtsuka, GABA Sensitivity in
Solitary Turtle Cones: Evidence for the Feedback Pathway from
Horizontal Cells to Cones...89

M.W. Hankins, J.S. Rowe and K.H. Ruddock, Properties of Amino
Acid Binding Sites on Horizontal Cells Determined by Electrophysiological Studies on the Isolated Roach Retina....................99

R. Nelson, T. Lynn, A. Dickinson-Nelson and H. Kolb,
Spectral Mechanisms in Cat Horizontal Cells..........................109

A. Gallego, Advances in Horizontal Cell Terminology
Since Cajal..122

K.-I. Naka and H. Sakai Functional Morphology of the Outer
Plexiform Layer..141

A. Bruun, B. Ehinger and K. Tornqvist, Neurotransmitters
in the Retina of the Mudpuppy, Necturus Maculosus......................152

S. Yazulla, C.L. Zucker, J.L. Mosinger, K.M. Studholme,
Pyriform Amacrine Cells in the Goldfish Retina: An EM Immuno-
cytochemical/Autoradiographical Study.................................161

W.K. Stell, Putative Peptide Transmitters, Amacrine Cell
Diversity and Function in the Inner Plexiform Layer...................171

M.B.A. Djamgoz, J.E.G. Downing, E. Wagner, H.-J. Wagner
and I. Zeutzius, Functional Organization of Amacrine
Cells in the Teleost Fish Retina.....................................188

N.N. Osborne, D.W. Beaton and S. Patel, The Serotonin-
Accumulating Cells in the Rabbit Retina..............................205

H. Kolb and R. Nelson, Functional Neurocircuitry of
Amacrine Cells in the Cat Retina.....................................215

P. Gouras and H.U. Evers, The Neurocircuitry of
Primate Retina...233

R. Weiler, Afferent and Efferent Peptidergic Pathways in
the Turtle Retina..245

H. Ikeda and J. Robbins, Postnatal Development of GABA
and Glycine Actions on the Surround Inhibition of Cat
Retinal Ganglion Cells in the Area Centralis.........................257

S. Vallerga and G.M. Ratto, Are Dendritic Beads Related to
Synaptic Loci..265

Subject Index..270

FOREWORD

This memorial symposium took place in Alicante, Spain on October 5, 1984 in conjunction with the 6th International Congress of Eye Research. It was held in commemoration of the 50th anniversary of the death of the great Spanish neurobiologist, Santiago Ramon Y Cajal (1852-1934). Cajal was 82 years old at the time of his death. Even at the end, he is described by the Canadian neurosurgeon Wilder Penfield in a preface to the English edition of Cajal's last book Neuronismo o Reticularismo that even though feeble from age "there burned within him the boundless enthusiasm of the born explorer and his eyes blazed through his shaggy brows" as he talked to his interviewer. His enthusiasm was understandable when one reads his autobiography Recuerdos de Mi Vida. His research was to him a delicious rapture, an irresistable enchantment. He writes that he pursued the delicate forms of nerve cells as an entomologist might pursue brightly colored butterflies in a garden. Cajal's garden was the brain and within its chambers he describes seeing hidden islands and virginal forms which seemed to be awaiting since the beginning of the world for a worthy contemplator of their beauty. Cajal was an extraordinary explorer of our inner universe, the mind. He pursued this quest not only with love but with enormous pride, dedication and truth.

Cajal devoted considerable time to understanding the neurocircuitry of the retina. His classic La Retine des Vertebres which appeared in La Cellule in 1892 was translated two years later into German by Richard Greeff and has since been translated into English simultaneously by Sylvia A. Thorpe and Mitchell Glickstein in 1972 and by Deborah Maguire and Robert W. Rodieck in 1973. The retina is part of the central nervous system and shares all of the complexity of the brain but because it directly faces the external visual world it provides more of a clue to its function than most other neural circuits. As Cajal must have realized the secret of the brain resides in its circuitry. He was fascinated by what he found with the light microscope. Imagine what his delight would have been with the electronmicroscope, the microelectrode and the dawning of electronic computer analogues of the circuits we are discovering today. Cajal would have been an enraptured participant of this symposium in his honor and in his native land.

Peter Gouras   Antonio Gallego
Columbia University   University of Madrid

PARTICIPANTS

M.B.A. Djamgoz (188) Cellular Neurobiology Laboratory, Imperial College, London, England

J.E. Dowling (1) Department of Cellular and Developmental Biology, Harvard University, Cambridge, Massachusetts

B. Ehinger (152) Department of Ophthalmology, University of Lund, Lund, Sweden

G. Falk (34) Biophysics Unit, Department of Physiology, University College, London WC1E 6BT England

A. Gallego (122) Instituto de Investigaciones Oftalmologicas, Universidad Complutense, Madrid, Spain

P. Gouras (233) Columbia University, New York, N. Y.

H. Ikeda (257) Vision Research Unit of Sherrington School, The Rayne Institute, St. Thomas' Hospital, London, England

A. Kaneko (89) National Institute for Physiological Sciences, Okazaki, Japan

H. Kolb (215) Physiology Department, University of Utah, Salt Lake City, Utah

K.-I. Naka (141) National Institute for Basic Biology, Okazaki, Japan 444

K. Negishi (77) Department of Neurophysiology, Neuroinformation Research Institute (NIRI), University of Kanazawa School of Medicine, Ishikawa, Japan

R.A. Normann (19) University of Utah, Salt Lake City, Utah

R. Nelson (109) Laboratory of Neurophysiology, National Institute of Neurological and Communicative Disorders and Stroke, Bethesda, Maryland

N. N. Osborne (205) Nuffield Laboratory of Ophthalmology, University of Oxford, Oxford, England

M. Piccolino (66) Instituto di Neurofisiologia del C.N.R., Pisa, Italy

K.H. Ruddock (99) Imperial College, London, England

M. Slaughter (51) Department of Biophysical Sciences, State University of New York, Buffalo, N. Y.

W.K. Stell (171) University of Calgary, Department of Anatomy, Calgary, Alberta, Canada

S. Vallerga (264) Instituto di Cibernetica e Biofisica del C.N.R., Camogli, Italy

R. Weiler (244) Zoological Institute, University of Munich, Munich, West Germany

S. Yazulla (161) Department of Neurobiology and Behavior, State University of New York, Stony Brook, N. Y.

Neurocircuitry of the Retina
A Cajal Memorial

Some New Approaches and Directions in Retinal Research

John E. Dowling, Eric M. Lasater, Lucy H. Y. Young
Department of Cellular and Developmental Biology
Harvard University
Cambridge, Massachusetts 02138

Several new and powerful techniques have recently been introduced into neurobiology that promise to enhance significantly our understanding of neuronal cell structure, function and chemistry. Included among these are 1) primary culturing of adult neurons, 2) patch-clamping of neurons to record membrane currents and potentials, and 3) the production of monoclonal antibodies specific to neuronal cell surfaces. We are using all three techniques in our laboratory and here we review some of these experiments, emphasizing the kinds of information these approaches provide.

The experiments to be described relate to the horizontal cells of teleost fish, which are particularly large and have been a favorite source for study since Gunnar Svaetichin first recorded from them some 30 years ago (Svaetichin, 1953; Svaetichin and MacNichol, 1958). A number of groups, including our own, have described short term (up to 7-14 days) primary culturing of horizontal cells from carp, goldfish and skate (Tachibana, 1981; Lasater and Dowling, 1982; Shingai and Christensen, 1983; Lasater, Dowling and Ripps, 1984). We have recently found that the horizontal cells from the white perch (Roccus americana) retina cultured particularly well (Dowling et al, submitted; Lasater and Dowling 1985) and we begin by describing horizontal cells in primary cultures from this animal.

Horizontal Cells in Culture
        The retina of the white perch is a typical teleost retina with numerous rods, large single and double cones and four layers of horizontal cells. To isolate cells, retinas are incubated in L-15 tissue culture medium containing 1.7 mg/ml papain activated with L-cysteine for 40 minutes (Lasater and Dowling, 1982). After washing in fresh L-15, the retina is broken apart by trituration with Pasteur pipettes. Following the settling of cells in the culture dishes (2-4 hrs), 4 types of horizontal cells can be distinguished (Fig. 1). The type H1 and H2 cells appear similar to the H1 and H2 horizontal cells of the pikeperch retina (Hassin, 1979); they are distally positioned in the retina and are probably both cone-related cells. The H3 cell is likely to be a cone-related cell while type H4 may be a cone or rod-related horizontal cell.

An obvious question is how much alteration occurs to a horizontal cell when it is isolated from the retina. Figure 2 shows a freshly isolated H2 cell that looks extraordinarily similar to an H2 cell stained in the intact retina. We have also observed that freshly isolated H1 and H3 cells in culture closely resemble H1 and H3 cells in the intact retina. We have not observed sufficient number of H4 cells in the intact retina to judge whether these cells are morphologically similar to isolated H4 cells and we have no information concerning fine structural or molecular changes that may occur in any of these cells when they are isolated.

With time in culture the morphology of the horizontal cells changes. After 6-12 hours in culture, all horizontal cell types tend to withdraw their finer processes and to round up partially. Horizontal cells from other species have also been observed to undergo such shape changes in culture (Lasater and Dowling, 1982; Lasater, Dowling and Ripps, 1984). There is variation in the extent that individual perch horizontal cells

Neurocircuitry of the Retina, A Cajal Memorial
A. Gallego and P. Gouras, Editors

2

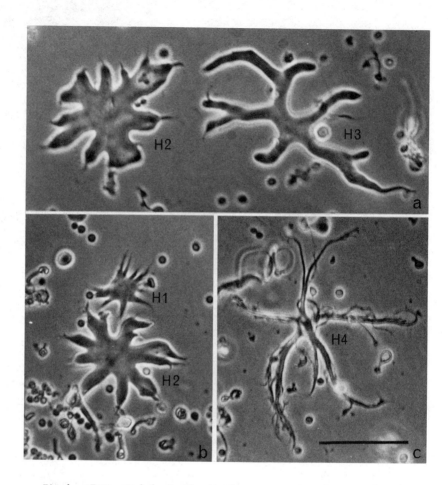

Fig 1. Four morphologically distinct types of horizontal cells
(H1-H4) are observed in cultures of the white perch retina. The
four types appear to correspond to the four layers of horizontal
cells typically seen in radial sections of this retina. The H1
cells are most distally positioned while the H2 cells are found in
the second layer. The H3 and H4 cells are more proximally
located. The H1, H2, and H3 cells are likely to be cone
horizontal cells while the H4 cell may be a rod horizontal cell.
Calibration bar = 50 μm.

change in shape, but despite the alteration and variation in cell
morphology after a few days in culture, it is still possible to identify
the four cell types (see, for example, Fig. 4). After 2-4 days in
culture, the horizontal begin to extend new fine processes outward,
particularly from preexisting processes (Fig. 3a and b). By 6-8 days, the
new processes are very prominent and they continue to grow, becoming
indistinguishable from the processes from which they derive. Process
growth continues over time, not only by the horizontal cells, but by other

3

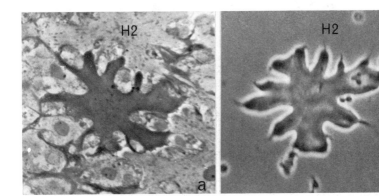

Fig. 2. Freshly isolated white perch horizontal cells closely resemble in morphology their counterparts in the intact retina. a) An H2 cell non-specifically stained in an immunoperoxidase stained preparation. b) A freshly isolated H2 cell observed in culture. This cell is the H2 cell illustrated in Fig. 1a.

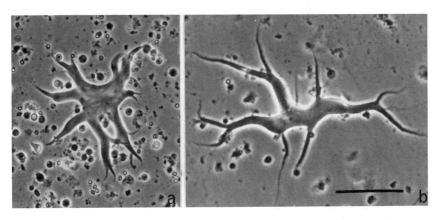

Fig. 3. Process outgrowth from white perch retinal cells in culture. a) An H1 cell 6 days in culture; b) An H2 cell 15 days in culture. Bar = 50 μm.

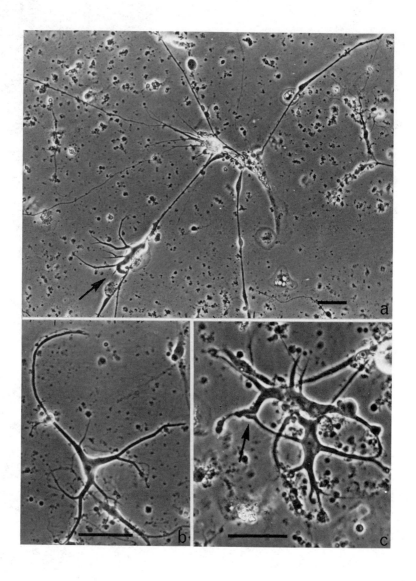

Fig. 4. Longer term retinal cell cultures. A low power micrograph showing extensive process growth by retinal cells 18 days in culture. The arrow indicates a horizontal cell which is intertwined with a cell that appears glial in origin; b) An isolated horizontal cell 18 days in culture; c) Two intertwined cells, believed to be horizontal cells that have been in culture 18 days. The arrow indicates an obvious contact made by one cell onto the other. See text. Bars = 50 μm.

cells, both neuronal and glial. After 14-21 days in culture (Fig. 4a & b) processes several hundreds of micrometers long are frequently seen and it is often difficult to recognize types of cells or even whether a cell is neuronal or glial. Very often the cell processes appear intertwined and obvious contacts between cells are observed (arrow Fig. 4c). These latter observations raise the interesting question of whether neurons in culture make functional synaptic connections. We have succeeded in showing that electrical coupling occurs between horizontal cells in short term (1-7 days) culture (see below) but we think it likely that this coupling reflects electrical junctions formed in vivo and that survived the isolation process.

Electrical Coupling Between Cultured Horizontal Cells

Virtually all of our physiological experiments on cultured horizontal cells have so far involved cells isolated for only 1-7 days. For recording potentials and current flow across the membrane, we have found whole cell patch clamping to be ideal (Neher et al., 1978; Sakmann and Neher, 1983). The perch cells in culture tend to be flat, which makes intracellular recording with conventional micropipettes difficult. With patch-clamp pipettes, which remain on the surface of the cell and have large tips and low resistances, it is relatively easy to voltage-clamp and current-clamp the cells, as well as to pass large currents and small molecules into them.

We have recently employed whole-cell patch clamping on cultured white perch horizontal cells to test for electrical coupling between pairs of these cells and to examine the effects of dopamine on this coupling. We briefly describe these experiments to illustrate the power of this recording method for such investigations as well as to emphasize the value of employing cells in culture to examine certain questions.

In white perch cell cultures of relatively high density, pairs of cells that overlap to some extent are quite frequently seen (Fig. 5). The overlapping cells may be of the same type or of different type. Occasionally three or more overlapping cells are observed. Most of our observations so far have been on pairs of H2 or H3 cells (Fig. 5). To record from these cells, patch-electrodes with relatively large tip diameters (i.e. resistances of 5-8 mΩ) were placed on both cells of a pair. Gentle suction was applied to the interior of the pipette to form a gigohm-seal between electrode and cell membrane. Following a short (30 second) wait for equilibration purposes, stronger suction was applied to break through the cell membrane and to establish intracellular contact. In a typical experiment, one cell was voltage-clamped and the other current clamped. Current pulses were passed into the voltage-clamped driver cell to shift the membrane potential by 20mV. Potential changes were monitored in the current-clamped follower cell to assess the extent of coupling.

The left side of Fig. 6a shows the results of an experiment with a pair of H2 cells in which small current pulses were applied to the driver cell that shifted the membrane potential by 10 mV. A potential change of nearly 10 mV occurred in the follower cell, indicating that the two cells were tightly coupled. Reversing the polarity of the current pulses did not alter the amplitude of the potential shifts observed in the follower cell. On the right hand side of Fig. 6a, a larger current pulse was injected into the driver cell that shifted the holding potential by 20 mV. A potential of 19.0 mV was recorded in the follower cell. The coupling coefficient is defined as the ratio of the voltage recorded in the follower cell divided by the voltage shift occurring in the driver cell

6

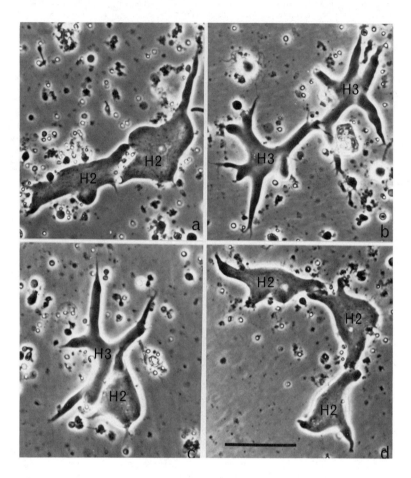

Fig. 5. Overlapping horizontal cells in culture. a) Pair of type H2
cells; b) Pair of type H3 cells; c) Pair consisting of a type H2 (right)
and a type H3 cell; d) Three overlapping type H2 cells. In short term
culture (1-5 days) the type H2 cells have only a few short blunt processes
while the type H3 cells typically have 4-6 elongated processes.
Bar = 50 μm.

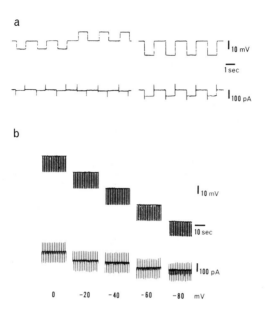

Fig. 6. Coupling between a pair of cultured H2 cells. a) The lower traces show current records from the voltage-clamped driver cell, while upper records show voltage records from the current-clamped follower cell. Current pulses were applied to the driver cell to shift the membrane potential by 10 mV (left record) or 20mV (right record). Since the cells were tightly-coupled, the shift in potential in the follower cell was close to that induced by the current pulses in the driver cell. In this case, the coupling coefficient (voltage shift recorded in follower cell/voltage shift induced in driver cell) was 0.95. Note that a similar voltage change was induced in the follower cell by both inward, hyperpolarizing and outward, depolarizing pulses (left record). The nonlinear increase in the amount of current needed into the driver cell to induce a doubling of the change in membrane potential (compare lower traces, left and right records), was caused by the activation of a voltage sensitive conductance (anomolous rectifier) in the driver cell when the membrane potential was shifted from -60 to -80 mV. b) Coupling between horizontal cell pairs at various membrane voltages. The holding potential of the driver cell (bottom trace) was varied between 0 and -80 mV while current pulses were injected into the driver cell that hyperpolarized the cell by -20 mV. The voltage-pulses recorded in the follower cell (top) varied between 18.5 and 19.5 mV showing that at all membrane potentials, the cells remained well-coupled. Note the resting potential of the follower cell varied in concert with changes in the holding potential of the driver cell. The current trace baseline, as well as the size of the injected current pulses, varied in the driver cell at the various holding potentials, because of the activation of both steady and transient voltage-sensitive conductances. The brief deflections at the beginning and end of the current pulses represent capacitative transients in this and the following figures.

(Harris et al., 1983); for this pair of cells it was 0.95, a typical result. In a sample of 89 overlapping pairs of cells of the same type (53 type H2's, 24 type H3's, 9 type H1's and 3 type H4's), 93% showed evidence of coupling and of these 71% had coupling coefficients of 0.6 or better. On the other hand, of 16 pairs of overlapping cells of different types (i.e. Fig. 5c) 81% showed no evidence of coupling, and of the three that showed coupling, it was very weak. In one instance, a coupling coefficient was determined for three overlapping H2 cells (Fig. 5d). The electrodes were positioned on the two end cells, and current pulses were passed through the three cells. The coupling coefficient in this instance was found to be 0.9.

Fig. 6b shows that the coupling between horizontal cells in culture does not depend on the potential of the coupled cells. In this experiment, the holding potential of the driver cell was varied between 0 and -80 mV, while current pulses were applied that transiently shifted the membrane voltage by -20 mV. Because of the tight coupling between the cells, the steady membrane potential of the follower cell altered in concert with the shift of the holding potential in the driver cell (upper traces). However, the hyperpolarizing potentials recorded in the follower cells were between 18.5 and 19.5 mV regardless of the membrane potential. The lower traces show that the amount of current required to shift the membrane potential 20 mV in the driver cell varied somewhat because of voltage-sensitive conductances activated at the various holding potentials (Tachibana, 1983). The differences in baseline level of the current traces also reflect the activation of voltage-sensitive conductances.

To determine the resistance and conductance of the junctions between well-coupled cells (i.e. with coupling coefficient of 0.9), pulses were applied to the current-clamped cell in four experiments and the amount of current passing into the voltage-clamped cell measured. The resistances of these junctions were determined to be 42, 26, 35 and 45 megohms, indicating junctional conductances of 238, 384, 285, and 200 nanosiemens respectively. Typical input resistances of single isolated perch horizontal cells determined by whole cell patch clamping ranged between 500 and 1,000 megohms. Thus the resistances of the junctions is less than 15% of the input resistance of the cells, consistent with coupling ratios of 0.9 for these pairs of horizontal cells.

It has been proposed that dopamine, via cyclic AMP, modulates electrical coupling between horizontal cells (Teranishi et al., 1983; Cohen and Dowling, 1983; Piccolino et al., 1984) and we have begun to test this hypothesis. We have observed that the application of short pulses (0.5 - 1 sec) of Ringer's containing dopamine to coupled cells significantly altered the strength of coupling (Fig. 7). Typically, a change in coupling was observed within 10-15 seconds after application of the drug, peak effects occurred after 2-4 minutes, and recovery required an additional 5-10 minutes. After the application of pulses of Ringers containing relatively high concentrations of dopamine (100 - 200 μM), the coupling coefficient typically decreased by up to 90% (i.e. to 0.10). As the coupling decreased, the driver cell was no longer able to maintain the follower cell at the holding potential and the membrane potential of the follower cell hyperpolarized to approximately -80 mV, the usual resting potential of horizontal cells in culture. During recovery, the coupling coefficient increased to its former value and the resting potential of the follower cell depolarized to the holding potential of -60 mV.

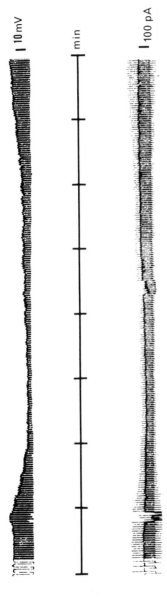

Dopamine 200 µM

Fig. 7. Effects of dopamine on cell coupling. A 1 sec pulse of Ringer's containing 200 µM dopamine was applied to the pair of H2 cells at the arrow. Coupling began to decrease after about 15 sec as shown by the smaller voltage changes observed in the follower cell. As uncoupling proceeded, the membrane potential of the follower cell hyperpolarized from −60 mV, the holding potential of the driver cell, to approximately −78 mV. Also the amount of current flowing into the driver cell decreased as uncoupling proceeded because of the increase in the cell's input resistance. After about 2 min, the cells were maximally uncoupled and the coupling coefficient was less than 0.15. The coupling gradually recovered over the next 5–6 min. A movement artifact is seen in both traces at the time of dopamine application.

Another effect of the uncoupling action of dopamine is seen in the current record of the driver cell (Fig. 7). As uncoupling occurred, the current required to shift the membrane potential -20 mV decreased, reflecting the increased input resistance of the cell, i.e. increased junctional resistance. When pulses of Ringer's containing lower concentrations of dopamine were applied (25 or 50 uM), the effects on coupling were correspondingly decreased, suggesting that the uncoupling response to dopamine was graded. In all, we observed uncoupling effects of dopamine on 18 pairs of cells; of these 12 pairs of type H2 cells, 5 pairs of type H3 cells and one was a pair of type H1 cells. Dopamine was not applied to any of the 3 pairs of H4 cells recorded from in this study.

The effects of dopamine on modulating the electrical coupling between horizontal cells appear to be relatively specific. This is shown by the experiment illustrated Fig.8 in which L-glutamate was applied to pairs of coupled horizontal cells. This agent, at a concentration of 100 μM induced a large, transient inward current flow ($\sim$300 PA) into the cells, as shown in the record of the voltage-clamp driver cell (lower trace). The inward current caused a transient membrane potential depolarization, as shown in the record of the current-clamped follower cell. However, the coupling between the cells was affected very little; i.e. the coupling coefficient decreased transiently from about 0.9 to 0.8 and then rapidly recovered.

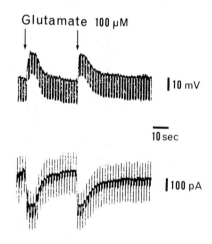

Glutamate 100 μM

10 mV

10 sec

100 pA

Fig. 8. Effects of L-glutamate on horizontal cell coupling. L-glutamate induced an inward current flow in the driver cell of about 300 pA. In addition, at the peak of the presonse, the input resistance of the driver cell was decreased, as reflected in the larger current pulses needed to hyperpolarize the cell 20 mV. Because of the large inward flow of current induced by L-glutamate, the voltage clamp on the driver cell was unable to maintain the holding potential on the follower cell. Thus the follower cell depolarized by about 15 mV. Note, however, the coupling ratio between the cells changed little as a result of the L-glutamate application.

These experiments thus demonstrate that electrical coupling occurs between horizontal cells in culture. Furthermore, it appears that the coupling observed in cultured horizontal cells is similar to that seen in the intact retina. That is, cells of the same morphological type are strongly coupled, but cells of different morphological types are not coupled (Witkovsky and Dowling, 1969; Kaneko, 1971). In addition, we have observed that pairs of coupled horizontal cells in culture are responsive to dopamine, at concentrations (25-200 μM) known to activate adenylate cyclase in horizontal cells (Van Buskirk and Dowling, 1981). Earlier experiments had shown that such concentrations of dopamine alter the receptive field size of horizontal cells recorded in the intact retina, suggesting that dopamine modifies the electrical coupling between horizontal cells (Negishi and Drujan, 1979; Teraishi et al., 1984; Piccolino et al., 1984). The present experiments employing pairs of isolated cells and whole cell patch-clamp recording methods provide direct evidence that this neurotransmitter decreases the conductance of these electrical synapses, and that these techniques provide the means for assessing this effect quantitatively.

Monoclonal antibodies specific to horizontal cells

With the development of methods to isolate fish horizontal cells, it has also been possible to separate these neurons from the other retinal cells while maintaining their viability. This can be done by velocity sedimentation with Ficoll gradients and this procedure yields fractions highly enriched in horizontal cells (Van Buskirk and Dowling, 1981). Such fractions can be used to immunize mice, thus eventually producing monoclonal antibodies specific to these elements.

We have succeeded in producing monoclonal antibodies against carp horizontal cells using this approach (Young and Dowling, 1984). So far sixteen hybridomas have been identified that secrete antibodies specific to horizontal cells. The hybridomas were classified into three groups with respect to the staining of horizontal cells produced by their antibodies at the light microscopic level using standard indirect immunofluorescent and ABC-immunoperoxidase staining techniques. The three cone horizontal cell subtypes and one rod horizontal cell subtype found in the carp retina are located in well-defined layers (Fig. 9). The type I cone horizontal cells (CH1) are located most distally in the inner nuclear layer, while the type II and type III cone horizontal cells (CH2 and CH3) and rod horizontal cells (RH) are located proximal to the CH1 horizontal cells. One of the hybridomas was classified in group I, i.e. staining by its antibody appeared to be associated with all horizontal cells. Fourteen of the hybridomas were classified in group II, i.e. staining by these antibodies was associated only with the distally positioned CH1 horizontal cells, while one hybridoma was in group III, i.e. staining by its antibody was associated with a proximal non-CH1 type of horizontal cell. Figs. 9b-d show immunoperoxidase staining patterns elicited by the three different groups of antibodies; (b) shows staining of most if not all horizontal cell perikarya with an antibody from a group I hybridoma; (c) shows staining of the perikarya of the most distal horizontal cells, the CH1 cells, with an antibody from a group II hybridoma; (d) shows staining of horizontal cell perikarya proximal to the CH1 cells, by an antibody from a group III hybridoma.

In all three micrographs of Fig. 9, some staining deeper in the inner nuclear layer can be seen, which corresponds to the location of the axon-like processes that extend from the cell perikarya and terminate close to the inner plexiform layer. The staining of these processes is

12

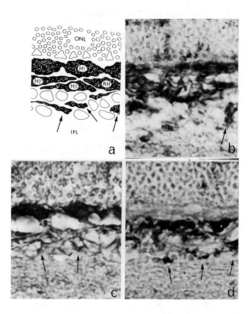

Fig. 9. a) Schematic diagram indicating the location of the subtypes of horizontal cells in the inner nuclear layer of carp retina. The type 1 cone horizontal cells (H1) are located most distally and their cell bodies form a distinct band. Type II and type III cone horizontal cells (H2 and H3) and the rod horizontal cells (RH) are located proximal to the CH1 cells and their cell bodies are less distinctly layered. Arrows indicate axonal processes that extend from the CH cells toward the inner plexiform layer (IPL). ONL, outer nuclear layer. (b-d) Staining of all subtypes of horizontal cells. c) Staining of CH1 cells only. d) Staining on non-CH1 horizontal cells, which are located proximally to a clearly unstained CH1 layer. Axonal processes located deeper in the inner nuclear layer are indicated by arrows. Bar = 10 μm.

shown particularly clearly in Fig. 9c and d (arrows). In Cyprinids, only cone horizontal cells appear to extend axon-like processes (Stell, 1975) suggesting that the cells stained in (d) are either CH2 or CH3 horizontal cells, or both.

Group II hybridomas were most commonly isolated probably because the majority (approximately 65%) of the horizontal cells in the Cyprinid retina are of the CH1 type (Stell and Lightfoot, 1975). Of the antibodies secreted by these hybridomas, a number appeared to recognize different antigens or antigenic determinants on the CH1 cell because they demonstrated different staining patterns. Figure 10a and b show staining by one of these antibodies, (HC-II.7, using an indirect immunofluorescence staining technique. The staining extends all along the CH1 cell body layer and, in addition, there is some fainter staining deeper in the inner nuclear layer (arrowheads), i.e. this antibody appears to stain both the cell perikaryon and axon process. At higher magnification (Fig. 10b), it can be seen that in the CH1 cell body layer staining is confined to cell contours, suggesting that the specific antigen is on the cell surface.

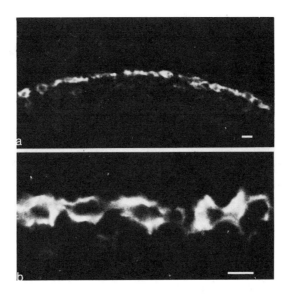

Fig. 10. Immunofluorescent staining of frozen sections of retina by HC-II.7, a CH1 antibody. a) Staining extends all along the CH1 cell body layer and there is some faint staining in the inner nuclear layer (arrowheads). b) At higher magnification, the staining appears to be confined to the cell surface. (a and b, bar = 10 μm).

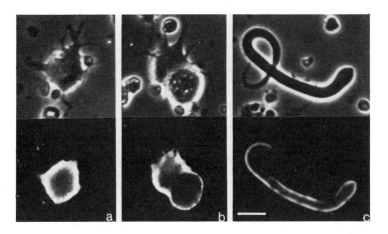

Fig. 11. Immunofluorescent staining of CH1 horizontal cells in culture by antibody HC-II.7. a) Staining is present mainly on the perikaryon and is generally absent from the dendritic processes of the cell. b) Two adjacent horizontal cells, both of which show staining. c) A labeled axon terminal. Note unstained background cells in all three micrographs. Bar = 10 μm.

To analyze further the location of the horizontal cell-specific antigens, and to identify directly staining of the so-called axon processes of the cone horizontal cells, we routinely tested our antibodies on isolated horizontal cells in freshly prepared or 24-hr cell cultures of carp retina. Figure 11 shows immunofluorescence labelling of fixed isolated horizontal cell perikarya (a and b) and an axon terminal (c) by antibody, HC-II.7. Staining in all cases appeared to be confined to the cell surface. This is shown particularly clearly in the lower part of (b) and the axon terminal in (c) in which the micrograph focus was approximately at the cell equator. We have also observed that living cells show similar immunofluorescence staining, again indicating that the specific antigens are localized on the cell surface. Not all antibodies stained all parts of the cultured CHl horizontal cells; some reacted only with the cell perikarya and did not stain the axonal processes.

Evidence that the antigen recognized by antibody HC-II.7 is a plasma membrane protein was provided by a biochemical characterization of the antigens. Plasma membranes from enriched horizontal cell mixtures were isolated and the membrane proteins were iodinated using a mild iodination procedure to ensure minimal loss of immunological activity. Following reaction with antibody, the proteins were precipitated and run on a polyacrylamide gel. With antibody HC-II.7, as shown in Fig. 12, a single band of molecular weight 48-50 KD appeared on the resulting autoradiogram.

Adult carp horizontal cells ordinarily do not survive more than 7-10 days in culture, even when grown on polylysine-coated coverslips. After 3-4 days, vacuoles appear in the cytoplasm of many cells and the number of adhering cells decreases rapidly thereafter. After 7 days in culture, the majority of those horizontal cells still attached to the coverslip have rounded and processes extending from the cells are only rarely seen.

Horizontal cells maintained on HC-II.7 antibody-coated coverslips, on the other hand, were more numerous, had more processes and survived longer than cells grown on control or polylysine-coated coverslips. For example, immediately after settling (3 hrs), there was a 20-25 fold increase in the number of horizontal cells attached to HC-II.7 coated-coverslips as compared to control coverslips coated with an unrelated IgG$_1$ monoclonal antibody, and a 4-5 fold increase as compared to polylysine-coated coverslips. Furthermore, at least 85% of the horizontal cells observed in the HC-II.7-coated coverslips also survived longer, with a large fraction living more than two weeks. At least half of the cells retained processes which were usually observed only for the first few days in cultures grown on polylysine-coated coverslips, and only for the first few hours on cells grown on control coverslips. The processes on the cells showed qualitative differences as well; horizontal cells in HC-II.7 cultures tended to have a complex network of processes, in contrast to cells maintained on polylysine treated coverslips which typically had only 1-3 processes. The majority of horizontal cells grown on antibody HC-II.7 did not develop vacuoles until past day 15. Table 1 provides a detailed comparison of horizontal cell survival in culture when maintained on control, polysine-, or antibody HC-II.7-coated coverlsips over the course of 21 days. Finally horizontal cells maintained on antibody HC-II.7-coated coverslips were tested electrophysiologically, and they showed normal resting potentials (-60 to -80 mV) and vigorous responses to L-glutamate and its analogue, kainate (Lasater and Dowling, 1982).

T A B L E 1

Relative cell-adhesion enhancement provided by antibody HC-II.7 and polylysine

Relative Number of Horizontal Cells/Percentage With Processes

	3 hr	1 day	3 days	5 days	7 days	9 days	11 days	15 days	21 days
Control	X/50	0.85X/40	0.6X/30	0.4X/20	0.25X/15	0.1X/5	0.05X/5	0	0
Polylysine	5X/60	5X55	3.5X/40	2X/30	1.5X/25	1.0X/10	0.5X/10	0.3X10	0.1X/10
HC-11.7	20-25X/85	20X/80	15X/70	10-12X/60	10X/60	8X/50	6-7X/50	5X50	3X/50

Enriched horizontal cell fractions were plated on coverslips coated with antibody HC-II.7, polylysine, or an unrelated IgG_1 (control). X was assigned to represent the number of horizontal cells (10-40) counted in a field of fixed size from control (3 hr) cultures, and the number of horizontal cells counted in antibody HC-II.7 and polylysine cultures were calculated and recorded relative to control. The number after the slash gives the percentage of cells that had processes.

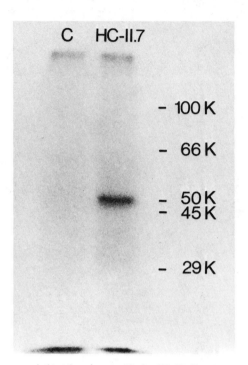

Fig. 12. Immunoprecipitation by antibody HC-II.7. A protein molecule of 50 kD   is seen on autoradiograph of NaDodSO$_4$/polyacrylamide gel electrophoresis of the immunoprecipitation produce obtained with antibody HC-II.7. Normal mouse serum was used for control (c).

In undertaking these experiments, we had three questions in mind. First, is it possible to raise monoclonal antibodies to a specific type of neuron, namely the retinal horizontal cell; second, is it possible to raise antibodies that will react only with the surfaces of these cells; and third is it possible to raise antibodies that will react only with horizontal cell subtypes. Our experiments indicate positive answers to all three of these questions, and they have provided other interesting observations as well. That is we have raised monoclonal antibodies that appear to recognize 1) all horizontal cells in the retina but no other type of retinal neuron, 2) specific subtypes of horizontal cells, and 3) discrete regions of one subtype of horizontal cell. Furthermore, of the hybridomas which have been studied most extensively, all appear to secrete antibodies specific to the horizontal cell surface. This is the case whether the antibodies were reacted with cells fixed in the intact retina, cells isolated and fixed, or isolated cells unfixed and living. These data thus suggest that there are a) surface antigens common to all horizontal cells but not to other retinal neurons; b) surface antigens specific to subtypes of horizontal cells and c) surface antigens found only on certain parts of horizontal cells.

MacLeish et al., 1983; (see also Leifer et al., 1984) using salamander neurons, were the first to show that certain antibodies can enhance mature neural cell growth in culture. With antibody HC-II.7, we have shown that a cell-subtype specific antibody can enhance selectively the appearance of horizontal cells in culture and prolong their survival. Horizontal cells maintained on antibody HC-II.7 coated coverslips have been tested electrophysiologically and they showed normal resting potentials and strong responses to drugs such as L-glutamate and its analogue, kainate. How the antibody exerts these effects is not clear. The enhancement of horizontal cell survival in culture does not appear to be a nonspecific effect of mouse immunoglobulins, as no improvement was found when preimmune serum, or an unrelated $IgG1$ monoclonal antibody was used to coat coverslips. As was pointed out by MacLeish et al., (1983) it will be important to determine whether the antibody is simply serving as a better substrate for the cells, i.e. provides better cell adhesion, or is doing something more specific to the isolated neurons.

Monoclonal antibodies similar to those we have produced will be useful for a variety of purposes. For example, they can be used to identify cells in culture when, for example, such cells have altered their morphology substantially (i.e. Fig. 4). Furthermore, such antibodies can provide a cell tag, enabling the isolation of subtypes of cells. Finally, such molecules can serve as probes to identify and to characterize functional groups on the cell surface, thus extending our understanding of the molecular basis of neuronal cell function.

In summary, we have described a few of the newer techniques presently available to explore neuronal cell structure and function, and how these techniques can be applied to studies of the retina. For example, our results indicate that retinal cell cultures are particularly favorable preparations for the study of the biophysical, pharmacological, molecular and, perhaps, developmental properties of individual classes of retinal neurons. Furthermore, with techniques such as patch clamping, and the use of monoclonal antibodies as cell surface probes, it is now possible to gain insight into areas of retinal cell function heretofore inaccessible. With the use of these approaches, and others, we will be able to add considerably to our understanding of retinal cell function over the next few years.

Acknowledgements

This research was supported in part by national Institutes of Health grants, EY 00811 and EY 00824. Marian Pak helped with the identification of the perch horizontal cells and prepared the section of the perch retina shown in Fig. 2. Patricia Sheppard prepared the figures and Stephanie Levinson typed the manuscript.

18

References
Dowling, J.E., Pak, M.W. and Lasater, E.M. (submitted).
Cohen, J.E. and J. E. Dowling, Brain Res. 264, 307 (1983).
Harris, Al.L., D. C. Spray and MV.L. Bennett, J. Neurosci. 3, 79, (1983).
Hassin, G., J. Comp. Neurol. 186:529 (1979).
Kaneko, A., J. Physiol. 213: 95 (1971).
Lasater, E.M. and J.E. Dowling, Proc. Natl. Acad. Sci. 79, 936 (1982).
Lasater, E.M. and J.E. Dowling, Proc. Natl. Acad. Sci. 82, (1985).
Lasater, E.M., Dowling, J.E. and Ripps, H. J. Neurosci. 8, 1966 (1984).
Leifer, D., S. A. Lipton, C.J. Barnstable and R. H. Masland, Science 224, 303 (1984).
MacLeish, P.R., C.J. Barnstable and E. Townes-Anderson, Proc. Natl. Acad. Sci. 80, 7014 (1983).
Negishi, K. and B. Drujan, Neurochem. Res. 4: 313 (1979).
Neher, E., B. Sakmann and J. H. Steinback, Pflugers Arch. 275: 219, (1978).
Piccolino, M., J. Neyton and H.M. Gerschenfeld, J. Neurosci. 4:2477 (1984).
Sakman, B. and E. Neher (eds) in: Single-Channel Recording, Plenum Press, New York (1983).
Shingai, R. and Christensen, B.N. Neurosci. 10, 893 (1983).
Stell, W.K., J. Comp. Neurol. 159:503, (1975).
Stell, W.K. and D.O. Lightfoot, J. Comp. Neurol. 159:473 (1975).
Svaetichin, G, Acta Physiol. Scand. 29, Suppl. 106:565 (1953).
Svaetichin, G. and E. F. MacNichol, Ann. N.Y. Acad. Sci. 74: 385 (1958).
Tachibana, M., J. Physiol. 345:329 (1983).
Teranishi, T., K. Negishi and S. Kato, Nature 301:243 (1983).
Teranishi, T., K. Negishi and S. Kato, J. Neurosci. 4:1271 (1984).
Van Buskirk, R. and J.E. Dowling, Proc. Natl. Acad. Sci. 78:7825 (1981).
Witkovsky, P. and J.E. Dowling, Z. Zellforsch. 100:60 (1969).
Young, L.H.Y. and J.E. Dowling, Proc. Natl. Acad. Sci. 81:6255 (1984).

Chromatic Interactions Between Cones of Differing Spectral Classes:
Anatomical and Electrophysiological Studies in Turtle

Richard A. Normann[1], Ido Perlman[2] and Helga Kolb[1]
Department of Physiology, School of Medicine[1]
University of Utah
Salt Lake City, Utah

Department of Physiology Faculty of Medicine[2]
Technion, Israel

The neural interactions which culminate in the perception of unique "colors" when one views monochromatic stimuli of various wavelengths has remained an intriguing problem despite the extensive studies which have been directed towards this question using psychophysical, biochemical, anatomical and physiological techniques. Because cone photoreceptors provide the input to this system, these neurons have been intensively studied. This knowledge has provided the basis for our understanding of subsequent retinal and central color processing. In this article, I will briefly review what has been learned about color information processing by cones, and I will focus on our recent anatomical and physiological experiments which have revealed new pathways by which signals arising in one spectral class of turtle cones may influence cones of differing spectral classes. Because of the number of intracellular studies which have been conducted in cones from the turtle retina, this paper will deal mainly with turtle cones.

Trichromacy in the Turtle Retina

Since the earliest observations of Young (1802a,b) it was believed that there might be three color channels in the human retina, each channel being sensitive to a different part of the visible spectrum. This hypothesis was supported by a variety of psychophysical studies and by densitometric measurements in patients with defective color vision (see Brindley (1970) for a review) and was directly verified as soon as intracellular recordings became possible in the vertebrate retina. Tomita, Kaneko, Murakami, and Paulter (1967) measured the action spectra of a large population of cone photoreceptors in the carp retina and found that these spectra could be classified into three groups with peak sensitivities at 462 nm (blue sensitive cones), 529 nm (green sensitive cones) and 611 nm (red sensitive cones). These values were in accord with the peaks in the absorption spectra measured microdensitometrically in goldfish cones by Marks (1965). Baylor and Hodgkin (1973) measured the spectral sensitivities of turtle cones and discovered that the turtle retina, like the carp and goldfish was trichromatic, with blue, green and red sensitive cones manifesting peaks in their spectral sensitivity curves at 460 nm, 550 nm and 630 nm, respectively. Liebman and Granda (1971), Liebman (1972) and Lipetz (1984) applied microspectrophotometric techniques to the turtle cones and their data confirms Baylor and Hodgkins results. However, while the peaks of the absorption spectra and the spectral sensitivities are similar, the shapes of the spectra differ; the spectral sensitivity curve is considerably narrower than the absorption spectra of the photopigments contained in the cone's outer segments. Also, Baylor and Hodgkin observed that the short wavelength end of the spectra measured in each class of cones varied considerably from cone to cone. They ascribed these differences to the presence of the intensely colored oil droplets located at the base of the outer segments (Ives, Normann and Barber, 1983). The finding of trichromacy in the turtle retina provided further impetus to use the turtle retina as a model of color processing in the human retina.

Univariance and Cone Photoreceptors

One concept which has advanced our understanding of color information processing in the retina is the principle of univariance. This principle states that for any given state of adaptation, the effect of light on a cone is a function only of the number of quanta absorbed by the cone (Naka and Rushton, 1966). One consequence of univariance is that an individual cone should not be able to distinguish the "color" of the quanta which stimulate it and the photoresponses evoked by monochromatic stimuli of any wavelength should be indistinguishable from each other (when compared on a constant absorbed quantal basis). The early intracellular studies on cone photoreceptors (Baylor and Hodgkin, 1973) seemed to indicate that this principle was obeyed by cones, however, subsequent work has indicated that there are stimulus conditions where deviations from this principle will occur.

Deviations from Univariance

Cone photoreceptors were originally believed to be strictly presynaptic neural elements whose sole input was light energy. The intracellular studies of Baylor, Fuortes and O'Bryan (1971), however, indicated that cones were also postsynaptic to other retinal neurons. Cones appeared to receive excitatory input from neighboring cones and inhibitory input from horizontal cells. Neither of these interactions, however, was believed to alter the univariant nature of the red cone photoresponse. Baylor and Fuortes (1970), and later, Detwiler and Hodgkin (1979) showed that the excitatory interaction between cones appeared to be limited to cones of like spectral class; red cones only received input from neighboring red cones and green cones only receive input from neighboring green cones.

Cones are also postsynaptic to horizontal cells via a negative feedback pathway (Baylor and Fuortes, 1970). However, the inhibitory pathway from luminosity horizontal cells to red cones would not be expected to alter the univariant nature of the red cone photoresponse. This expectation is based upon the action spectra measured in luminosity type horizontal cells by Fuortes and Simon (1974) and by Yazulla (1976) which was shown to be very similar to that of the red cone. Presumably, the red cone population provides the main input into the luminosity horizontal cells. Accordingly, the extent of the horizontal cell feedback will only be a function of the magnitude of the red cone response. Since the red cone photoresponse is expected to be univariant, the horizontal cell response will also be univariant as will its feedback effect as reflected in the red cones.

Because luminosity type horizontal cells also provide inhibitory feedback onto green cones (and possible blue cones), these cones would not be expected to obey the principle of univariance; green cones experience two inputs, each of which has a different spectral sensitivity. One input is due to photoisomerizations of the green sensitive photopigment located in their outer segments, and one results from negative feedback from red sensitive luminosity type horizontal cells. Nonunivariant photoresponses were first observed in green sensitive cones in the turtle retina by O'Bryan (1973), and the departure from univariance was largest when large diameter spots were used (conditions which provided maximal stimulation of the very large receptive fields of the horizontal cells).

Nonunivariant photoresponses have also been reported to occur in double cones by Richter and Simon (1974). Double cones were originally believe to be a population composed of red sensitive cones (principle members) and green sensitive cones (accessory members) which were closely apposed along much of their lengths. If this close apposition provides a pathway for mixing of signals between the red and green members, one would expect this class of cones to manifest nonunivariant photoresponses. Richter and Simon measured the spectral sensitivities of a number of double cones and noted that the shapes of the spectra were a function of the chromatic adaptation used. Red backgrounds shifted the peak of the spectra towards the short wavelength end of the spectrum, and green backgrounds shifted the spectra towards the red end of the spectrum. However, recent microspectrophotometric measurements by Lipetz (1984) provide strong evidence that the photopigments contained in the principle and accessory members of the double cones are both red sensitive. The findings of Richter and Simon are difficult to reconcile with these recent observations but indicate that there is a population of red cones in the turtle retina which receive a strong, excitatory short wavelength input.

To better understand the role of cones in color information processing, we have conducted a series of anatomical and electrophysiological experiments which were designed to reexamine the question of univariance of red cones (Normann, Perlman, Kolb, Jones and Daly, 1984). We have discovered that red cones are not univariant even when stimulated with small diameter spots (which produce only minimal excitation of horizontal cells). Our data is consistent with the notion that red cones are connected not only to neighboring red cones but also to neighboring green cones, and that this interaction is excitatory in nature. Our anatomical studies indicate that this interaction may be mediated by invaginating and/or basal junctions between the pedicle of one cone and the telodendritic processes which radiate from neighboring cones. Before describing our physiological observations, we will first describe these anatomical pathways.

Anatomical Studies

Our anatomical evidence for a color mixing pathway at the distal part of the retina is based upon light and electron microscopic studies of Golgi stained turtle cones. Figure 1 shows a light micrograph of the synaptic ending (pedicle) of such a Golgi stained cone. The pedicle is a spherical shaped structure from which radiate numerous basal processes called telodendria (Cajal, 1892). These telodendria can be better appreciated in whole mount views of Figure 2. Each cone has five to six of these telodendria, each extending about 10 to 15 microns from the pedicle. Telodendria terminate in the pedicles of neighboring cones (Lasansky, 1971; Normann, et al., 1984; Kolb and Jones, 1985).

In order to learn the spectral classes of the cone from which the telodendria radiate (source cone) and the cone to which the telodendria project (target cone), we have examined serial ultrathin sections of these Golgi stained cones and followed the telodendria from source to target cones. Since each spectral class of cone can be recognized in the electron microscope by the density, size and location within the outer nuclear layer of its oil droplets (Kolb and Jones, 1982), we were able to identify the spectral classes of source and target cones. Figure 3 shows a Golgi stained red single cone as seen by electron microscopy. Based upon serial reconstructions of telodendria from nine red and three green cones, we have learned that the telodendria of red cones project to neighboring red cones and also to neighboring green cones, and the telodendria of green cones project to neighboring red cones.

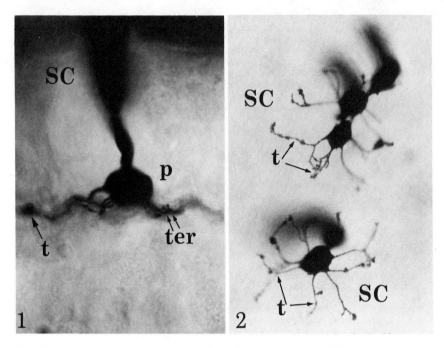

Fig. 1. Light micrograph of a Golgi stained single cone (SC) seen in vertical section. Numerous telodendria (arrow t) bearing clusters of terminals (ter, small arrows) radiate from the base of the cone pedicle (p). X1500.

Fig. 2. Golgi stained single cones (SC) as seen in retinal whole mount. The radiating delodendria (t arrows) are better appreciated in this view and their clusters of terminals are more apparent. X1200.

Not only have we determined the spectral nature of the source and target cone telodendritic projections, we have also examined the nature of the contacts made by these processes. Telodendria terminate at the pedicles of target cones and make invaginating and/or narrow-cleft basal junctions (Kolb and Jones, 1985); junctions very similar to those made between cones and bipolar cells.

An example of an invaginating junction is shown in Fig. 4. In this example, the source cone was determined to be a "green" cone and the target cone was determined to be a "red" cone. The synapse appears to be a typical triad with a synaptic ribbon located in the red cone at the apex of the synaptic ridge, two horizontal cell lateral processes located on each side of the ribbon, and the green cone telodendron forming the central element. The telodendria do not project completely to the ribbon. In fact, telodendria forming central elements are typically separated from the ribbon by a cap of horizontal cell lateral processes (Fig. 4). Lasansky (1971) described similar central endings for cone telodendria in the turtle outer plexiform layer and he suggested that they were receiving

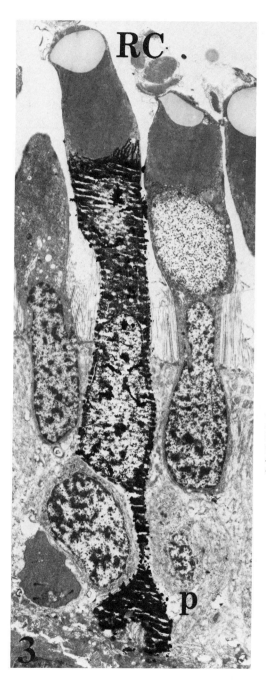

Fig. 3. Electron micrograph of a complete Golgi stained red single cone (RC) in the turtle retina. The large opaque oil droplet identifies this as a red cone. Paraboloid, cell body and pedicle are stained with a dense deposit of silver chromate. X3000.

24

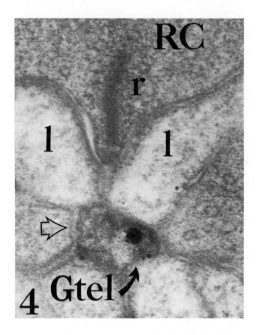

Fig. 4. Golgi stained telodendron (Gtel, arrow) of a green cone ends as a central element in a target red cone (RC). The central element makes a narrow gap junction with the target cone pedicle (open arrow) and lies under the synaptic ribbon (r) with an intervening cap of horizontal cell lateral elements (1's). X75000.

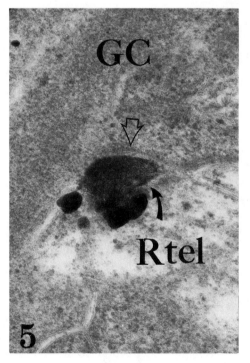

Fig. 5. Golgi stained telodendron of a red cone (Rtel, arrow) ends at a target green cone (GC) at a narrow-cleft basal junction (open arrow). X70000.

input from the horizontal cells rather than from the target cones. We have not seen any specialized junctions between source central elements and horizontal cell lateral elements but we note that central elements make a narrow-cleft basal junction with the target cone (open arrows, Fig. 4). So, based upon the similarity of this synapse with the invaginating hyperpolarizing bipolar synapse seen in another species (Nelson and Kolb, 1983), we conclude that this anatomical pathway may provide a means by which cones of one spectral class transmit excitatory signals to cones of differing spectral classes.

The telodendria of neighboring cones also contact the target cone base at narrow-cleft basal junctions distant from the horizontal cell lateral elements as shown in Fig. 5. Here a red cone telodendron is making this type of basal junction with a neighboring green cone pedicle. This basal junction has little density on the presynaptic membrane, and a narrower cleft between the pre- and postsynaptic membranes than that of the wide cleft "striated" basal junctions between cones and bipolar cells originally described by Lasansky (1971). These narrow-cleft basal junctions are made by source telodendria on target cones either as a single projection to the target cone base, or en route to becoming a central contact (Kolb and Jones, 1984).

A third type of junction has been observed to occur between telodendria as they pass close to each other in the neuropil of the outer plexiform layer. This type of junction is quite extensive and has a septalaminar appearance typical of electrical synapses or gap junctions (Kolb and Jones, 1984). We suspect that these large gap junctions occur between telodendria of like spectral class cones. Possibly, these junctions may be a specialized pathway which enhances the spatial integration of cones of like spectral class.

The final type of cone contact we have observed occurs in the visual streak of the retina. Here, the density of cones is so great that neighboring cones often abut against each other. In the region of their pedicles, small punctate gap junctions are often seen (Kolb and Jones, 1984). This type of contact occurs between all neighboring cones, irrespective of spectral class.

It is clear from this brief description of our anatomical studies that there are at least two pathways by which signals originating in one class of cone can be transmitted to cones of different spectral class. One pathway resembles conventional chemical synapses (the invaginating and basal types of junctions) and the other pathway appears to be via electrical junctions (telodendron to telodendron gap junctions and pedicle to pedicle gap junctions). We have summarized these pathways in the cartoon of Fig. 6.

Fig. 6. Summary diagram of connections between different spectral classes of photoreceptors in the turtle retina. Telodendria pass from red to green and from green to red cones and make what appear to be chemical synapses at narrow-cleft basal junctions. All photoreceptors are joined by punctate gap junctions between their pedicles in the visual steak region of the retina. Larger gap junctions occur between telodendria as they pass each other in the neuropil of the outer plexiform layer.

26

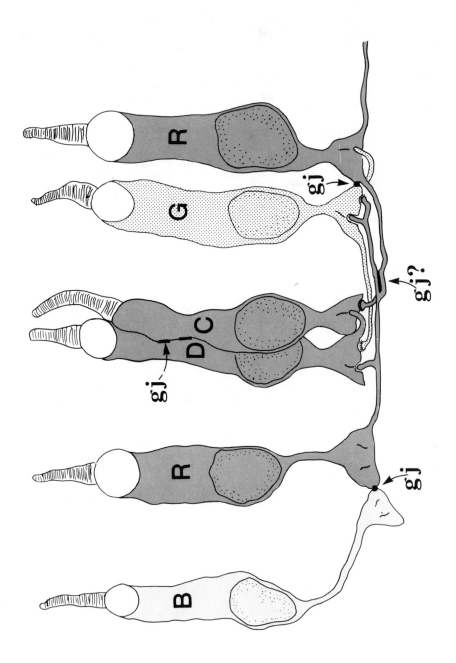

Physiological Studies

The extensive anatomical pathways just described by which cones of one spectral class make synaptic contacts with cones of differing spectral classes strongly suggests that cones of the turtle retina should not obey the principle of univariance. We describe below a series of tests of this principle; each of which provides physiological evidence for mixing of signals between cones of differing spectral classes.

The most straightforward test would be to examine the responses of a red cone to red and green test flashes which produced an equal number of photoisomerizations in the cone's outer segment. While it would be extremely difficult to adjust the intensities of these red and green flashes such that this goal was achieved, one can simply adjust the intensity of one of the two flashes (ie., the red intensity) such that the amplitude of the red response matches the amplitude evoked by the green flash. If univariance maintains, the kinetics of these matched responses should be identical. Further, increasing the intensities of both of these matching red and green stimuli by identical factors should result in larger amplitude responses which again should be indistinguishable in all aspects. The results of this type of experiment are shown in Fig. 7 where we have plotted the amplitudes of red cone photoresponses as a function of the intensity of the red (filled circles) and green (open circles) test flashes which evoked each response. These intensity response curves differ significantly. The responses evoked by the red stimuli can be well approximated by the smooth curve which is a plot of the Naka-Rushton relation (1966), $V= Vmax*I/(I+\sigma)$, where V is the amplitude of the response evoked by intensity I, Vmax is the maximum response which can be evoked in the cone, and σ is the intensity which evokes a half maximal response (1/2 Vmax). This curve, however, provides a poor fit to the responses evoked by green stimuli; the intensity response curve is much broader and appears to be composed of two portions, a relatively shallow portion evoked by dim flashes and a faster rising portion which is evoked by brighter test flashes. While this very simple test of univariance indicates that the red cone receives an additional short wavelength input, it could be argued that this additional input arises via the negative feedback pathway from luminosity type horizontal cells. However, the data of Fig. 7 were obtained with 320 um diameter test flashes, a spot size large enough to fully illuminate the cones excitatory receptive field yet small enough to minimize horizontal cell feedback effects.

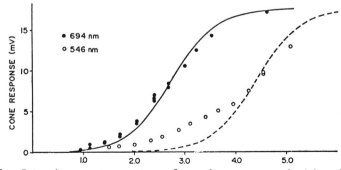

Fig. 7. Intensity response curves of a red cone measured with red (694 nm) and green (546 nm) test flashes. Test flashes were of 62 msec. duration and were 320 um diameter. Intensities are expressed as the total number of quanta (either 546 nm or 694 nm) in the stimulus/square micron of retinal area.

28

Chromatic Adaptations

A more revealing test of univariance would be to use the technique of chromatic adaptation to preferentially desensitize one class of cones. Background illumination (chromatic adaptation) of any color will desensitize all cones (Normann and Perlman, 1979), with the degree of desensitization in each spectral class of cones given by the rate of photoisomerizations each class of cone experiences. Red backgrounds will produce a greater rate of isomerization of red cones, and therefore will produce a greater desensitization of red cones than either green or blue cones. Similarly, green backgrounds will produce a greater desensitization of green cones than red or blue cones. However, if cones were univariant and responded only to isomerizations in their own outer segments, chromatic adaptation should have no effect on either the shape of the intensity response curves measured with red and green test flashes, or the separation between these curves on the log intensity axis. Accordingly, the ratio of sensitivities to red and green test flashes which are superimposed upon any chromatic background should also be independent of the intensity and color of the background illumination.

The results of such a chromatic adaptation experiment are shown in Fig. 8 where red cone sensitivities to red and green test flashes were measured in the dark adapted condition and under conditions of 2.9 mm diameter red and green background illumination. The traces in Fig. 8A show "linear range" photoresponses in the dark adapted retina evoked by red (694nm, solid trace) and green (546nm, dashed trace) flashes. We have

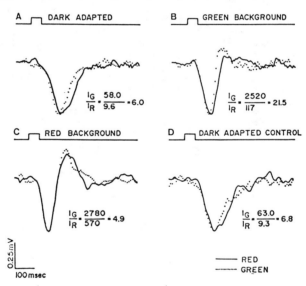

Fig. 8. The effect of chromatic background illumination on red cone linear range responses elicited by red and green stimuli. The numbers to the right of each pair of responses are the intensities of the green and red stimuli used to evoke each linear response, and the ratio of these intensities. A) Linear responses evoked in the dark adapted retina before the application of chromatic backgrounds. B) Linear responses in green (500 nm) background of 4.19×10^{6} quanta/sec/square micron. C) Linear responses in red (700nm) background of 6.96×10^{4} quanta/sec/square micron. D) Control linear range responses recorded after these periods of chromatic adaptation.

studied linear range responses in order to measure cone sensitivities to red and green test flashes, a measurement which is only meaningful if the conditions of linearity apply. Baylor and Hodgkin (1973) have shown that for dim flashes, the cone satisfies the condition of linearity; halving the intensity of a dim flash reduces the entire response by one half. Because these responses were linear, they were slightly scaled with our computer to produce a perfect amplitude match. Even in the linear range the responses do not match perfectly in kinetics; the red response returns to baseline more slowly than does the response to the green flash. This difference in kinetics was seen in most cones studied, and can also be seen (although to a much lesser extent) in similar measurements made by Baylor and Hodgkin (Fig. 6 of their 1973 paper). These differences in kinetics have been studied in greater detail in another series of experiments which have been described in a recent report (Perlman, Normann, Itzhaki and Daly, 1985). The red and green flash intensities which evoked these equal amplitude responses, and the ratio of these intensities are shown to the right of the traces. In this red cone, the sensitivity to red flashes was 6.0 times higher than the sensitivity to green flashes.

A pair of matched amplitude linear range photoresponses evoked by red and green test flashes which were superposed upon a bright green (500 nm) background is shown in Fig. 8B. As is evident from the numbers to the right of these traces, the cone has been desensitized by the background and it now takes more intensity to evoke these 0.5 mV responses. However, while the red intensity had to be increased by a factor of 12.2 over its dark adapted value, the green intensity had to be increased by a factor of 43.4 over its dark adapted value. The ratio of red flash sensitivity to green flash sensitivity under conditions of green background illumination was 21.5, a value 3.6 times the dark adapted value.

When this experiment was repeated with red and green test flashes superposed on a red (700 nm) bright background, the responses shown in Fig. 8C were obtained. In this case, the intensities of the red flash had to be increased by a factor of 59.3 over its dark adapted value, while the intensity of the green flash was increased only by a factor of 47.9 over its dark adapted value. As for the green backgrounds, the ratio of red to green flash sensitivities measured with the red background (4.9) was not equal to the value measured in the dark; the red background has decreased the ratio by a factor of 0.82 over the dark adapted ratio. The pair of traces in Fig. 8D are dark adapted control responses recorded after the periods of chromatic adaptation.

These results indicate that red cones do not obey the principle of univariance. Furthermore, the data suggests that the red cone receives an additional short wavelength input which is excitatory in nature. In the dark adapted retina, red flashes mainly excite the red cone. Green flashes strongly excite green cones and to a lesser degree the red cones. However, the green cone excitation is coupled to the red cone, increasing its response to green flashes. Green backgrounds preferentially decrease green cone sensitivity, and thus reduce the green cone component of the red cone response to a green flash. This results in the increase in the ratio of the red flash to green flash sensitivity observed with green backgrounds. A similar argument can explain the decrease in this ratio observed with red backgrounds.

The results shown in Figs. 7 and 8 were selected from experiments performed on 14 separate red cones. While the additional short wavelength input was seen in all experiments, the extent of the additional input varied from cone to cone. The degree to which each red cone deviated from univariance was quantified by dividing the ratio of red to green flash sensitivities at each background intensity, $(S694/S546)L$, by the ratio measured in the dark adapted state, $(S694/S546)D$. Also, since the degree to which a given background will desenitize any particular cone is a function of that cone's dark adapted sensitivity, the "strength" of each chromatic background was defined in terms of the decrease in cone sensitivity (measured with red light) caused by the background intensity, relative to the cone's dark adapted red flash sensitivity, $(S694)L/(S694)D$.

Our results in all cones studied are summarized in Fig. 9 where we have plotted the deviation from univariance of each cone as a function of the strength of the background for 20 backgrounds. This plot shows the effects of both red backgrounds (open circles) and green backgrounds (filled circles). Results obtained from a univariant cone when plotted in this manner would be represented as the horizontal line $((S694/S546)L = (S694/S546)D)$. Figure 9 indicates that 1) all 14 cones studied deviated from univariance, 2) the degree of the effect is a function of the background intensity and varies from cone to cone, and 3) the nature of the interaction is excitatory. Since the amount of short wavelength input into the red cone varies from cone to cone, it is tempting to suggest that part of the variation in the red cone spectral sensitivity curves recorded by Baylor and Hodgkin (1973) could reflect differences in this input.

The excitatory nature of the short wavelength input into the red cones provides the most compelling argument against horizontal cell involvement

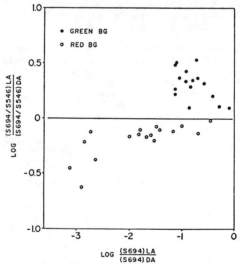

Fig. 9. The deviation from univariance of 14 red cones as a function of the color and strength of background illumination. The deviation is expressed in terms of the effect of the chromatic background on the red to green sensitivity ratio relative to the dark adapted ratio. A cone obeying the principle of univariance will exhibit a constant red to green sensitivity ratio, independent of the state of adaptation. Data points from such a cone would fall on the horizontal line in this plot. The strength of the background is expressed as the change in the cone sensitivity to red stimuli induced by the background.

in this mixing of signals between cones. In all studies which have investigated horizontal cell feedback onto cones, this pathway has been found to be inhibitory in nature. This observation, coupled with the relatively small diameter test flashes used in this study (which produce only minimal horizontal cell responses) indicates that this signal mixing must occur via a direct pathway between cones of differing spectral classes.

The Spectral Sensitivity Curve of the Additional Input

Because of the paucity of blue cones in the retinal mosaic, one would expect that the spectral sensitivity curve of the additional short wavelength input to red cones resembles that of green cones (peaking around 550 nm). We have verified this prediction by measuring the spectral sensitivity curve of red cones in the dark adapted retina and under conditions of chromatic adaptation with red and green background illumination. Linear range sensitivity was measured using test flashes of monochromatic light at seven wavelengths spanning the visible spectrum. Figure 10A shows the dark adapted action spectrum (open circles) and

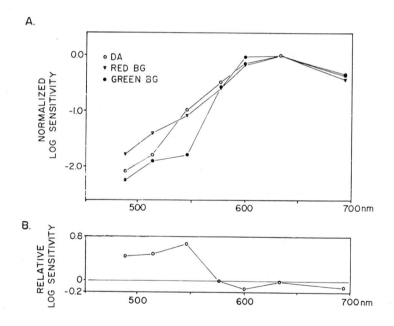

Fig. 10. A) Spectral sensitivity curves of a red cone under dark adapted and light adapted conditions. Each spectral sensitivity curve (generated from measurements of linear sensitivity at seven wavelengths which span the visible spectrum) was shifted vertically to normalize for maximum sensitivity at 633 nm. B) Difference spectrum of the short wavelength input to red cones obtained by subtracting the spectrum measured in the presence of green background illumination from that measured in the presence of red background illumination.

spectra measured under red (triangles) and green (filled circles) background illumination. The dark adapted action spectrum is similar in shape to those reported by Baylor and Hodgkin (1973) and peaks between 600 and 650 nm. The light adapted spectra have been shifted vertically so that they coincide with the dark adapted spectrum at 633 nm. The three action spectra do not superpose upon each other as one would expect if univariance were obeyed. As was seen in Fig. 8, the green background reduces the relative sensitivity to green flashes more than expected while red backgrounds augment the relative sensitivity to green flashes. We have constructed an action spectrum of the additional short wavelength input to red cones by subtracting the curve measured under green chromatic adaptation from that measured under red chromatic adaptation. The resulting difference spectrum is plotted in Fig. 10B and, as predicted, peaks at around 550 nm, the wavelength of maximum sensitivity of the green cones.

Estimating the Extent of the Green Cone Input

The results of Fig. 10B can be used to get a very rough estimation of the extent of this additional short wavelength input to red cones. The dark adapted spectral sensitivity curve reflects photon absorption which occurs in both the red and green cones and is broader than expected from the absorption spectrum of the red cone photopigment. However, since green background illumination produces a greater desensitizing effect on green than red cones, the spectral sensitivity curve measured under green backgrounds more closely approximates the red cone spectral sensitivity curve (uncontaminated by green cone input). By normalizing these two curves such that they coincide at 633 nm, we can estimate the green cone contribution to the dark adapted red cone response to a green stimulus. This normalization circumvents the desensitizing effects of the backgrounds and indicates what the red cone sensitivity to 546 nm light would be if the green input is minimized. Specifically, from the normalized curves, the dark adapted red cone is 0.8 log units more sensitive to 546 nm quanta than is the green adapted red cone. This implies that for the red cone shown in Fig. 10, the additional green cone input is increasing sensitivity to green test flashes by a factor of 6.3, or that 86% of the "linear" response of this red cone to green test flashes originates in neighboring green cones. It is clear that the green cones provide a significant input into the red cone. It should be noted that the relative contribution of green cones to the red cone's response varied between cells. The value calculated above represents an example of a red cone with a substantial green cone input. In other cones, the interaction was less pronounced but was always observed.

If this pathway is as significant as estimated, one wonders why the pathway has not been described before. Baylor and Hodgkin (1973) measured linear range responses of red cones to red and green test flashes, and as mentioned earlier, their results show similar, but less obvious differences in the kinetics of the responses. Detwiler and Hodgkin (1979) directly studied cone-cone interactions by simultaneously impaling two nearby cones and observing the response of one cone to currents passed through the microelectrode into the other cone. While these workers were able to replicate Baylor and Fuortes' original work (1970) showing electrical coupling between cones of like spectral class, they were unable to demonstrate any coupling between cones of differing spectral class. We suggest that this pathway is best revealed with the chromatic stimuli and adaptations used in this study and are most apparent when "linear range" responses are studied. Since red cones are surrounded by and coupled to a larger number of red than green cones, the coupling between red cones would be expected to appear "stronger" than between red and green cones.

Accordingly, two electrode experiments may not be well suited to the study of color mixing. Currents injected into a single red cone will be shunted to neighboring red cones and provide only a subtle input to nearby green cones. Monochromatic green flashes on top of a red background, on the other hand, will stimulate the entire population of nearest green cones, and their summated input onto an impaled (and desensitized) red cone can be clearly seen.

Just as it has been difficult to appreciate the evolutionary advantages of excitatory electrical coupling between cones of like spectral class, it is equally difficult to understand why the turtle retina mixes signals between cones of differing spectral classes. If this interaction were inhibitory, the advantages would be clear; the animal would experience enhanced color contrast. Red-green borders would be augmented, and the shapes of the spectral sensitivity curves would be narrower, allowing the turtle better discrimination between colors which differ in wavelength by only a subtle degree. However, the interaction appears to be excitatory. Thus, red-green borders will lose contrast, and the animal will have a more difficult task differentiating between colors.

References

Baylor, D.A. and Fuortes, M.G.F. J. Physiol. 207,77 (1970).
Baylor, D.A., Fuortes, M.G.F. and O'Bryan, P.M. J. Physiol. 214,265 (1971).
Baylor, D.A. and Hodgkin, A.L. J. Physiol. 234,163 (1973).
Brindley, G.S. Physiology of the Retina and Visual Pathway. (The Williams and Wilkins Co., Baltimore, 1970).
Cajal, S.R. La retine des vertebres. La Cellule. Translatee by Thorpe, S.A., Glickstein, M. in The Structure of the Retina. Thomas, Springfield (1972).
Detwiler, P.B. and Hodgkin, A.L. J. Physiol. 291, 75 (1979).
Fuortes, M.G.F. and Simon, E.J. J. Physiol. 240, 177 (1974).
Ives, J.T., Normann, R.A. and Barber, P.W. J. Opt. Soc. Am., 73, 1725 (1983).
Kolb, H. and Jones, J. J. Comp. Neurol. 209, 331 (1982).
Kolb, H. and Jones, J. J. Neurocyt. 13, 567 (1984).
Kolb, H. and Jones, J. J. Neurophysiol in press (1985).
Lasansky, A. Phil. Trans. Roy. Soc. B 262, 365 (1971).
Liebman, P.A. and Granda, A.M. Vis. Res. 11, 105 (1971).
Liebman, P.A. in Handbook of Sensory Physiology, Vol. VII/I, (Springer-Verlag, Berlin, (1972) p 481.
Lipetz, L.E. in The Visual System: A Symposium to Honor Edward F. MacNichol. Alan R. Liss, Inc., New York 1984.
Marks, W.B. J. Physiol. 178, 14 (1965).
Naka, K.I. and Rushton, W.A.H. J. Physiol. 185, 536 (1966).
Nelson, R. and Kolb, H. Vis. Res. 23, 1183 (1983).
Normann, R.A. and Perlman, I. J. Physiol. 286, 491 (1979).
Normann, R.A., Perlman, I., Kolb, H., Jones, J. and Daly, S.J. Science 224, 625 (1984).
O'Bryan, P.J. J. Physiol. 235, 207 (1973).
Perlman, I., Normann, R.A., Itzhaki, A. and Daly, S.J. Vis. Res. (1985) (in press).
Richter, A. and Simon, E.J. J. Physiol. 242, 673 (1974).
Tomita, T., Kaneko, A., Murakami, M. and Pautler, E.L. Vis. Res. 7, 519 (1967).
Yazulla, S. Vis. Res. 16, 727 (1976).
Young, T. Phil Trans. 1802, 12 (1802).
Young, T. Phil. Trans. 1802, 387 (1802).

The Transmission of Rod Signals to Horizontal and Bipolar Cells

Gertrude Falk
Biophysics Unit, Department of Physiology
University College
London WC1E 6BT, England

One of the most impressive features of the dark-adapted rod visual system, known from psychophysical experiments (Hecht et al., 1942; Brumberg et al., 1943; van der Velden, 1944) is its ability to perform as a near-ideal detector of light, capable of detecting the absorption of a few photons. High sensitivity is already present at the retinal ganglion cell level for, as observed by Barlow et al., (1971), the absorption of a photon within its receptive field has a high probability of eliciting extra impulses in some ganglion cells.

What then is the contribution of the outer plexiform layer, where rods make synaptic contact with bipolar and horizontal cells, to the high performance of the retina? Other questions follow. What is the gain at the synapse? What is the signal produced in a bipolar cell by the absorption of a single photon in its receptive field? What is the signal-to-noise ratio and what is the contribution of the synapse to this ratio? What is the transmitter from rods to second order cells? In order to gain information on these questions, the retina of the spotted dogfish was chosen for study. It has the advantage that it contains almost exclusively rods and the bipolar and horizontal cells, with which they make synaptic contact, are relatively large so that stable prolonged recording with microelectrodes becomes feasible.

In Neumayer's paper of 1896 on the fine structure of the elasmobranch retina, he noted that Ramon y Cajal (1893) had published the results of a comprehensive investigation on the structurtal relationships in the retina of all classes of vertebrates with the exception of elasmobranchs. In his study of elasmobranch retina, Neumayer was at pains to follow Cajal's methods and nomenclature as regards the layers of the retina and the structures within them. The structure of the dogfish retina has been more recently studied by Stell and Witkovsky at the light and electron microscopical level (Stell and Witkovsky, 1973a,b; Witkovsky and Stell, 1973a,b).

Results

The flash responses to a light spot or full-field illumination of cells immediately postsynaptic to rods is illustrated in Fig. 1: off-centre (hyperpolarizing) bipolar cell, (A and B), horizontal cell (C) and on-centre (depolarizing) bipolar cell (D).

Several features (apart from polarity) stand out immediately. The responses are of different time course. The responses of off-centre bipolar cells to dim flashes are much briefer than the other cells and become oscillatory when both centre and surround are illuminated. The wave-form of dark-adapted on-centre cell responses was unaffected by simultaneous illumination of the centre and surround (Fig. 1D). Light responses of either off- or on-centre cells were not inverted by a light stimulus presented as an annulus. Off-centre bipolar cells were not frequently encountered in the rod-dominated dogfish retina. They constituted only about 3% of all bipolar cell recordings (out of about 600 cells) and will not be further analyzed. In what follows bipolar cells will refer to those of the on-centre type.

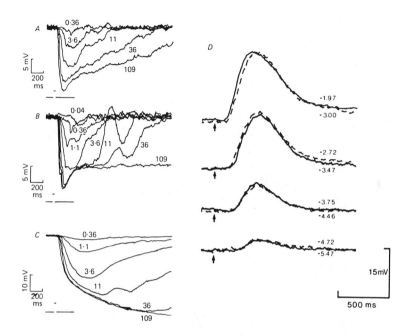

Fig. 1 Responses of postsynaptic cells to brief flashes of varying light intensities. A, B responses of an off-centre bipolar cell to a spot 210 um in diameter centred on the cell and to full-field illumination, respectively. C responses of a nearby horizontal cell to full-field illumination. Numbers by the records give light intensity as the mean number of photoisomerizations/rod. Timing of the flash is shown below each set. D responses of an on-centre bipolar cell to a centred spot, 200 um in diameter (continuous trace), and to large field illumination (dashed trace). The arrow indicates the time at which a 15 ms flash was given. The unattenuated light intensity was equivalent to 1275 Rh**/flash. The numbers above and below each response gives the attenuation in log units for the spot and for diffuse illumination.

Synaptic Gain

It is clear that there is a considerable signal processing in the outer synaptic layer. In order to examine this more closely, a comparison is made in Fig. 2 of the responses of an on-centre bipolar cell and a neighbouring horizontal cell which was penetrated spontaneously soon after the responses in Fig. 2A were recorded. In order to facilitate comparison, we define the flash sensitivity, S_F, as the peak amplitude of the response to a dim flash divided by the mean number of photoiso-merizations per rod evoked by the flash (abbreviated as Rh**) so that S_F has the dimensions of mV/Rh**. The flash sensitivity of the bipolar cell in Fig. 2 was 360 mV/Rh** while for the horizontal cell it was 4.5 mV/Rh**. The dimmest flash in Fig. 2A which gave a response of about 1.5 mV in the bipolar cell was 0.004 Rh**, i.e. one photoisomerization in one out of 250 rods. In order to produce a

36

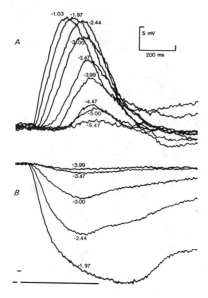

Fig. 2. Comparison between flash
responses of an on-centre bipolar
cell (A) and a neighbouring horizontal cell (B). The unattenuated
light intensity was 1200 Rh**/flash.
The numbers near each record indicate
log attenuation of the light. Bipolar
cell membrane potential in the dark
- 55 mV; horizontal cell - 45 mV.
(From Ashmore and Falk, 1979).

comparable response in the horizontal cell about 80 times as much light
horizontal cells about 8 mV/Rh**. Since the flash sensitivity for rods is
about 1-2 mV/Rh**, these results indicate that there is gain in signal
transmission from rods to bipolar or to horizontal cells and that the
average gain in the rod-bipolar cell synapse may be as high as 200-300
(Ashmore and Falk, 1980a).

Synaptic Filtering

There are obvious differences in the time course of bipolar and
horizontal cells. In order to highlight these differences, the dim flash
responses of the horizontal-bipolar cell pair shown in Fig. 2 have been
superimposed and normalized to the same peak amplitude (Fig. 3). It is
clear that the bipolar cell response to a flash has a much longer delay,
peaking at a later time, but that the maximum rate of rise of the response
has a more rapid rate of rise and rate of fall. The form of the
horizontal cell response is not very different from what has been
described for rod responses in a number of different vertebrate species.
The flash response of rods, horizontal cells and bipolar cells can be
described by an electrical analogue, that of a response to a very brief
pulse applied to a filter made up of a buffered cascade of low-pass
filters (Fuortes and Hodgkin, 1964; Penn and Hagins, 1972; Schwartz, 1976)
Ashmore and Falk, 1980A). The electrical analogues describing the
response of each cell type differ only in the number of stages and the
time constants of the filter stages. Schnapf and Copenhagen (1982),
recording from both rods and horizontal cells in the turtle retina,
reported that if the rod signal were passed through a filter containing
one low-pass stage and one high-pass stage, a good approximation to the
horizontal cell response was obtained.

Because of their size, it has not been possible to record from dogfish
rods. However, Ashmore and Falk (1979, 1980a) showed that the input-
output relations at the rod-bipolar cell synapse were far more complicated
than at the rod-horizontal cell synapse. The synaptic filter required

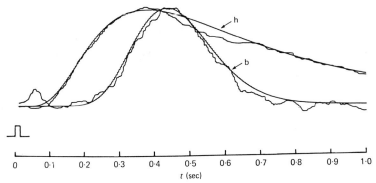

Fig. 3. Comparison of the time course of the small signal flash response of the bipolar (b) and horizontal cell (h) shown in Fig. 2. The responses have been superimposed and normalized to the same peak and amplitude. The smooth curves fitted to the responses were an empirical fit based on an electrical analog. (From Ashmore and Falk, 1980a).

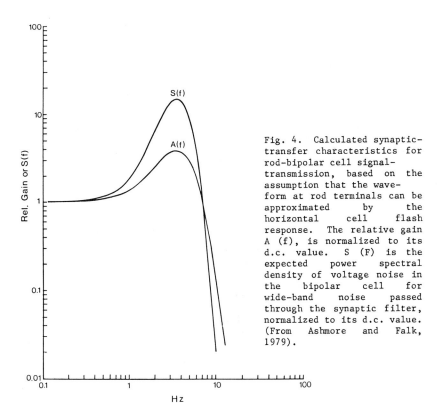

Fig. 4. Calculated synaptic-transfer characteristics for rod-bipolar cell signal-transmission, based on the assumption that the waveform at rod terminals can be approximated by the horizontal cell flash response. The relative gain A (f), is normalized to its d.c. value. S (F) is the expected power spectral density of voltage noise in the bipolar cell for wide-band noise passed through the synaptic filter, normalized to its d.c. value. (From Ashmore and Falk, 1979).

more delay stages as well as high-pass stages. Some characteristics of
the filter are shown in Fig. 4. The curve labelled A(f) represents the
gain of the system, normalized to its D.C. level, for different frequency
components of an incoming signal from the rods. It will be seen that the
gain rises up to a peak near 4 Hz before declining steeply at higher
frequencies. The peak is due to the high-pass filter stages. This has
important consequences for transmission of rod signals since the coupled
rod network itself performs high-pass filtering (Detwiler et al., 1978,
1980; Attwell and Wilson, 1980) so that rod signals speed up as they
spread through the network from the site of photon absorption. The
synaptic filter enhances rod signal-transmission by greater amplification
by the bipolar cell of the attenuated, but faster signals arising from the
more distant rods. The tuned filter characteristic at the rod-bipolar
synapse transforms the relatively slow rod signal into a less "sluggish"
one and thereby improves temporal resolution. The curve labelled $\underline{S}(f)$ and
will be referred to in the section on noise in bipolar cells.

What is the Effect of a Single Photon

Since the rod-bipolar cell synapse operates at high gain, it seemed
possible to estimate the voltage change produced by a single isomerization
occurring within the bipolar cell's receptive field. The single-photon
event was determined by two methods (Ashmore and Falk, 1980b, 1982). Both
rely on an analysis of fluctuations in voltage which arise from the
quantal nature of light.

Response to Flashes. In this method, a series of very dim flashes, which
are within the linear range of response, are presented and the variance
and mean of the response determined at each light intensity. Since the
absorption of light quanta follows a Poisson distribution, the variance in
number will be equal to the mean number of quanta absorbed. Figure 5
shows the results of one such experiment. It will be seen that both the
variance and means increase linearly with light intensity but that the
variance has a non-zero value in the dark, due to the presence of dark
noise. The ratio of the slope of the variance increase with light to the
slope of the mean gives x_1, the single-photon signal, 190 uV, for this
cell. The mean value for 13 cells was 250 uV. In order to test the idea
that the fluctuations were due to the variable number of photons in the
light stimulus itself plus dark noise, "frequency-of-seeing" curves were
constructed (Fig. 6), analogous to those used by Hecht et al., (1942).
The data were well fitted by the culumative Poisson sum,

In these experiments the flash sensitivity was also determined and
since the flash sensitivity $S_F = Nx_1$, the number of rods, N, which
converge onto a bipolar cell was determined, with a mean value of 1600.
With an inter-rod spacing of 3.9 μvm, if rods were arranged in a square
lattice, they would occupy a circular patch whose mean diameter would be
160 um with a range of 90 - 330 μm. If arranged in a hexagonal array the
mean diameter would be 150 um. This value is larger than the dendritic
spread determined by Procion yellow injection (Ashmore and Falk, 1980a)
and larger than the range of dendritic spread for bipolar cells which
appear to be of a similar type in the retina of the smooth dogfish
(Witkovsky and Stell, 1973a). It is possible that the receptive field
exceeds the dendritic span either because of rod-rod coupling or because
of coupling between bipolar cells. Witkovsky and Stell (1973b) found
sparse gap junctions between bipolar cell axon terminals in the dogfish
retina.

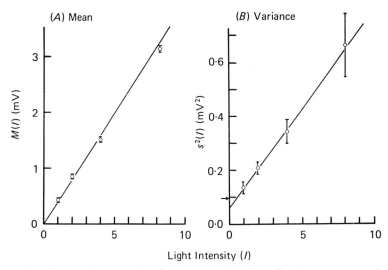

Fig. 5. Determination of the peak amplitude of the response of an on-centre bipolar to a single photoisomerization, within its receptive field, from an analysis of the mean A and variance B in response to repeated flashes of dim light. Light intensity has been normalized so that I = 1 corresponds to 2.64×10^{-3} Rh**/flash. Error bars in A indicate S.E. of the mean and in B the S.D. of the variance estimate. The arrow in B shows the variance measured in the dark. The lines are least-square fits to the data. The ratio of the slopes of the lines gives the single-photon signal, x_1 = 186 uV. x_1 determined for this cell from an analysis of steady-state voltage noise was 168 μV (cell 6 of Table 1 of this paper. (From Ashmore and Falk, 1980b).

Voltage Noise in On-Centre Bipolar Cells

Another powerful technique for determining the single-photon signal, first used by Hagins and Srebro (Hagins and Srebro, 1965; Hagins, 1965), is to analyze the statistical fluctuations in the steady state by means of the power spectral density of the noise. Thus, if a single isomerization in a rod produces a response in the bipolar cell, $\underline{x}$ (t), then for a Poisson process, the mean response resulting from the linear superposition of many photoisomerizations will be

$$V = \lambda \alpha_1^2 t_1 \tag{1}$$

where is the mean rate of photoisomerizations, x_1 is the peak amplitude of the photon shot event and t_1 is the integration time. The variance of the voltage fluctuations will be

$$\sigma_1^2 = \lambda \alpha_1^2 t_1 / \mathcal{Q}_1 \tag{2}$$

where Q_1, is a constant which depends on the shape of $\underline{x}$ (t).

40

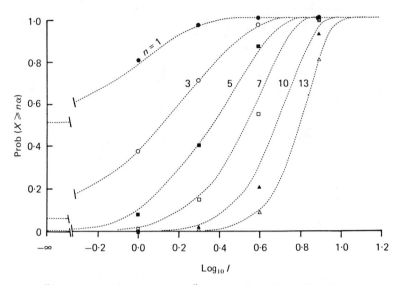

Fig. 6. "Frequency-of-seeing curves". Data from the cell illustrated in Fig. 6, plotted as the probability that the peak response amplitude equals or exceeds a criterion level equal to n times x_1 (= 186 uV) plotted against log of the normalized light intensity. The dotted curves are the theoretical Poisson sums for each integral number n, taking into account dark noise. (From Ashmore and Falk, 1980b).

Typical responses to long pulses to light of different intensities, both in the linear and non-linear range, are illustrated in Fig. 7. It will be noted that the noise present in darkness is suppressed by bright light but that the noise increases at low light levels. Power spectra were computed (Fig. 8). The spectra were interpreted as the sum of two independent components: one component consists of photon noise plus photon-like events which occur even in darkness while the other was assumed to be synaptic noise due to chemical transmission (Falk and Fatt, 1972; Ashmore and Falk, 1979, 1982). The way in which noise spectra were decomposed into components is illustrated in Fig. 9 and described more fully by Ashmore and Falk (1982). $S_1(f)$ corresponds to the power spectral density of photon noise; $S_2(f)$ was assumed to be synaptic noise. Integration of each component over frequency gives the variance of the component.

The single-photon signal. At low light intensities the photon-noise increased linearly with light, as did the mean depolarization (Fig. 10A). The single-photon signal x_1 was determined from eqns. (1) and (2) and the values are given in Table 1. There was good agreement between the values obtained from observing fluctauations in response to brief flashes and from power spectral analysis (Ashmore and Falk, 1980b, 1982).

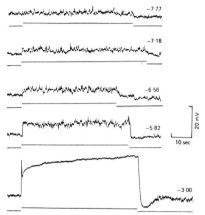

Fig. 7. Noise changes in a bipolar cell with steps of light of varying intensity diffusely illuminating the retina. Duration of the light is shown by the traces, under each second. The $\log_{10}$ of attenuation of the light (unattenuated intensity 7.9 x 10^4 Rh**/s) is shown above each record. (From Ashmore and Falk, 1980a).

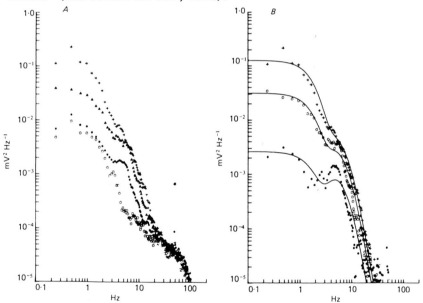

Fig. 8. Power spectral density of voltage noise of an on-centre bipolar cell. A, raw spectra at different light intensities (Rh**/s) before subtraction of electrode and instrumentation noise. ●, dark;▲7.4 x 10^{-3}; +, 83 x 10^{-3};○, 37. B, after subtraction of extraneous noise; ●, dark; ○, 7.4 x 10^3 Rh**/s; +, 83 x 10^3 Rh**/s. The continuous curves were constructed by the method described in the text and illustrated in Fig. 9. Cell 2 of Table 1. (From Ashmore and Falk, 1982).

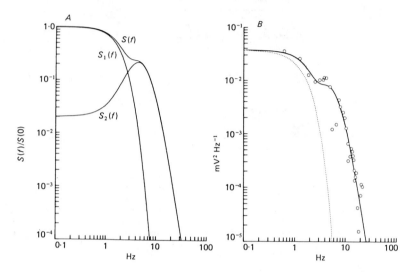

Fig. 9. Decomposition of the power spectrum S(f) of bipolar cell noise into 2 components, shown in A. B shows the difference spectrum in dim light for cell 8 in Table 1. The continuous curve is the fit with the parameters in A. The dotted line shows the expected spectrum of photon noise, based on the time course of the average response to dim flashes. (From Ashmore and Falk, 1982).

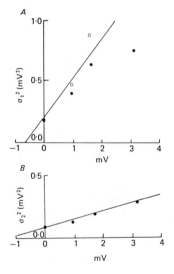

Fig. 10. Plots of the variance of photon noise (A) and synaptic noise (B) against membrane depolarization in dim light. Open circles in A are points which have been corrected for non-linearity, as described by Ashmore and Falk (1982).

T A B L E 1

Properties of the Single-Photon Signal and the Unitary Synaptic
Event in On-Centre Bipolar Cells

Cell	V_{max} (mV)	S_F (mV/Rh*)	x_1 (uV)	N	d (um)	x_2 (uV)	$\frac{V_{max}}{x_2}$	$\frac{V_{max}}{x_2 t_2}$ sec^{-1}	n_o
1	29	126	191	656	103	5.9	4920	2.7×10^5	382
2	35	128	226	566	100	8.1	4330	6.1×10^5	1070
3	30	1858	463	4010	260	71	425	9.3×10^3	29
4	17	330	45	8530	375	6.4	2650	5.8×10^4	31
5	31	450	288	1560	162	6.4	4830	2.6×10^5	528
6	17	136	168	810	116	17	1000	2.2×10^4	43
7	19	154	169	911	125	-	-	-	-
8	21	110	71	1550	161	4.5	4660	6.5×10^5	422
9	35	14	44	322	74	0.0	41000	2.2×10^6	605
10	25	42	57	732	111	4.5	5580	3.3×10^5	105
11	12	15	39	385	80	-	-	-	-
12	32	19	21	908	124	3.3	9680	2.1×10^5	28
13	19	-	160	-	-	-	-	-	-
Mean	24.3	281	150	1790	151	12.7	7750	4.7×10^5	329

Table 1 V_{max} is the maximum response to a bright flash of light. S_F is the flash sensitivity. x_1 is the single-photon signal; N the number of rods which converge onto a bipolar cell calculated from S_F/x_1; d the diameter of a circular field occupied by N rods if arranged in a hexagonal lattice. S_2 is the amplitude of the unitary synaptic event (probably the miniature postsynaptic potential) calculated from the limiting slope, near the dark, of the linear relation between synaptic noise variance and depolarization by light, taking into account the appropriate shape factor Q_2. V_{max}/x_2, when corrected for non-linear summation, gives the mean number of events which control the membrane potential in the dark and $V_{max}/(x_2 t_2)$, if corrected for non-linear summation, the rate of synaptic events in the dark. n_o gives the number of synaptic events suppressed when there is a single photoisomerization in the receptive field of a bipolar cell. The numbering of cells corresponds to Tables 1 and 2 in Ashmore and Falk (1982) where other cell properties are given. The mean potential in the dark was -44mV.

Synaptic Noise

It will be noted in Figs. 8 and 9 that the component $S_2(f)$ attributed to synaptic noise has similar features to the characteristics of the synaptic filter (Fig. 4). It was found that at low light intensities, synaptic noise increased linearly with the mean depolarization (Fig. 20B). The peak amplitude of the unitary synaptic event x_2 was calculated from the slope of the variance vs. mean graph and the appropriate Q_2, the shape factor. The results are given in Table 1. The mean amplitude of x_2 in the dark was 13 μV (hyperpolarization).

The mean number of simultaneous events in the dark. The mean number of transmitter events controlling the potential of the bipolar cell in the dark would be given by the maximum response to bright light V max (when it is assumed that all transmitter release is suppressed) divided by the unitary event x_2, if there were linear summation. However, there is a correction required for non-linear summation which is R_D/R_L, the ratio of the cell's input resistance in darkness and in bright light. The value of V_{max}/s_2 is given in Table 1. The mean value was 7750. The correction factor for non-linear summation is about 2.5 (Ashmore and Falk, 1980a), so that the mean number of simultaneous elementary transmitter events would be 19,000.

These events will be contributed by all the rods which make synaptic contact with a bipolar cell. From the size of the dendritic field of the bipolar cell (Witkovsky and Stell, 1973a) and the spacing of rods (Ashmore and Falk, 1980b), it is estimated that about 300-500 rods make synaptic contact. (The number of rods which signal to bipolar cells may be greater than those actually making synaptic contact by a factor of 4 because of rod-rod coupling.) The mean number of simultaneous synaptic events/rod in the dark is therefore estimated to be about 50. The integration time, t_2, calculated from the time course of the unitary synaptic event (Ashmore and Falk, 1982) has a mean value of 27 ms, so that the dark rate of synaptic events/rod would be about 1800/s.

The number of transmitter events suppressed by a single photon

If the depolarization of the rod bipolar cell results from the suppression of synaptic transmitter release, then the number of transmitter events, n_0, suppressed by each photon absorbed within the rod pool of the bipolar cell can be shown to be equal to the ratio of the slopes of the zero-frequency asymptotes of the S_1 and S_2 spectral components against response, when both response and variance change linearly with light. This number had a mean value of 330 (Table 1). During the response to a single photon, the number of transmitter events controlling the dark membrane potential would have been 1900 x t_1/t_2 = 2.6 x 10^5. Hence the single photon would have suppressed the release of 330/2.6 x 10^5 = 0.12% of the number during a response. This figure is consistent with a previous estimate of 1/400 for the fractional change in the conductance of the light modulated channels at the peak of the single-photon response (Ashmore and Falk, 1980b).

Signal-to-Noise

The dark noise in bipolar cells consisted of photon-like events plus synaptic noise. The equivalent background or "dark light" was estimated by Ashmore and Falk (1977, 1982) who measured the noise variance as a function of known light intensities. They found that in the dark-adapted state photon-like events occur at a rate equivalent to a background in which one rhodopsin molecule per rod is isomerized every 560 sec at $17°C$. The results were consistent with direct observations made by Baylor et al., (1980) on toad rods and with psychophysical estimates (Barlow, 1956) taking into account differences in temperature and rhodopsin content. These dark photon-like events were assumed to arise from thermal isomerization of rhodopsin with a rate constant of 10^{-11} s at $20°C$, with a half-life for rhodopsin of the order of 2000 years. However, these values may be an underestimate of the stability of rhodopsin, for an increase in photon-like dark events occurs following relatively weak rhodopsin bleaches (Lamb, 1980; Ashmore and Falk, 1981). This increase in noise may be related to some step in phototransduction and it seems possible that such events may occur in the fully dark-adapted retina.

Synaptic noise variance in the dark tended to be lower than the noise due to photon-like events by a factor of about 0.7. An estimate of the signal-to-noise was made from the ratio of the amplitude of the single-photon signal to the r.m.s. value of the dark noise. This amounted to about 0.7 (Ashmore and Falk, 1980b, 1982). This would suggest that the absorption of about 5 photons in the receptive field of a bipolar cell within an integration time of 300-400 ms might be reliably signalled to a ganglion cell.

The Rod Neurotransmitter
Membrane conductance changes. The equivalent circuit of a postsynaptic cell is shown in Fig. 11A. The element g_r is a variable conductance controlled by the neurotransmitter and E_r is the reversal potential for this conductance path. E_o and G_o refer to a non-synaptic path. There is ample evidence to sustain Trifonov's original hypothesis (Trifonov, 1968) that rods release transmitter at a high rate in the dark and the hyperpolarization by light reduces that release. Figure 11B shows that, as the release of rod transmitter is decreased by light, the input resistance of an on-centre bipolar cell decreases. The rod transmitter reduces synaptic conductance with a reversal potential more positive than the dark potential (Kaneko, 1971; Toyoda, 1973; Nelson, 1973; Ashmore and Falk, 1980a). On the other hand, Trifonov et al., (1974) have shown in an ingenious way that the photoreceptor neurotransmitter opens ionic channels of horizontal cells and that the reversal potential is near zero potential, implying that the channels are fairly non-selective for cations (as are those of on-centre bipolar cells).

Transmitter candidates. L-Glutamate, L-aspartate and a number of their analogues mimic the action of the rod neurotransmitter on horizontal and bipolar cells in the intact retina (Shiells et al., 1981; see also the contributions of others in this volume). The action of one such analogue, kainate, on an on-centre bipolar cell is illustrated in Fig. 12A. In this experiment synaptic transmission was blocked by adding 2mM Co^{2+} to the perfusate. In the absence of the transmitter (which closes semi-selective Na^+ channels), the cell depolarized and this was accompanied by a fall in input resistance. When kainate was added to the perfusate, the cell hyperpolarized and the input resistance increased. In contrast horizontal cells were depolarized by kainate, quisqualate, L-glutamate and L-aspartate.

One extremely interesting analogue of glutamate is 2-amino-4-phosphonobutyric acid (APB) which hyperpolarized on-centre bipolar cells, increases membrane resistance and blocks the response to light, indicating that it acts on the same channels as does the rod neurotransmitter (Fig. 12B). However, it is without affect on membrane potential or light response of rod horizontal cells. This provides a very strong indication that the binding sites for the rod neurotransmitter of horizontal and on-centre bipolar cells have different properties (considered in more detail, by Slaughter and Miller in this volume).

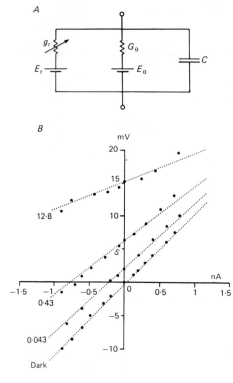

Fig. 11. Changes in input resistance of an on-centre bipolar cell arising from a change in transmitter concentration produced by a light flash. A is an equivalent circuit of a postsynaptic cell. The conductance of transmitter-controlled channels is represented by a variable conductance g_r which ranges between zero and a maximum conductance G_r. E_r is the reversal potential for this path. E_o and G_o represent the source potential and conductance of non-synaptic sites and C is the capacitance of the cell membrane. B shows the current-voltage relation of a bipolar cell in darkness and at the peak of responses to flashes of different intensity ($Rh^* /$ flash), given by the numbers to the left of each one. The ordinate is the voltage displacement from the dark level. Potential in the dark – 37 mV; E_r, obtained from the point of intersection of the lines and the potential in the dark, was – 10 mV. Input resistance in the dark 10.3 MΩ; in bright light light 4.3 MΩ. (Adapted from Ashmore and Falk, 1980a).

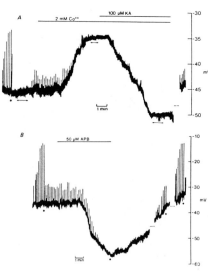

Fig. 12. Hyperpolarization of on-centre bipolar cells by kainate (KA) and APB, superfusing a dogfish eyecup. In A, Co^{++} was first used to block synaptic transmitter release, resulting in depolarization of the cell and a large decrease in cell input resistance consistent with the idea that the rod neurotransmitter closes semi-selecive NA channels (resistance measurements made during the intervals indicated by arrows). KA hyperpolarized the cell and increased the cells input resistance. B, APB hyperpolarized the cell and blocked responses to light even of high intensity (delivered at time shown by the dot). Input resistance was increased by APB. (Adapted from Shiells et al., 1981).

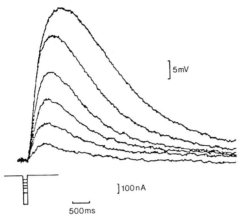

]5mV

]100nA

500ms

Fig. 13. Ionophoretic responses to close application of L-glutamate to a rod horizontal cell on the surface of a retinal slice. The duration and size of the ionophoretic pulses are indicated in the lower part of the record (Shiells, unpublished).

The study of L-glutamate and 1-aspartate action in the superfused retina is complicated by uptake mechanisms for these putative transmitters (Marc and Lam, 1981; Ishida and Fain, 1981). We have more recently used ionophoresis onto cells located on the surface of relatively thin radial slices of retina under visual control via an intra-red camera attached to a microscope (Falk and Shiells, 1984a; Shiells and Falk, in preparation). Figure 13 illustrates the depolarizations produced by brief ionophoretic pulses of L-glutamate on a rod horizontal cell. Such cells in the slice responsed to light with hyperpolarizations of up to 60 mV, much like cells in the intact retina. Ionophoresis from multibarrel pipettes indicated that L-glutamate and kainate were equipotent while aspartate was about 1/10 as potent. Since kainate is effective at about 1 uM, the conclusion is that glutamate too acts at a concentration of uM or less, as there may still be some uptake of glutamate near the surface of the slice when glutamate diffuses (Falk and Shiells, 1984a,b). A cooperativity of 2 molecules of agonist acted to open an ionic channel in rod horizontal cells. Cooperativity could be demonstrated when transmitter background was reduced by a step of light (Sheills and Falk, in preparation). These experiments suggest that glutamate and kainate act on synaptic rather than extra-synaptic sites on rod horizontal cells. Definitive experiments with aspartate are not as yet complete. The finding that D-aspartate acts as a competitive antagonist to L-glutamate, kainate and L-aspartate adds additional, but not conclusive support to the idea of a common site of action. Antagonism by D-aspartate to L-glutamate and kainate depolarization of isolated horizontal cells of the goldfish retina was reported by Ishida (1984). These isolated cells differ form those in the retinal slice in that they do not respond to L-aspartate and they appear to be about 1/10 as sensitive to L-glutamate compared with kainate (Dowling et al., 1983; Ishida, 1984). It remains to be determined whether these differences are species specific, rod-cone specific or the result of enzymic degradation or loss of membrane receptors during cell isolation.

Discussion

Synaptic Gain

One very surprising result is that the voltage gain in synaptic transmission from rods to on-centre bipolar cells is at least 200 while the gain at the rod-horizontal cell syanpse is about 8. These figures are arrived at from the ratio of flash sensitives of rods and post-synaptic cells in the linear range of their flash responses in the dark-adapted state. A mean flash sensitivity of 1 mV/Rh* was assumed, based on measurements in other species (Fain, 1975; Copenhagen and Owen, 1976; Detwiler et al., 1980).

The maximum gain A_{max} at the optimum operating point of the synapse can be derived as given in more detail by Falk and Fatt (1972; 1974a,b). A general expression for the maximum gain at a synapse where the transmitter opens ionic channels is

$$A_{max} = \frac{bp\ (a-1)}{4\quad a}\ (E_r - E_o) \qquad (3)$$

where $a = 1 + G_r/G_o$ and G_r is the total conductance of synaptically controlled channels, G_o the conductance of non-synaptic channels E_r and E_o the voltage sources in the equivalent circuit of a postsynaptic cell in Fig. 11. The parameter b is an empirical constant whose reciprocal is the potential change at the presynaptic terminal necessary to give an e-fold change in transmitter release. p is a constant $\gg 1$, depending on the number n of transmitter molecules required to open an ionic channel and if released in packets, the extent to which transmitter packets may interact. At the neuromuscular junction, where transmitter release is quantized, it is likely that p is close to one since the lifetime of a packet of acetylcholine is determined by a process (hydrolysis) which is more rapid than diffusion so that the effect of a packet on conductance remains localized (Hartzell et al., 1975). It is only when cholinesterase is inhibited that potentiation occurs. Although the present results indicate that there may be a cooperativity of two for the transmitter at the rod-horizontal cells, there is no information on the rate of uptake or destruction of transmitter compared with diffusion.

Voltage dependence of transmitter release. Synaptic gain would be higher if there were a steeper dependence of rod transmitter release on membrane potential than is found at other synapses. The value of b p can be estimated from equation (3) for the rod-horizontal cell synapse. Trifonov et al., (1974) have estimated E_r = OmV. E_o has the value of - 120 mV, the internal potential observed in dogfish horizontal in bright light or when transmitter release is suppressed by Co^{2+}. This presumably corresponds to the K^+ equilibrium potential for measurements of the ionic concentration of the vitreous gave a K^+ concentration of 2.3-2.5 mM while (Na^+) was 250mM. The expected internal concentration of K^+ would be about 250mM if osmotic equilibrium is to be maintained, giving a ratio of about 100 for internal (K^+) to external (K^+). The value of a is not known. However, it is likely that $a \gg 1$ since is was observed that application of glutamate analogues could drive the internal potential of horizontal cells to a value close to the estimated value of E_r (Shiells et al., 1981). With A_{max} = 8, on average (Ashmore and Falk, 1980a), bp would have the value 0.27 mV^{-1}. Since p ranges between 1-2, an e-fold change in transmitter release would be produced by a 4-8 mV change in rod membrane potential, comparable to values reported for a number of different synapses (e.g. Liley, 1956; Kusano et al., 1965; Katz and Miledi, 1967; Martin and Ringham, 1975).

It may also be noted that the maximum gain for a synapse at which the transmitter opens ion channels occurs when the internal potential is

$$E = (a+1) \ (E_r - E_o)/2A \qquad (4)$$

When $a \gg 1$, eqn. (4) reduces to the result given by Falk and Fatt (1972), that the optimum potential of the postsynaptic cell, set by transmitter action, lies midway between the reversal potential and E_o. It is interesting, therefore, that the average potential in the dark of rod horizontal cells is -59 mV (Ashmore and Falk, 1980a), virtually identical with the theoretical potential for maximum gain.

These considerations make it unlikely that the high gain at the rod-on-centre bipolar cell synapse could arise from an unusually steep relation between potential at rod terminals and transmitter release, unless it is assumed that the synapses with horizontal cells and bipolar cells are effectively segregated or that they have different transmitters. These possibilities seem improbably from electron microscopical and pharmacological evidence.

Falk and Fatt (1974a,b) have shown that it is possible, in principle, to have a higher gain at a synapse at which the trasmitter closes ion channels. However, a kinetic scheme which yields a relation between conductance change g and concentration of transmitter (T) (assumed to be proportional to the rate of transmitter release) of the form

$$\Delta g = -G_r \ \frac{[T]^n}{[T]^n + K^n} \qquad (5)$$

where K is an apparent dissociation constant, such as was used (except for a change of sign) in deriving egns, (3) and (4), yields identical equations. In order to obtain higher gain, it seems necessary to suppose that receptor sites may continue to bind transmitter even when a large fraction are occupied. Both the temporal properties of the bipolar cell signal and the noise spectrum also suggest a more elaborate kinetic scheme than is found at other synapses.

Acknowledgements

Much of the work cited was done in collaboration with Prof. Paul Fatt, Dr. Johathan Ashmore and more recently, Dr. Richard Shiells. I am grateful to Prof. Robert Werman for correspondence regarding synaptic gain and cooperativity and to Dr. Christopher Fry and Miss Beryl Moon for measurements of Na and K concentrations in dogfish vitreal fluid. Original work was generously supported by the Medical Research Council, the Science and Engineering Research council and the Rank Prize Funds.

References

Ashmore, J.F. and Falk, G. Nature, 270, 69 (1977).
Ashmore, J.F. and Falk, G. Vis. Res. 19, 419 (1979).
Ashmore, J.F. and Falk, G. J. Physiol., 300, 115 (1980a).
Ashmore, J.F. and Falk, G. J. Physiol., 300, 151 (1980b).
Ashmore, J.F. and Falk, G. J. Physiol., 332, 273 (1982).
Attwell, D. and Wilson, M. J. Physiol., 309, 287 (1980).
Barlow, H.B. J. Opt. Sco. Am. 26, 634 (1956).
Barlow, H.B., Levick, W.R. and Yoon, M. Vis. Res. Suppl., 3, 87 (1971).
Baylor, D.A., Matthews, G. and Yau, K.-W. J. Physiol., 309, 591 (1980).
Brumberg, E.M., Vavilov, S.I. and Sverdlov, Z.M. J. Phusiol., 7, 1 (1943).
Copenhagem D.R. and Owen, W.G. J. Physiol., 259, 251 (1976).
Detwiler, P.B., Hodgkin, A.L. and McNaughton, P.A. J. Physiol. 300, 213,

Dowling, J.E., Lasater, E.M., Van Buskirk, R. and Watling, K.J. Vis. Res. 23, 421 (1983).

Fain, G.L. Science 187, 838 (1975).

Falk, G. and Fatt, P. in Handbook of Sensory Physiology. VII/1. H.J.A. Dartnall, ed. (Springer Verlag, Berlin 1972) pp. 200-240.

Falk, G. and Falk, P. Vis. Res. 14, 739 (1974a).

Falk, G. and Fatt, P. in Lecture notes in Biomathematics Vol 4, M. Conrad, W. Guttinger and M. Dal Cin, eds (Springer Verlag, Berlin 1974b) pp. 171-204.

Falk, G. and Shiells, R.A. J. Physiol, 357, 8P (1984a).

Falk, G. and Shiells, R.A. International Union of Physiological Sciences, Jerusalem, p. 278 (1984b).

Fuortes, M.G.F. and Hodgkin, A.L. J. Physiol., 172, 239 (1964).

Hagins, W.A. Cold Spring Harb Sympos Quant Biol., 30, 403 (1965).

Hartzell, H.C., Kuffler, S.W. and Yoshikami, D. J. Physiol., 251,427 (1975).

Hecht, S. Shlaer, S. and Pirenne, M. J. Gen. Physiol. 25, 819 (1942).

Ishida, A.T. Brain Res. 298, 25 (1984).

Ishida, A.T. and Fain, G.L. Proc. Nat. Acad. Sci. 78, 5890 (1981).

Kaneko, A. Vis. Res. Suppl., 3, 17 (1971).

Katz, B. and Miledi, R. J. Physiol., 192, 407 (1967).

Kusano, K., Livengood, D.R. and Werman, R. J. Gen. Physiol., 50, 2579 (1967).

Liley, A.W. J. Physiol., 134, 427 (1956.

Marc, R.E. and Lam, D.M.K. Proc. Nat. Acad. Sci. 78, 7185 (1981).

Martin, A.R. and Ringham, G.L. J. Physiol., 251, 409 (1975).

Nelson, R. J. Neurophysiol., 36 519 (1973).

Neumayer, L. J. Arch. Mikrosk. Anat., 48, 83 (1896).

Penn, R.D. and Hagins, W.A. Biophys. J. 12, 1073 (1972).

Cajal, Ramon y. La Cellule Vol. 9 (1893).

Schnapf, J.L. and Copenhagen, D.R. Nature 296, 862 (1982).

Schwartz, E.A. J. Physiol., 257, 379 (1976).

Shiells, R.A., Falk, G. and Naghshineh, S. (Nature 294, 592 (1981).

Stell, W.K. and Witkovsky, P. J. Camp. Neurol., 148, 33 (1973a).

Stell, W.K. and Witkovsky, P. J. Camp. Neurol., 148, 1 (1973b).

Toyoda, J. Vis. Res. 13, 283 (1973).

Trifonov, Yu A. Biofizika 13, 809 (1968).

Trifonov, Yu A., Byzov, A.L. and Chailahian, L.M. Vis. Res. 14, 229 (1974).

van der Velden, H.A. Physica, 11, 179 (1944).

Witkovsky, P. and Stell, W.K. J. Comp. Neurol., 148 47 (1973a).

Witkovsky, P. and Stell, W.K. J. Comp. Neurol., 150 147 (1973b).

The Role of Glutamate Receptors in Information Processing
in the Distal Retina

Malcolm M. Slaughter, Robert F. Miller*
State University of New York
Buffalo, N. Y. 14214

Washington University*
St. Louis, MO 63110

Although visual information processing occurs at many levels from retina to cerebral cortex, a surprising degree of differentiation occurs in the distal retina. The photoreceptors, through pigment diversity within rods and cones, produce selective responses to light of varying wavelengths and intensities. These responses are permuted synaptically by conversion of the monotonic photoreceptor response to a multiplicity of waveforms that vary in their polarity, amplification, and latency. The foundations for many parameters of vision are derived from this first synapse in the visual pathway. Through synaptic divergence, second order neurons give rise to such fundamental processes as the segregation of ON and OFF channels, the development of surround inhibition, the interaction of rod and cone signals, and the encoding of color specificity. This is accomplished through a combination of anatomical, physiological, and pharmacological specializations both presynaptically and postsynaptically.

We have been particularly interested in the role of neurotransmitters and their receptors in the generation of these multiple modalities. To begin to address this topic, we examined the mechanisms of cell communication between photoreceptors and the three classes of second order neurons. Although the responses of ON bipolars, OFF bipolars, and horizontal cells are different, these neurons share similar synaptic loci and recent evidence indicates that they all respond to the same photoreceptor neurotransmitter, presumably glutamate (Murakami et al., 1972, 1975; Bloomfield and Dowling, 1982; Slaughter and Miller, 1983a). It therefore seemed reasonable to suppose that at least part of the diversity of responses originated in a differentiation in postsynaptic receptor-ionophore complexes.

The experimental protocol relied on evaluating chemical analogs of glutamate and aspartate. The basis for this analysis was established by the reports of Curtis and Watkins (1960, 1963) which demonstrated that the potency of excitatory amino acids depended on the presence of a carbon chain containing two carboxyl and one amino groups. These three moieties, which are all charged at physiological pH, presumably represent the sites bound by the postsynaptic receptor. These workers were also able to show that as the carbon chain length between these groups increased the agonist activity first increased, then decreased, indicating a preferred separation for receptor activation. The ideal chain length for agonists was equivalent to that of aspartate or glutamate. They found that the effectiveness of excitatory amino acid antagonists, like agonists, also depended upon the presence of two carboxyl and one amino groups, although the preferred chain length for blocking activity was found to be one or two carbons longer than glutamate.

This discovery has led to the probing of acidic amino acid receptors by using analogs of varying chain length or ligands containing modification of the carboxyl or amino groups. This approach has been particularly fruitful in characterizing the presumed aspartate receptor, which is activated selectively when a methyl group is added to the amino nitrogen of aspartate (N methyl aspartate) or blocked when the D form of longer chain asparate analogs are used (eg. D alpha amino adipate, D alpha

Neurocircuitry of the Retina, A Cajal Memorial
A. Gallego and P. Gouras, Editors

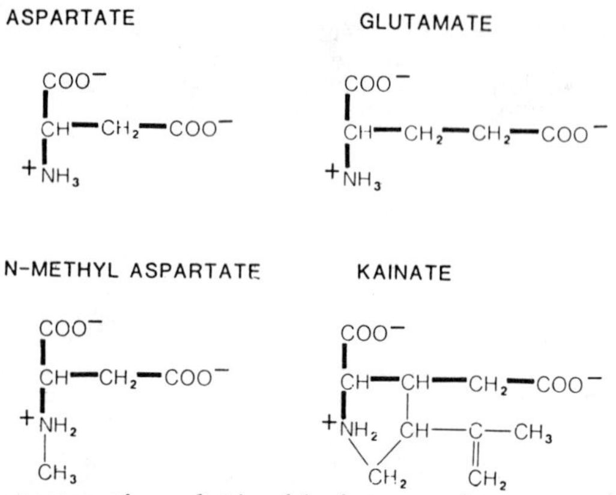

ASPARTATE   GLUTAMATE

```
COO⁻                    COO⁻
 |                       |
CH—CH₂—COO⁻            CH—CH₂—CH₂—COO⁻
 |                       |
⁺NH₃                    ⁺NH₃
```

N-METHYL ASPARTATE   KAINATE

```
COO⁻                    COO⁻
 |                       |
CH—CH₂—COO⁻            CH—CH—CH₂—COO⁻
 |                       |   |
⁺NH₂                   ⁺NH₂ CH—C—CH₃
 |                         \  ||
CH₃                        CH₂ CH₂
```

Fig. 1. Illustrates the relationship between glutamate and aspartate and their selective agonists, kainic acid and N methyl aspartic acid, respectively.

amino suberate, or D 2-amino-5-phosphonovalerate) (Watkins and Evans, 1981). Another procedure aimed at identifying excitatory amino acid receptor subtypes incorporates the active moieties of aspartate or glutamate into conformationally restricted molecules, usually ring structures. This has been most effective in the development of selective glutamate agonists such as kainic acid, quisqualic acid, and AMPA.

We have used these techniques to investigate acidic amino acid receptors on second order retinal neurons. Our initial experiments were directed at determining if either aspartate or glutamate was a likely photoreceptor transmitter candidate in the mudpuppy. In the carp retina, Murakami and his colleagues had reported that either amino acid could mimic the action of the photoreceptor neurotransmitter on horizontal cells (Murakami et al., 1972) and both types of bipolar cells (Murakami et al., 1975). At that time acidic amino acid pharmacology did not offer agents that could distinguish between aspartate and glutamate receptors. Subsequently, Wu and Dowling (1978) reported that alpha amino adipate blocked L-type horizontal cells, suggesting that the carp retina possessed aspartate receptors. Therefore we performed a preliminary screening using N methyl aspartate as an aspartate agonist and kainic acid as a glutamate agonist. The relationship of these agonists to glutamate and aspartate is illustrated in Fig. 1. Our findings, summarized in figures 2-4, indicated that kainic acid was much more potent than N methyl aspartate on all three types of second order neurons (Slaughter and Miller, 1983a). Kainic acid suppressed the light responses of these neurons by driving their membrane potential close to the dark membrane voltage, the potential evoked by the photoreceptor neurotransmitter which is released maximally in the dark. Kainic acid effects on horizontal cells and ON bipolars were seen with concentrations of 1 µM, while total suppression of the light response could be produced with 50-100 uM kainic acid. Concentrations of N methyl aspartate between 50 uM and 2mM did not mimic the effects of the photoreceptor neurotransmitter. Low magnesium, which enhances N methyl aspartate's action in some systems (Nowak et al., 1984), had no effect on these cells. These results suggested that bipolar and horizontal cells possess glutamate-like receptors rather than aspartate-like receptors. The ineffectiveness of several presumed aspartate antagonists, such as alpha

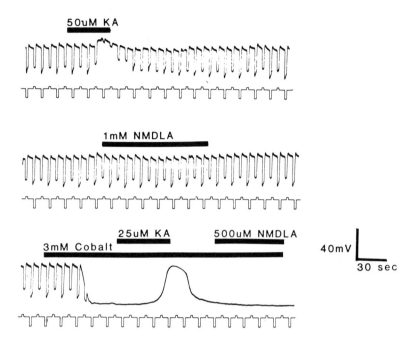

Fig. 2. Compares the action of kainic acid (KA) and N methyl aspartate
(NMDLA) on the membrane potential and light responses of a horizontal
cell. Kainic acid depolarizes this cell close to the dark membrane
voltage generated by the endogenous photoreceptor neurotransmitter.
Kainic acid is effective after chemical synaptic neurotransmission has
been blocked by cobalt, indicating a direct action on the horizontal cell.
N methyl aspartate has little effect. The dark bars above the
intracellular voltage traces indicate the duration of drug application and
the square pulses below the traces indicate light stimuli. Upward pulses
are small spots of light (200 μm) and downward deflections are annuli of
light (400 μm inner diameter, outer diameter greater than retina). From
the J. Neuroscience, 1983)

amino adipate and alpha amino suberate, supported this conclusion. This
preferential sensitivity to glutamate agonists has also been observed in
fish horizontal cells by Ishida and Fain (1981) using an uptake inhibitor,
by Lasater and Dowling (1981) using isolated horizontal cells in culture,
and by Rowe and Ruddock (1982a,b) using pharmacological analogs. However,
our experiments also provided a clue that there was a difference in the
excitatory amino acid receptors among the three second order neurons.
Kainic acid was not as potent on OFF bipolars as on ON bipolars and
horizontal cells while 1 mM N methyl aspartate had a slight depolarizing
action. Thus, the OFF bipolars appeared to have a different pharmacology
than the other second order neurons.

54

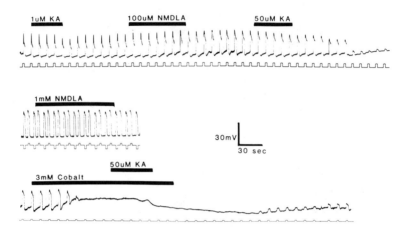

Fig. 3. Contrasts the effects of kainic acid and N methyl aspartate on ON bipolar cells. As in horizontal cells, kainic acid mimics the effect of the photoreceptor transmitter, even when synaptic neurotransmission is blocked by cobalt, while N methyl aspartate does not. (From J. Neuroscience, 1983)

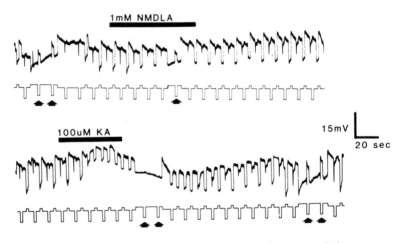

Fig. 4. Shows a recording from an OFF bipolar cell. N methyl aspartate has a slight depolarizing action, kainic acid is more potent although less effective than in the previous two figures. (From the J. Neuroscience, 1983)

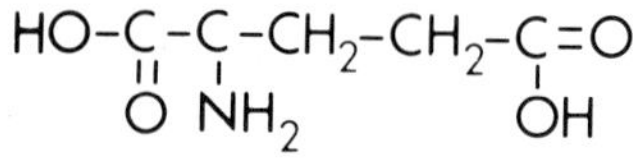

HO-C-C-CH$_2$-CH$_2$-C=O
   ‖ | |
   O NH$_2$ OH

GLUTAMIC ACID

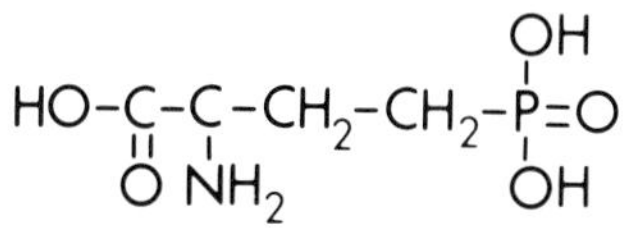

                          OH
HO-C-C-CH$_2$-CH$_2$-P=O
   ‖ | |
   O NH$_2$ OH

2-AMINO-4-PHOSPHONO-BUTYRIC ACID

Fig. 5. Illustrates the similarity between glutamic acid and 2-amino-4-phosphonobutyric acid.

At this juncture it is appropriate to point out one of the advantages of studying excitatory amino acid receptors in the distal retina. Glutamate, aspartate, and their analogs have direct excitatory effects and several secondary actions such as increasing extracellular potassium (Krnjevic et al., 1982), producing cell swelling and neurotoxicity (Olney, 1969; Yazulla and Kleinschmidt, 1980), and altering the uptake mechanisms responsible for neurotransmitter inactivation (Balcar and Johnston, 1972; Ishida and Fain, 1981). The auxillary actions often make comparisons between presumed receptor subtypes very difficult, particularly if these effects are localized and therefore affect some synapses while sparing others. The juxtapositon of the synaptic receptors of second order neurons in the amphibian distal retina (Dowling and Werblin, 1969); Lasansky, 1978) permits a clearer comparison of the differential effects of excitatory amino acid analogs on the three classes of neurons. As it turned out, the correlation between receptor subtypes and the three neuronal classes facilitated the characterization of these receptors.

Because our results indicated that bipolar and horizontal cells possessed glutamate-like receptors, we tested a variety of glutamate analogs. We used ring structure analogs in which the conformations were restricted and analogs in which one of the three presumed binding sites (amino or either carboxyl group) was modified. One of the latter analogs, in which the terminal carboxyl group was replaced by a phosphonic acid moiety, was 2-amino-4-phosphonobutyrate (APB) (see Fig. 5). Cull-Candy et al., (1976) reported that APB acted as a glutamate antagonist at the locust neuromuscular junction. In the mudpuppy retina, we found that it was a glutamate agonist that activated ON bipolar receptors, but not horizontal cell or OFF bipolar receptors (Fig. 6). Like the photoreceptor neurotransmitter, APB hyperpolarized ON bipolar cells by closing membrane channels. APB's action on the ON bipolar persisted in the presence of cobalt indicating a direct, rather than a polysynaptic, action. This combination of effects indicated that APB was acting on synaptic receptors and identified a distinct class of glutamate receptors (Slaughter and Miller, 1981). This study provided the first identification of this class

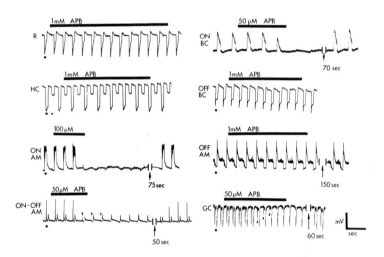

Fig. 6. Shows the effect of 2-amino-4phosphonobutyric acid (APB) on distal and proximal retinal neurons. In the distal retina, APB mimics the action of the photoreceptor transmitter only on ON bipolars. In the inner retina, ON responses are blocked. (From Science, 1981)

of glutamate receptors, which has subsequently been identified at various sites in the central nervous system (Butcher et al., 1983).

In the retina, the localization of APB's action to the ON bipolar synapse makes it a useful tool in analyzing retinal circuitry. Since the ON bipolars initiate the ON center response, APB eliminates the ON pathway throughout the retina. This action of APB has been confirmed in other retinas, including the dogfish (Shiells et al., 1981) and rabbit (Neal et al., 1981; Bloomfield and Dowling, 1982; Massey et al., 1983). It has led to a comparison of ON versus OFF pathways in the rabbit retina (Neal et al., 1981; Massey and Redburn, 1982) and in visual centers in the brain of monkey (Schiller, 1982) and cat (Horton and Sherk, 1984).

Another acidic amino acid analog, which acts as an antagonist, is cis 2,3 piperdine dicarboxylic acid (PDA), described by Davies et al., (1981). In the distal retina, the action of PDA was complementary to APB since it suppressed tyhe light responses of OFF bipolar and horizontal cells, while leaving ON bipolar responses relatively unaffected (Fig. 7). The action of this antagonist confirmed two preliminary conclusions: 1) that OFF bipolar and horizontal cell synaptic responses were mediated by excitatory amino acid receptors and 2) that ON bipolar receptors were distinct from those on other second order neurons. PDA has been described as a general excitatory amino acid antagonist, which blocks both aspartate and glutamate receptors. We have made similar observations in the proximal retina (Slaughter and Miller, 1983b). However, our previous experiments indicated that N methyl aspartate (presumed aspartate) receptors did not mediate light responses in the distal retina, so that the action of PDA could be ascribed to its glutamate receptor antagonism. Consistent with this conclusion, we found taht PDA could block the kainic acid generated

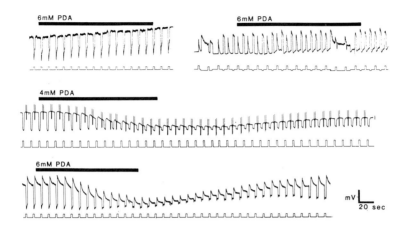

Fig. 7. Illustrates the action of cis 2,3 piperidine dicarboxylic acid (PDA) on neurons in the distal retina. Horizontal cell (middle trace) and OFF bipolar (lower trace) light responses are suppressed while photoreceptor (upper left) and ON bipolar (upper right) responses are unattenuated. (From Science, 1983)

depolarization of horizontal cells (Slaughter and Miller, 1983c). The effects of APB and PDA suggested that there were two classes of glutamate-like receptors on second order neurons: one associated with ON bipolars and another found in OFF bipolar and horizontal cells.

However, our initial studies using kainic acid indicated that OFF bipolar receptors were pharmacologically different than horizontal cell receptors. Another glutamate analog, D-o-phosphoserine, made this distinction more apparent (Slaughter and Miller, 1985a). This agent was able to suppress the light response of horizontal cells while leaving ON and OFF bipolar responses intact (Fig. 8). The center responses of both bipolar cells were unchanged or enhanced while the antagonistic surround, believed to be due to horizontal cell feedback, was suppressed (Fig. 8 arrows). Like PDA, D-o-phosphoserine was able to block the depolarization of horizontal cells by exogenously applied kainic acid, supporting the conclusion that it suppressed synaptic responses by blocking glutamate-like receptors. The selective actions of APB and D-o-phosphoserine indicate that there are three classes of glutamate receptors in the distal retina and that each receptor type is associated with a particular class of second order neuron.

We naturally were interested in the molecular mechanisms underlying the differentiation of the three glutamate-like synaptic receptors. In this regard, agonists are often more informative than antagonists because agonists both bind and activate the receptor-ionophore complexes. Although excitatory amino acid pharmacology is poorly developed compared to that of other neurotransmitters such as acetylcholine or norepinephrine, it has the advantage that most compounds are derived from the active components of glutamate or aspartate. This allows a comparison of presumed binding sites among the various ligands. Taking advantage of the potency and selectivity of APB, we began our analysis by focusing on the ON bipolar synaptic receptor (Slaughter and Miller, 1985b). We found

58

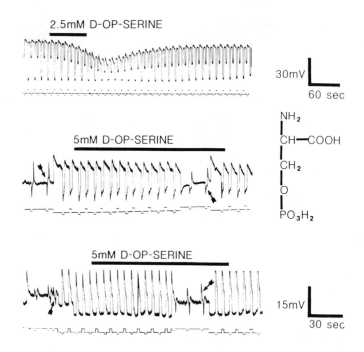

Fig. 8. Shows that D-o-phosphoserine selectively suppresses the light responses of horizontal cells. The surround responses of the bipolar cells are blocked (arrows) but the center responses persist. (From Nature, 1985)

that the L enantiomer of APB was approximately 10 fold more potent that the D stereoisomer. This indicated, not surprisingly, that the receptor preferentially interacted with the L form of agonists. We also tested a series of presumed aspartate receptor antagonists, such as D alpha amino adipate and D alpha amino suberate. They did not suppress the ON bipolar light responses, confirming our initial supposition that this receptor did not possess the pharmacological characteristics of an aspartate receptor. To verify that APB was acting as a glutamate analog and to disprove the possibility that the phosphonic acid group alone was responsible for the action of APB, we tested several acidic amino acid analogs that contained phosphonic acid components but varied in chain length. As illustrated in Fig. 9, 2-amino-3-phosphonopropionate, a phosphonic acid analog of aspartate, was inactive at the ON bipolar receptor. APB was a very potent agonist at the ON bipolar synapse and is the phosphonic acid analog of glutamate. 2-amino-5-phosphonovalerate, one carbon longer than APB, showed a moderate level of activity at the ON bipolar receptor. These results indicate that the phosphonic acid moiety alone is insufficient to activate the ON bipolar receptor and also demonstrates again that the glutamate-length analog is the most potent.

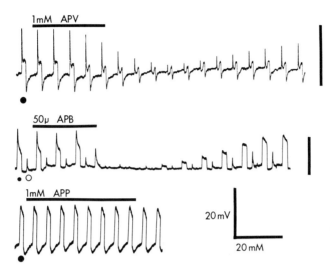

Fig. 9. Compares the actions of phosphonic analogs of aspartate (APP), glutamate (APB), and adipate (APV) on the light responses of ON bipolar cells. (From the J. Neuroscience, 1985)

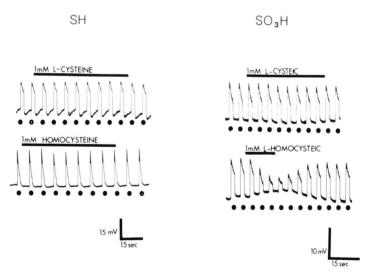

Fig. 10. Illustrates the effect of thiol and sulphonic acid analogs of aspartate and glutamate on ON bipolar light responses. (From the J. Neuroscience, 1985)

But these experiments did not clarify why APB activated only one class of glutamate receptors in the retina. To answer this question, we investigated the ramifications of the phosphonic acid substitution on the molecular properties of APB. The phosphonic acid moeity is more acidic than the corresponding carboxyl group of glutamate. We assessed the possibility that this explained the specificity of APB by testing glutamate and aspartate analogs that had sulphonic acid substitutions since these compounds would also be strongly acidic. Our results, shown in Fig. 10, using cysteic acid (an aspartate analog) and homocysteic acid (a glutamate analog), indicated that acidity alone did not explain the action of APB. Although, again, the glutamate analog was more potent than the aspartate analog, homocysteic acid was not as potent as APB. More significantly, we found that homocysteic acid depolarized a variety of neurons in both the inner and outer retina. Thus it lacked selectivity for the ON bipolar receptor.

Another possible explanation of APB's select action is that the size and charge on the phosphonic acid group makes the folded conformation of APB far less favorable than the folded form of glutamate. This suggests that APB's selectivity might reflect the preferential binding of the ON bipolar receptor to an extended configuration of glutamate. To pursue this possibility we examined several conformationally restricted excitatory amino acid analogs depicted schematically in Fig. 11. The two upper compounds are analogs of the extended conformation of glutamate in

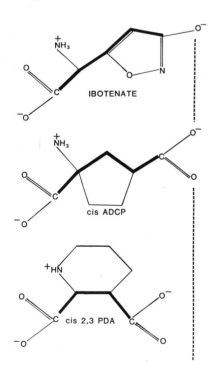

IBOTENATE

cis ADCP

cis 2,3 PDA

Fig. 11. Depicts the chemical formulas of three glutamate analogs (glutamate backbone in bold outline). This schematic shows that the top two compounds mimic extended forms of glutamate in which the terminal hydroxyl groups (dotted line) are approximately 5A from the alpha carbon. (From the J. Neuroscience, 1985)

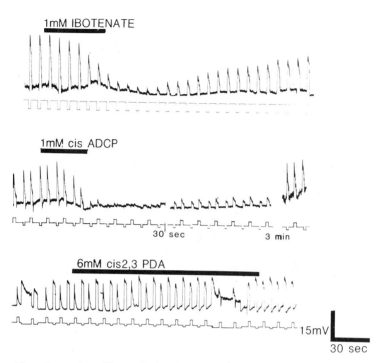

Fig. 12. Shows the effect of the three compounds depicted in the previous
figure on the light responses of ON bipolar neurons. The extended analogs
mimic the action of APB. (From the J. Neuroscience, 1985).

which the two carboxyl groups are separated by approximately 4A. The
lower molecule matches a more folded conformation of glutamate in which
the intercarboxyl distance does not exceed 3.5A. When we tested these
compounds while recording from ON bipolar cells (Fig. 12) we found that
the two extended glutamate analogs were effective agonists at the ON
bipolar, while the folded analog was inactive. These two extended
glutamate analogs were also selective for ON bipolar receptors in the
distal retina. This supports the hypothesis that the ON bipolar neurons
possess a distinct glutamate receptor that interacts preferentially with
an extended configuration of glutamate.

When we compared the three dimensional molecular structures of APB,
ibotenate, and ADCP (amino dicarboxy cyclopentane) we found one
conformation that all three molecules had in common. This was based on
comparing the position in space of the hydroxyl group of the terminal
carboxyl moiety relative to the alpha carboxyl and amino groups. Since
all the acidic amino acids have the same configuration at the alpha
carbon, this analysis localized the one variable binding site. The
extended conformation of glutamate that corresponds to this common configuration of the three analogs is shown at the top of Fig. 13. We have
found that all the agonists that are effective at the ON bipolar, such as
kainic acid, quisqualic acid, and AMPA, can match this spatial arrangement
of the three binding sites.

62

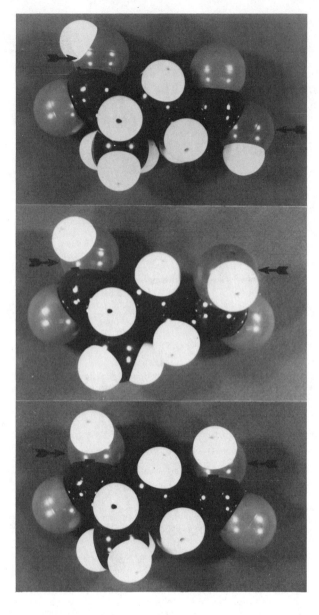

Off
Bipolar

On
Bipolar

Fig. 13. Pictures molecular models of glutamate in conformations that correspond to the proposed configurations that preferentially interact with the ON bipolar receptor (top), the horizontal cell receptor (middle), and the OFF bipolar receptor. Arrows indicate location of the two postulated carboxyl binding sites in each conformation.

A similar, though more limited analysis of the OFF bipolar and horizontal cell receptors suggests that they interact with fully or partially folded conformations of glutamate, respectively. Since these receptors were blocked by cis 2,3 piperidine dicarboxylic acid, they must bind to glutamate analogs in which the intercarboxyl distance is about 3.5A or less. A comparison of the structure of D-o-phosphoserine, which is selective for the horizontal cell receptor, with PDA suggests that the horizontal cell receptor interacts with glutamate analogs that have an intercarboxyl distance of 3.5A. Although PDA can assume more folded positions, with shorter intercarboxyl distances, the steric and charge forces in the constitutents of D-o-phosphoserine make more folded conformations unfavorable. This comparison suggests that glutamate in a partially folded conformation binds and activates the horizontal cell synaptic receptors. This molecular configuration of glutamate is shown in the middle of Fig. 13. The analysis of the horizontal cell receptor is limited by the fact that both D-o-phosphoserine and PDA are antagonists and, therefore, do not meet all the requirements for activation of the receptor. However, since they contain the three binding sites possessed by glutamate, it may be reasonable to propose that they are binding to the same spatial arrangement of sites that agonists bind. Another limitation is that neither agent is potent, both require millimolar concentrations to be effective. This may signify that they are not ideal matches for the horizontal cell receptors, although other explanations are also tenable. Within these limitations, the data indicates that the horizontal cell receptor preferentially interacts with glutamate when it is in a more folded form than that for the ON bipolar receptor.

The information on the OFF bipolar is even more limited. No selective agents have yet been found. The action of PDA on the OFF bipolar sets broad boundary conditions for the receptor. In addition, the ineffectiveness of D-o-phosphoserine, which can match many of the less folded conformations of PDA, implies that the OFF bipolar is interacting with a folded form of PDA. This is supported by the low potency of agents such as kainic acid and quisqualic acid, again suggesting that the receptor preferentially binds folded acidic amino acid analogs. The glutamate molecule shown at the bottom of Fig. 13 represents a folded conformation with an intercarboxyl separation of approximately 3A. The present data on OFF bipolar pharmacology is consistent with this configuration, although this is preliminary and confirmation awaits more specific OFF bipolar agonists and antagonists.

These findings place both retinal and glutamate pharmacology in a new perspective, suggesting a close relationship between synaptic pharmacology and neural anatomy and physiology. The morphological and functional differentiation that permits the separation of visual information channels is reinforced by the biochemical specifialization of synaptic receptors. For example, the two classes of bipolars have opposing voltage responses to light stimulation (Werblin and Dowling, 1969), they send processes to complementary sublamina in the inner plexiform layer (Famiglietti and Kolb, 1976; Famiglietti et al., 1977), and they appear to possess distinct types of glutamate receptors. The differences may both mediate and preserve the coding of light signals. In the mudpuppy retina, Miller and Dacheux (1976) have found that the photoreceptor neurotransmitter generates three synaptic ionic conductances: chloride channels are closed in ON bipolars, chloride channels are opened in horizontal cells, while sodium channels are activated in OFF bipolars. These differences in ionic conductance and in synaptic transfer functions (such as latency, time to peak, and signal amplification) in each class of second order neuron may be mediated in part by these receptors. Considering the close link between receptor binding sites and the ionic channel, these discrete ionic mechanisms may necessitate distinct receptors on each cell type.

In the analysis of retinal circuitry, the existence of pharmacologically distinguishable receptors offers the opportunity to determine syanptic inputs by the selective elimination of particular pathways. This has already led to the identidication of ON input to chlinergic amacrine cells in the rabbit retina (Neal et al., 1981; Massey and Redburn, 1982), to the evaluation of interplay between ON and OFF pathways in the lateral geniculate of the monkey (Schiller, 1981) and cat (Horton and Sherk, 1984) and to the source of ON responses in the monkey (Schiller, 1982) and cat (Sherk and Horton, 1984) striate cortex.

Acidic amino acids may represent the predominant excitatory transmitters between vertebrate neurons. In the retina, glutamate and aspartate appear to be key excitatory neurotransmitters in both plexiform layers (Ikeda and Sheardown, 1982; Slaughter and Miller, 1983a-c). A similar level of importance has been proposed for these transmitters in the brain and spinal cord, indicating that the receptors identified in the retina may be employed throughout the central nervous system. However, the conventional, tripartite classification of excitatory amino acid receptors into quisqualate receptors, kainate receptors, and N methyl aspartate receptors (Watkins and Evans, 1981; McLennan, 1981; Fagg and Foster, 1982) does not fully explain retinal pharmacology. In the distal retina, kainic acid and quisqualic acid do not differentiate the three types of glutamate receptors. Both drugs are equipotent on ON bipolar and horizontal cell receptors, which we have been able to distinguish with APB and d-o-phosphoserine. The OFF bipolar is far less sensitive to kainic and quisqualic acids, nor does it fit the pharmacology of the N methyl aspartate receptor. Based on our observations in the retina, glutamate receptors can be subdivided into at least three types, of which the APB receptor is the best characterized. An aspartate receptor has been identified in the proximal retina (Ikeda and Sheardown, 1982; Slaughter and Miller, 1983a), and conforms to the N methyl aspartate pharmacology of the previous classification scheme. The deficiency of the conventional glutamate receptor categorization has also been noted in the brain (Fagni et al., 1983), although the only point of correlation between retina and brain so far has been the APB receptor. Over the past few years, binding studies have demonstrated that APB receptors are widely distributed in brain (Butcher et al., 1982) while manipulations of the binding medium have shown that they represent a distinct class of glutamate receptors (Fagg et al., 1982; Mena et al., 1982). Whether the glutamate-like receptors found in horizontal cells and OFF bipolars are also widespread awaits future studies and hopefully more potent and selective agents to simplify receptor indentification.

In summary, a glutamate-like acidic amino acid appears to be a photoreceptor neurotransmitter. It acts at three discrete receptors which can be correlated with the three types of second order neurons. The pharmacological differentiation of these receptors may be explained by the preferential binding of each receptor type to a slightly different conformation of glutamate.

References

Balcar, V.J. and G.A.R. Johnston, J. Neurochem. 19, 2657-2666 (1972).
Bloomfield, S.A. and J.E. Dowling, Soc. Neurosci. Abstr. 8, 131 (1982).
Bloomfield, S.A. and J.E. Dowling, Invest. Ophthal. Vis. Sci. 24, 221 (1983).
Butcher, S.P., J.F. Collins and P.J. Roberts, Br. J. Pharmac. 80, 355-364 (1983)

Cull-Candy, S.G., J.F. Donnellan, R.W. James, and G.G. Lunt, Nature, 262, 408-409 (1976).

Curtis, D.R. and J. C. Watkins, J. Neurochem. 6, 117-141 (1960).

Curtis, D.R. and J. C. Watkins, J. Physiol. (Lond.) 166, 1-14 (1963).

Davies, J., R.H. Evans, A.A. Francis, A.W. Jones and J. C. Watkins, J. Neurochem. 36, 1305-1307 (1981).

Dowling, J.E. and F. Werblin, J. Neurophysiol 32, 315-338 (1969).

Fagg, G.E. and A.C. Foster, Neuroscience 9, 701-719 (1983).

Fagg, G.E. and A.C. Foster, E. E. Mena and C. W. Cotman, J. Neurosci. 2, 958-965 (1982).

Fagni, L., M. Baudry and G. Lynch, J. Neurosci. 3, 1538-1546 (1983).

Famiglietti, E.V., A. Kaneko and M. Tachibana, Science 198, 1267-1269 (1977).

Famiglietti, E.V., H. Kolb, Science, 194, 192-195 (1976).

Horton, J.C. and H. Sherk, J. Neurosci. 4, 374-380 (1980).

Ikeda, H. and M.J. Sheardown, Neuroscience 7, 25-36 (1982).

Ishida, A.T. and G.L. Fain, Proc. Natl. Acad. Sci. 78, 5890-94 (1981).

Krnjevic, K., M.E. Morris and R.J. Reiffenstein, Can. J. Physiol. Pharmacol. 60, 1643-1657 (1982).

Lasansky, A., J. Physiol. (Lond.) 285, 531-542 (1978).

Lasater, E.M. and J.E. Dowling, Proc. Natl. Acad. Sci. 97, 936-940 (1982).

Massey, S.S. and D.A. Redburn, Vis. Res. 23,1615-1620 (1983).

Massey, S.S. and D.A. Redburn and M.L.J. Crawford, Vis. Res. 23, 1607-1613 (1983).

McLennan, H. in: Glutamate as a Neurotransmitter, G. DiChiara and G.L. Gessa, eds. (Raven Press, New York 1981) pp. 253-262.

Mena, E.E., G.E. Fagg and C.W. Cotman, Brain Res. 243,378-381 (1982).

Miller, R.F. and R.F. Dacheux, J. Gen. Physiol. 67, 639-659 (1976).

Murakami, M., K. Ohtsu and T. Ohtsuka, J. Physiol. (Lond.) 227, 889-913 (1972).

Murakami, M., T. Ohtsuka and H. Shimazaki, Vis. Res. 15, 456-458 (1975).

Neal, M.J., J.R. Cunningham, T.A. James, M. Joseph and J.F. Collins, Neurosci. Lett. 26, 301-305 (1981).

Nowak, L., P. Bregestovski, P. Ascher, A. Herbert and A. Prochiantz, Nature 307, 462-465 (1984).

Olney, J.W. J. Neuropathol exp neurol. 28, 4550474 (1969).

Rowe, J.S. and K.H. Ruddock, Neurosci. Lett. 30, 251-256 (1982a).

Rowe, J.S. and K.H. Ruddock, Neurosci. Lett. 30, 257-262 (1982b).

Schiller, P.H. Nature 297, 580-583 (1981).

Sherk, H. and J.C. Horton, J. Neurosci. 4, 381-393.

Shiells, R.A., G. Falk and S. Naghshineh, Nature, 294, 592-594 (1981).

Slaughter, M.M. and R.F. Miller, Science 211, 182-185 (1982a).

Slaughter, M.M. and R.F. Miller, J. Neurosci. 3, 1701-1711 (1982b).

Slaughter, M.M. and R.F. Miller, Science, 219, 1230-1232 (1983c).

Slaughter, M.M. and R.F. Miller, Nature, 5, 224-233 (1985b).

Slaughter, M.M. and R.F. Miller, J. Neurosci. in press (1985b).

Watkins, J.C. and R.G. Evans, Ann. Rev. Pharmacol. Toxicol. 21, 165-204 (1981).

Werblin, F. and J.E. Dowling, J. Neurophysiol. 32, 339-355 (1969).

Wu, S.M. and J.E. Dowling, Proc. Natl. Acad. Sci. 75, 5205-5209 (1978).

Yazulla, S. and J. Kleinschmidt, Brain Res. 182, 287-301 (1980).

Modulation of Gap Junction Permeability by Dopamine and
GABA In the Network of Horizontal Cells of the Turtle Retina

M. Piccolino[1], P. Witkovsky[2], J. Neyton[3],
H.M. Gerschenfeld[3], C. Trimarchi[1]

Instituto di Neurofisiologia del C.N.R.[1]
Pisa, Italy
New York University Medical Center[2]
New York, New York
Laboratoire de Neurobiologie de l'Ecole Normale Superieure[3]
Paris, France

In 1959, Furshpan and Potter showed that signal transmission at the
crayfish giant motor synapse occurred by means of a direct flow of current
from one cellular element to another, that is through a mechanism
basically different from that operating at classical chemical synapses.
Since this first demonstration, a similar direct mode of cellular
communication has been recognized and characterized between neurons as
well as between non-nervous cells in a variety of vertebrate and
invertebrate preparations. In consequence the existence of both
electrical and chemical synapses has received general recognition (see
Bennett, 1977; Lowenstein, 1981 for reviewes).

The morphological and physiological evidence accumulated thus far
indicates that transmission in electrical synapses occurs at specialized
intercellular junctions (gap junctions) whose elementary functional units
are low resistance channels bridging the gap between the coupled cells
(Lowenstein, 1966; Revel and Karnovsky, 1967; Goodenough, 1979). Interest
in electrical synapses has been strengthened by the observation that
uncharged molecules of low molecular weight can pass across these
junctions, in addition to the ions that mediate electrical transmission.
Gap junctions are thus implicated in a variety of cellular processes,
including metabolic cooperation and the control of cell growth and
differentiation (Gilula et al., 1972; Lowenstein, 1979; Bennett et al,
1981; Caveney, 1985).

Transmission of electrical signals exhibits functional characteristics
which differ in important respects from those of chemical synapses.
Intercellular communication at electrical synapses occurs without delay
and without significant synaptic noise. It generally is bidirectional.
Although in particular cases electrical synapses show a complex behavior,
they have been considered as rather simple and rigid devices for cellular
communication which lack the integrative properties and functional
plasticity inherent to chemical synapses. Electrical synapses seem to be
functionally advantageous when a rapid, reliable passive spread of signal
is demanded, but they appear not to underlie finely graded neuronal
integration.

Recent work, however, has challenged the idea of the rigid nature of
electrical transmission by showing that, at least in certain instances,
the permeability of the gap junction is modifiable. For example, it has
been demonstrated that gap junction channels close when intracellular
(Ca^{2+}) or (H^+) increases (Rose and Lowenstein, 1976; Turin and Warner,
1980; Spray et al., 1981). Future work will show whether changes in
intracellular ionic concentrations are a general mechanism of cell
uncoupling under physiological conditions. It appears also that gap
junction uncoupling may be involved in pathological situations, for
example in the process of "healing over" when normal cells become
uncoupled from damaged cells after tissue lesions (Deleze, 1975; DeMello
et al., 1969).

Neurocircuitry of the Retina, A Cajal Memorial
A. Gallego and P. Gouras, Editors

Another general mechanism which has been uncovered recently is the modification of the permeability of gap junctions by the action of chemical transmitters. Initial evidence derived from studies of non-nervous tissues. In pancreatic acinar cells, for instance, it was found that acetylcholine reduced the permeability of gap junctions, probably by increasing the intracellular concentration of calcium ions (Findlay and Peterson, 1981). In this and related cases (e.g., DeMello, 1982), in which an influence of chemical transmitters on gap junctions in non-nervous cells has been detected, the action appears to be a side effect of the modifying agent, whose main role is to control other parameters of target cell function.

A more specific mechanism of neurotransmitter control of electrical junctions has been discovered recently in our laboratories in the course of electrophysiological studies on the retina of the turtle Pseudemys scripta elegans (Piccolino et al., 1982; Gerschenfeld et al., 1982; Piccolino et al., 1984). The results of these studies indicate that GABA and dopamine, two presumed retinal transmitters, modify signal transmission among the axon terminals of the axon-bearing horizontal cells (H1 type) by modifying the permeability of the gap junctions existing between these cells (Witkovsky et al., 1983). It was observed that the application of GABA antagonists, or of dopamine and its agonists, induced a narrowing of the receptive field profile of the axon terminals of type H1 horizontal cells (H1AT) and reduced the spread of both current and Lucifer Yellow dye in the H1AT network. The effects of the GABA antagonists were indirect and probably due to a modulation of the release of dopamine from a class of retinal neuron. In this article we will provide a short review of the results of these studies and we will present some new pharmacological data on this subject. Similar results have been obtained in the fish retina in an intact preparation by Negishi and collaborators, and in an isolated cell preparation by Dowling and collaborators (see elsewhere in this volume).

The effect of GABA antagonists
The initial observation concerned the effect of GABA antagonists on the receptive field profile of the light responses recorded intracellularly from a H1AT. H1AT's responded to illumination of their receptive field with graded hyperpolarizations whose amplitudes depend on the extent of the retinal area stimulated. Under normal conditions only large spots or large annuli of light elicit large amplitude responses. Local illumination of the H1AT receptive field centers with small light spots results in small responses even when the stimulus is sufficiently large to cover all the photoreceptors directly connected to the H1AT being recorded from (Leeper and Copenhagen, 1982; Piccolino and Witkovsky, 1984 for reviews). The large receptive area of the H1AT response is the functional consequence of a strong electrical coupling between these structures. The coupling is mediated by numerous, large area gap junctions located between neighboring H1AT's (Witkovsky et al., 1983). In consequence, the synaptic current generated in one H1AT by local illumination is diluted in the network and thus fails to induce a sizeable modification of the membrane potential. On the other hand, a large amplitude response is generated in one H1AT by flashing a large annulus on its receptive field surround, even though the stimulus does not illuminate the photoreceptors directly connected to that H1AT. The explanation is that in the case of annular illumination, a large amount of current spreads from the neighboring H1AT's to the central one through the gap junction channels.

When the receptive field properties of H1AT's were evaluated in the presence of bicuculline or picrotoxin, it was found that following the

68

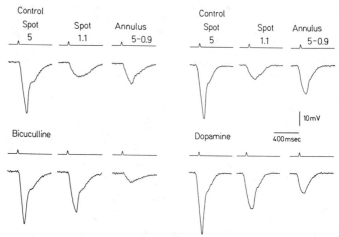

Fig. 1. Effects induced in the H1AT light responses by the application of
50 uM bicuculline (A) or by the application of 5 uM dopamine (B). In both
A and B the top tracings are the intracellular recordings of the responses
evoked in a H1AT by fixed intensity, white light stimuli in control Ringer
and the bottom tracings are the recordings of the responses induced by the
same stimuli following application of the drugs (as indicated). The
numbers near the stimulus trace above the top recordings indicate, in
millimeters, either the outer diameter of the spots or the outer and inner
diameter of the annulus. A and B refer to two different experiments.

application of these GABA antagonists, the responses elicited by small
central light spots markedly increased in amplitude, whereas those induced
by annuli of light decreased (Fig. 1a). This effect indicated that the
GABA antagonists reduced electrical coupling between neighboring H2AT's
and it was reasonable to suppose that these agents could have increased
the resistance of the gap junctions in the H1AT network. Another possible
explanation, however, was that the GABA antagonists decreased the
resistance of unspecialized H1AT membrane, i.e., membrane areas not
involved in the gap junctions. In a network of coupled elements the
coupling efficiency depends on the relation between two parameters;
junctional and extra-junctional resistance. A reduction of the coupling
can result from a decrease in extra-junctional resistance, since in that
case a large proportion of the synaptic input current would exit through
the unspecialized membrane of the stimulated elements. Thus the lateral
spread of signal would be reduce.

A study was carried out to discriminate between these two
alternatives; the results obtained strongly favored the idea that GABA
antagonists modified the coupling resistance. This conclusion was
supported by the results of two sorts of experiments. We analyzed first
the effect of the GABA antagonists on the electrical coupling between two
adjacent H1AT's simultaneously impaled with microelectrodes. It was found
consistently that, in conjunction with the receptive field changes
described above, the GABA antagonists induced an increase in the voltage
drop elicited in one H1AT by the injection of a constant current pulse
into the other H1AT (Fig. 2a). This behavior could be explained only by
assuming that the coupling reduction was the result of an increase in the
coupling resistance, as illustrated in Fig. 2B. The curves plotted in this

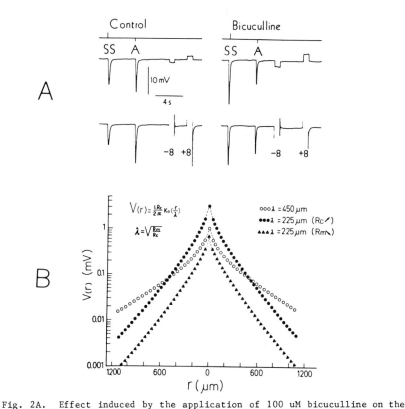

Fig. 2A. Effect induced by the application of 100 uM bicuculline on the
electrical coupling between two H1AT's located less than 80 uM apart.
Pulses of constant current (8 nA intensity of either polarity were
injected in the H1AT and monitored in the bottom tracings and the
resulting voltage drop recorded in the H1AT monitored in the upper
tracings. The responses induced in the two H1AT's by light stimulation
with either a 1230um small spot (SS) or with an annulus (A: outer diameter
3700 µm, inner diameter 1200 µm) are also illustrated. Notice the
increase of the voltage drop after bicuculline application and also the
change in the light response amplitudes (From Piccolino et al., 1982).
B. Spatial spread of current in a theoretical model simulating the H1AT
network. The voltage drop V(r) evoked by injecting a 1nA outward constant
current pulse at a point in the network is plotted on the ordinate against
the distance from the injection site on the abscissa. As indicated, the
network space constant λ is 450 um in the control curve (open circles),
and it is assumed to be reduced to 225 um by either a decrease in the Rm
(modelling the extra-junctional membrane resistance), or an increase of Rc
(modelling the coupling resistance). The values of (V(r) for r = 0 were
calculated from the equation at the top left of the figure which describes
the spatial decay of the potential in a bidimensional lamina (Lamb, 1976).
For 4 = 0, V(r) was calculated according to a "discrete" model (the
"square grid" model of Lamb and Simon, 1976) using experimental parameters
to fit the behaviour of the H1AT network (refer to the original paper,
Piccolino et al., 1984 for details.

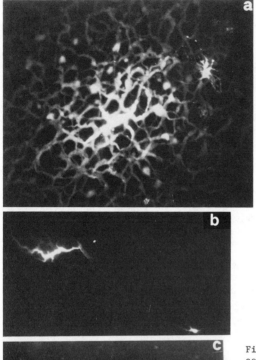

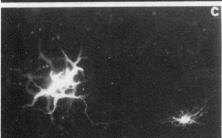

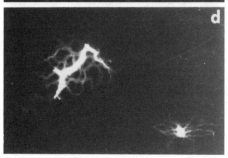

Fig. 3. Diffusion of intra-cellularly injected Lucifer Yellow in the network of the axon-bearing horizontal cells of the turtle retina. a, Control. b, After the application of 100 uM bicuculline. c, After the application of 100 uM picro-toxin. d, After the application of 10 uM dopamine. Notice the great extension of the dye spread from the injected axon terminal to neighbouring axon terminals and, moreover, the staining of the perikarya presumably by backfilling from the axon terminals. Notice in b to d the great restriction of the dye spread as compared to the control in a (from Piccolino et al., 1982, and Gerschenfeld et al., 1982, modified).

200 μm

figure represent the spatial decay of the electrotonic potential, as a function of the distance from the site of injection of an constant current. The H1AT network is modelled as a planar sheet (Jack et al., 1975; Lamb, 1976). Three different conditions are illustrated: a control condition in which the space constant of the sheet is 450 um, and two test conditions in which λ is reduced to one half, either by a <u>decrease</u> in extra-junctional resistance, R_m, or by an increase in the tangential or coupling resistance of the network, R_c. In the first case the amplitude of the electrotonic potential is smaller than the control irrespective of where within the planar sheet it is measured. In contrast, when R_c increases, the electrotonic potential is larger than control for distances 500 um or less from the injection site, but smaller than control for distances greater than 500 um. Since, in our experiments, the separation of injected cell from the cell in which the voltage was recorded was 100 um or less, only an increase in R_c can account for the results obtained. The interpretation of our finding, moreover, does not depend on the choice of a continuous sheet model to represent the H1AT network. Different "discrete" models lead to essentially similar predictions (Detwiler and Hodgkin, 1979).

More direct evidence in support of the control of gap junction permeability derived from experiments in which the coupling was studied by the injection of Lucifer Yellow. This fluorescent dye is capable of permeating the gap junction channels and has been used widely to study cell coupling (Stewart, 1978; 1981). Under control conditions the injection of Lucifer Yellow into one H1AT leads to an intense staining of an intricate network of H1AT's, due to diffusion of the dye across the gap junctions (Fig. 3a). In contrast, only the injected H1AT appeared well stained when the dye was introduced in the presence of either bicuculline or picrotoxin (Fig. 3, b,c). Lucifer Yellow does not permeate the ionic channels of the extra-junctional membrane and so our results may be safely interpreted to mean a reduced permeability of the gap junctions connecting neighboring H1AT's.

Effect of Dopamine
Some years ago, Negishi and Drujan (1979) reported that dopamine induced a narrowing of the receptive field profile of the horizontal cells of the carp retina, an effect which was very similar to our results in turtle retina with GABA antagonists. We wondered whether dopamine would act similarly on the H1AT of the turtle retina, and, if so, whether the effect was attributable to a reduction of gap junction permeability. We used a protocol similar to that employed in the study of bicuculline and picrotoxin actions; we observed that dopamine application resulted in a decrease of the response to light annuli (Fig. 1b). Dopamine, moreover, modified the spread of both current and Lucifer Yellow dye within the H1AT network (Fig. 3d). The effects of dopamine were mimicked by a number of dopamine agonists such as apomorphine, epinine and ADTN. In addition, we obtained evidence that dopamine acted through type D1 receptors. Application to the retina of sulpiride and domperidone, dopamine antagonists devoid of action upon D1 receptors, did not prevent the receptive field changes induced by dopamine and its agonists. On the other hand, flupentixol and piflutixol, which are powerful antagonists at D1 receptors, completely blocked the dopamine effects. This characterization of the dopamine receptors has been confirmed in more recent experiments in which other specific dopaminergic drugs have been studied. It was found that the dopamine effects were mimicked by the specific D1 agonist, SKF 38393, but not by the D2 agonists, RU 24213 and L 141865. The dopamine action, moreover, was blocked by the specific D1 antagonist, SCH 23390 (Piccolino and Witkovsky, 1985).

D1 receptors are those dopamine receptors coupled to an adenylate cyclase, and whose binding with specific ligands leads to an increase of intracellular cyclic AMP concentration (Kebabian and Calne, 1979). A dopamine-dependent adenylate cyclase has been found in the retina of all vertebrates studied and recent evidence suggests that it is present on the membrane of the horizontal cells themselves (Brown and Makman, 1972; Schorderet, 1977; Dowling and Watling, 1981; Van Buskirk and Dowling, 1981). We therefore investigated whether dopamine action could be mediated by cyclic AMP as a second messenger. We applied to the retina drugs able to increase the intracellular level of cyclic AMP by different mechanisms not involving the activation of the dopamine receptors. Both forskolin, a direct activator of the cyclase, and IBMX, an inhibitor of the phosphodiesterase that hydrolyzes cyclic AMP, mimicked the effects of dopamine on H1AT coupling (Gerschenfeld et al., 1982).

On the basis of this and other experimental evidence, it was concluded that dopamine modified the permeability of the gap junctions in the H1AT network by activating an adenylate cyclase whose probable location was on the membrane of the H1 horizontal cells themselves. As a corollary of this hypothesis, cyclic AMP is thought to play the role of an intracellular messenger leading to the reduction of gap junction channel permeability.

GABA-Dopamine Interactions

The similarity between the effects of the GABA antagonists and the effects of dopamine and its agonists led us to investigate whether a relation existed between the actions of these two classes of drugs. Our experiments results indicated that the action of GABA antagonists on the H1AT network is indirect and very probably mediated by an activation of retinal dopaminergic neurons. Thus, we found firstly that the effects of bicuculline and picrotoxin were prevented by pre-application of effective dopamine antagonists, eg., flupentixol. Secondly, bicuculline and picrotoxin were ineffective in modifying H1AT coupling when the retinas were treated for a long time with α-methyl-para-tyrosine, an inhibitor of tyrosine hydroxylase, the rate limiting enzyme of dopamine synthesis. Both these results can be explained by assuming that under normal conditions, GABA, released by a subclass of retinal neuron, reduces the release of dopamine from dopaminergic neurons whose terminals are situated in close proximity to the horizontal cells. GABA antagonists would interfere with this action and thus lead to an increase of dopamine release. This in turn would modify the coupling among H1AT's. Our model is consistent with the results of a recent biochemical study carried out in the fish retina in which it was shown that bicuculline application led to an increased dopamine release (O'Connor et al., 1984). The possibility that GABA has an inhibitory action on dopamine neurons also is suggested by experiments performed on rat retina. There it was found that GABA agonists reduced the activity of tyrosine hydroxylase (Morgan and Kamp, 1980). Interestingly, this effect occurs also in isolated cell preparations, suggesting that the action of GABA on dopamine terminals probably is a direct one (Marshburn and Iuvone, 1981).

The notion that GABA antagonists act on the H1AT network indirectly, and probably through the activation of dopaminergic neurons, is supported also by our most recent results. We found that the application to the retina of tetrodotoxin (TTX), the blocker of sodium channels involved in spike generation, completely prevented the effects of bicuculline. In contrast, TTX did not modify the action of dopamine.

Retinal Dopaminergic Neurons

In the previous discussion of the GABA-dopamine interactions we have tacitly assumed that the turtle retina is endowed with dopaminergic neurons that release their transmitter near to the horizontal cells. This point merits further discussion. In the vertebrate retina two classes of dopaminergic neuron have been recognized: dopaminergic amacrine cells and dopaminergic interplexiform cells (Ehinger, 1983). Dopaminergic amacrines have been found in all retinas investigated, whereas dopaminergic interplexiform cells have been identified only in certain species (e.g., fish, rat, cat, some monkeys, humans) but not in others (Ehinger et al., 1969; Nguyen-Legros et al., 1981; Oyster et al., 1983; Dowling and Ehinger, 1975; Frederick et al., 1982). Dopamine-containing interplexiform cells are obvious candidates for the cells controlling horizontal cell coupling, since their distal terminal arborizations are close to the horizontal cells. A study of dopaminergic cells in turtle retina, however, employing ^{3}H-dopamine uptake, amine fluorescence and immunocytochemical localization of an anti-tyrosine hydroxylase antiserum revealed dopaminergic amacrine cells but no dopaminergic interplexiform cell (Witkovsky et al., 1984). It is at least conceivable that dopamine, released by amacrine cells, could reach HlAT's by diffusion. This possibility receives support from morphological studies of other dopaminergic systems where it is found that the dopaminergic neurons may make only rare synapses on their recipient neurons. It has been postulated that diffusion for relatively long distances underlies the effect of the released dopamine on the target cells (Beaudet and Descarries, 1978).

Our recent pharmacological studies provide additional, indirect evidence that, in turtle retina, dopaminergic neurons modulate horizontal cell coupling. We found that a reduction of the electrical and dye coupling in the HlAT network was induced by the application of amphetamine, a drug capable of releasing dopamine from the dopaminergic terminals, but devoid of a direct effect on dopamine receptors. The action of amphetamine could be blocked by treatment of the retina with α-methyl-para-tyrosine as well as by dopamine antagonists. Moreover, dopa, the direct precursor of dopamine, mimicked the effect of dopamine on HlAT coupling; its action was reduced by benserazide, an inhibitor of its conversion to dopamine, as well as by dopamine antagonists. Finally, an indication of the existence of neurons capable of releasing dopamine derives from recent experiments employing veratridine. This drug is an activator of the fast sodium channels implicated in spike production (Narahashi, 1974). We found that the effects induced by veratridine on the HlAT's were similar to those of dopamine and could be blocked by dopamine antagonists. Moreover, they were blocked by TTX, indicating that they probably are attributable to the spike-inducing action of veratridine.

The results obtained with veratridine and with TTX, and the observation that TTX blocked the action of bicuculline, indicate that the dopaminergic amacrines of turtle retina are spike-generating cells. This indication, although based on indirect evidence, is consistent with the known spike-generating properties of many inner retinal neurons. Moreover, if we assume that the conclusion drawn from the experiments on rat retina, according to which GABA acts directly on dopaminergic neurons, is applicable also to turtle retina, then it is clear that TTX could block the action of bicuculline only by acting directly on the dopaminergic neuron.

Concluding Remarks

Since the first demonstration of the existence of dopamine-containing neurons in the retinas of rat and rabbit obtained by Malmfors and Haggendal (Malmfors, 1963; Haggendal and Malmfors, 1965), a large amount of experimental evidence has been accumulated which suggests that dopamine plays a transmitter role in the vertebrate retina. Dopaminergic neurons have been found in the retinas of all species investigated and the retinal dopaminergic system has been characterized through numerous biochemical and pharmacological studies. It has been shown that the retina is endowed with specific mechanisms for dopamine synthesis, uptake and release, all of which are modified by light stimulation (Ehinger, 1983). It also has been shown that there are specific dopamine receptors, mostly of the D1 type, in the retinas of many vertebrates.

Indications of a possible physiological role of dopamine in human visual function emerged from studies revealing abnormal visual responses after impairment of the dopamine system. Human subjects affected by Parkinson's disease or receiving dopamine antagonists, show abnormal visual evoked potentials (VEP) in response to pattern stimulation (Bodis-Wollner et al., 1982). Similar alterations were found in rats treated with α-methyl-para-tyrosine. Interestingly, these animals showed no modification of the potentials elicited by direct electrical stimulation of the optic nerve, which suggests a possible involvement of the retinal dopamine system in the observed VEP abnormalities (Dyer et al., 1981). This possibility also is consistent with the results of other studies on human subjects in which administration of various dopaminergic agents was found to modify electroretinographic responses (Filip and Balic, 1978; Fornaro et al., 1980).

On the basis of the studies of the dopamine action on the horizontal cells discussed in this article (see Negishi et al., this volume), it is now possible to formulate an hypothesis for a role of the retinal dopamine system in visual function. In this regard we need to refer to the evidence suggesting that horizontal cells are involved in neural interactions subserving the analysis of spatial contrast. Horizontal cells have a recurrent output onto cone photoreceptors through a sign-inverting synapse (Baylor et al., 1971). This feedback syanpse is responsible for the depolarizing surround responses elicited in cones by illumination of their receptive field periphery. Local illumination of the receptive field center with small light spots evokes, in cones, a purely hyperpolarizing response. The failure of small spots to elicit a measureable depolarizing component is explained by the fact that horizontal cells respond poorly to small light spots due to their large summation area. The feedback depolarizing influence of horizontal cells becomes apparent only with large spots or annuli of light, and thereby contributes to a mechanism of peripheral antagonism in the cone receptive field. As a consequence, cones acquire a spatial selectivity reminiscent of the behavior of contrast detectors. From a quantitative point of view this spatial selectivity is tuned according to the integration area of the horizontal cell. Any modification of the receptive field profile of the horizontal cells, such as that induced by dopamine, will result in a modification of the spatial selectivity of cones and, as a consequence, of the visual system as a whole. It might be expected therefore that interference with the retinal dopamine system could result in a modification of the spatial contrast function of the visual system. Recent experiments on human subjects are consistent with this possibility. The administration of dopaminergic drugs to normal subjects was found to induce a selective modification of the spatial contrast sensitivity function, as evidenced by an improvement of sensitivity in the middle spatial frequency range (Domenici et al., 1984). On the other hand, patients affected by Parkinson's disease showed a selective loss of contrast sensitivity in the same range of spatial frequencies (Bodis-Wollner et al., 1984).

In a more general context, the studies reviewed in this article strongly suggest that the permeability of gap junctions between nerve cells can be modulated by the action of specific neurotransmitters through a mechanism yet to be fully elucidated. At this point we wish only to emphasize that, by means of neurotransmitter control, electrical synapses may acquire some of the functional plasticity typical of chemical synapse without losing their specific functional characteristics.

Acknowledgement

The authors thank G.C. Cappagli for technical assistance, P. Taccini for preparing the illustrations and Dr. E. Meller for generously supplying some of the drugs utilized. Supported in part by grant EY 03570 to P.W.

References:

Baylor, D.A., Fuortes, M.G.F., O'Bryan, P.M., J. Physiol., (Lond) 214, 265-294 (1971).
Beaudet, A., Descarries, L., Neuroscience 3, 851-860 (1978).
Bennett, M.V.L. in "Cellular Biology of Neurons" Handbook of Physiology, Vol 1, The Nervous System E.R. Kandel ed (Williams and Wilkins, Baltimore, Maryland 1977) pp.357-416.
Bennett, M.V.L., Spray, D.C., Harris, A.L., Trends Neurosci. 4, 159-163 (1981).
Bodis-Wollner, I., Yahr, M.D., Mylin, L., Thornton, J. Ann. Neurol. 11, 478-483 (1982).
Bodis-Wollner, I., Mitra, S., Bobak, P., Guillory, S., Mylin, L. Invest. Ophth. Vis. Sci. 25, Suppl. 313 (1984).
Brown, J.H., Makman, M.H. Proc. Natl. Acad. Sci. 69, 539-543 (1972).
Caveney, S. Ann. Rev. Physiol. 47, 319-335 (1985).
Deleze, J. in "Electrophysiology of the Heart" B. Taccardi and G. Marchetti eds (Pergamon Press, London 1965).
De Mello, W.C. Physiologist 25, 197 (1982).
De Mello, W.C. Motta, G., Chapeau, M. Circ. Res. 24, 475-487 (1969).
Detwiler, P.B., Hodgkin, A.L., J. Physiol (Lond) 291, 75-100 (1979).
Domenici, L., Trimarchi, C., Piccolino, M., Fiorentini, A., Perception 13, A38 (1984).
Dowling, J.E., Ehinger, B., Science 188, 270-273 (1975).
Dowling, J.E., Watling, K.J. J. Neurochem. 36, 569-579 (1981).
Ehinger, B. in Progress in Retinal Research N. Osborne and G. Chader eds Vol 2, pp 213-232 (1983).
Ehinger, B., Falck, B., Laties, A.M., Z. Zellforsch. mikrosk. Anat. 97, 295-297 (1969).
Filip, V., Balik, J.C. Int. Pharmacophyschiatr. 13, 151-156 (1978).
Fornaro, P., Castrogiovanni, P., Perossini, M. Placidi, G.F., Cavalacci, G., Acta Neurologica 2, 293-299 (1980).
Findlay, I., Petersen, O.H., Cell Tissue Res. 225, 633-638 (1982).
Frederick, J.M., Rayborn, M.E., Laties, A.M., Lam, D.M.K., Hollyfield, JG., J. Comp. Neurol 210, 65-79 (1982).
Furshpan, E.J., Potter, D.O., J. Physiol. (Lond) 145, 289-325 (1959).
Gerschenfeld, H.M., Neyton, J., Piccolino, M., Witkovsky, P Biomedical Res. Suppl. 3, 21-32 (1982).

Gilula, N.B., Reeves, O.R., Steinbach, A., Nature (London) 235, 262-265 (1972).
Goodenough, D.A., Invest. Ophthal. 18, 1104-1122 (1979).
Haggendal, J., Malmfors, T., Acta Physiol Scand. 64, 58-66 (1965).
Iuvone, P.M., Galli, C.L., Garrison-Gund, C.K., Neff, N.H., Science, 202, 901-902 (1978).
Jack, J.J.B., Noble, D., Tsien, R.W., Electrical current flow in excitable cells. Clarendon Press, Oxford (1975).
Kebabian, J.W., Calne, D.B. Nature, 277, 93-96 (1979).
Lamb, T.D., J. Physiol. (Lond) 263, 239-255 (1976).
Lamb, T.D., Simon, E.J., J. Physiol. (Lond), 263, 257-286 (1976).
Leeper, H.F., Copenhagen, D.R., in "The S-potential" B. Drujan and M. Laufer eds (A. Liss, New York 1982) pp. 77-104.
Lowenstein, W.R., Ann. N. Y. Acad. Sci. 137, 441-472 (1966).
Lowenstein, W.R., Biochem. Biophys. Acta 560, 1-65 (1979).
Lowenstein, W.R., Physiol. Rev. 61, 829-913 (1981).
Malmfors, T., Acta Physiol. Scand. 58, 99-100 (1963).
Marshburn, P.B., Iuvone, P.M., Brain Res. 214, 335-347 (1981).
Morgan, W.W., Kamp, C.W., J. Neurochem. 34, 1082-1086 (1980).
Narahashi, T. Physiol. Rev. 54, 813-889 (1974).
Negishi, K., Drujan, B.D., J. Neurosci. Res. 4, 311-334 (1979).
Nguyen-Legros, J. Berger, R., Vigny, A., Alvarez, C., Neurosci. Lett. 27, 255-259 (1981).
O'Connor, P., Dorison, S., Watling, K.J., Dowling, J.E., Invest. Ophthal. Vis. Sci. 25 Suppl 3, 86 (1984).
Oyster, C.W. Takahashi, E.S., Brecha, N.C., Ciluffo, M., Invest. Ophthal. Vis. Sci 25 Suppl 3, 87 (1984).
Piccolino, M., Neyton, J. Witkovsky, P., Gerschenfeld, H.M. Proc. Natl. Acad. Sci., 79, 3671-3675 (1982).
Piccolino, M., Neyton, J.,   Gerschenfeld, H.M. J. Neurosci 4, 2477-2488 (1984).
Piccolino, M., Witkovsky, P., in Comparative Physiology of Sensory Systems. L. Bolis, R.D. Keynes and S.H.P. Maddrell (eds) (Cambridge University Press, Cambridge, U.K. 1984) pp. 371-404.
Piccolino, M., Witkovsky, P., Invest. Ophthal. Vis. Sci. Suppl 26, (1985).
Revel, J.B., Karnovsky, M. J. Cell Biol. 33, 7-12 (1967).
Rose, B., Lowenstein, W.R., J. Membrane Biol. 28, 87-119 (1976).
Schorderet, M., Life Sci. 20, 1741-1748 (1977).
Spray, D.C., Harris, A.L., Bennett, M.V.L., Science 211, 712-714 (1981).
Stewart, W.W., Cell 14, 741-759 (1978).
Stewart, W.W., Nature 292, 17-21 (1981).
Turin, L., Warner, A.E. J. Physiol (Lond) 300, 489-504 (1980).
Van Buskirk, R., Dowling, J.E., Proc. Natl. Acad. Sci. USA 78, 7825-7829 (1981).
Witkovsky, P., Owen, W.G. Woodworth, M. J. Comp. Neurol. 216, 359-368 (1983).
Witkovsky, P., Eldred, W., Karten, J. J. Comp. Neurol. 228, 217-225 (1984).

Dopaminergic Interplexiform Cells and Their Regulatory
Function for Spatial Properties of Horizontal Cells
in the Fish Retina

K. Negishi, T. Teranishi and S. Kato
Department of Neurophysiology, Neuroinformation
Research Institute (NIRI), University of Kanazawa
School of Medicine, 13-1 Takara-machi, Kanazawa
Ishikawa, Japan

Interplexiform cells with processes extending towards both the outer
(OPL) and inner plexiform layers (IPL) are found in many vertebrate
retinas (Gallego, 1971; Boycott et al., 1975). Histofluorescence studies
have revealed that dopamine (DA)-containing cells are generally present at
the innermost level of the inner nuclear layer (INL)(Ehinger, 1976). In
the retina of the cebus monkey and of various teleost fishes, however,
interplexiform cells contain DA (Dowling and Ehinger, 1975, 1978; Negishi
et al., 1981c). The processes of these DA cells have mutual synaptic
contacts between amacrine cells in the IPL an are presynaptic to
horizontal and bipolar cells in the INL (Dowling and Ehinger, 1975).
Therefore, the DA interplexiform cells provide a centrifugal pathway from
the IPL to OPL (Dowling and Ehinger, 1975, 1978).

In the fish retina, as one of the second-order neurons, horizontal
cells form two or three layers of subclasses immediately below the
photoreceptor cell layer. Each of the cell subclasses generates a certain
type of light-induced response (S-potential). The cells of each subclass
are electrically coupled via gap junctions between their somata and also
between their axon terminals (Yamada and Ishikawa, 1967; Naka and Rushton,
1967; Keneko, 1971; Tonosaki et al., 1984). It has been assumed that the
large spatial summation property of S-potentials (Tomita et al., 1958;
Norton et al., 1968; Negishi and Sutija, 1969) is due to lateral spread
via gap junctions. A fluorescent dye (lucifer yellow, LY) injected into a
horizontal cell normally diffuses to several neighboring cells via gap
junctions (Steward, 1978; Piccolino et al., 1982; Teranishi, 1983; Kaneko
and Stuart, 1984). Exogenously applied DA alters the spatial properties
of S-potentials, increasing in amplitude the center response to the spot
while decreasing the surround response to annular illumination (Negishi
and Drujan, 1978, 1979). These effects result in shrinkage of the
potential summation area (receptive field) of horizontal cells (Cohen and
Dowling, 1983) and have been attributed to the action of DA on membrane
resistance, particularly at the gap junctions (Negishi and Drujan, 1979;
Laufer, 1982; Piccolino et al., 1983). Our further studies (Teranishi et
al., 1983, 1984; Negishi et al., 1983) on photopic (cone-connected)
horizontal cells in the carp retina have shown that DA also restricts
intracellular LY to single injected cells, an effect similar to that of DA
on the lateral spread of S-potentials with which a dopaminergic blocker
haloperidol interferes.

Rapid and reversible effects of carbon dioxide (CO_2) and amonia (NH_3)
on the membrane potential of horizontal cells have been observed in
isolated fish retinas; CO_2 hyperpolarizes while NH_3 initially depolarizes
and subsequently hyperpolarizes the cells, accompanied by a diminution of
S-potentials (Laufer et al., 1961; Negishi and Svaetichin, 1966; Negishi,
1984). On the other hand, CO_2 and NH_3 have been shown to rapidly change
the intracellular pH (pH_i) of snail neurons (Thomas, 1974). Subsequently,
it has been demonstrated that the reduced pH_i with CO_2 abolishes ionic
communication between invertebrate cells (Turin and Warner, 1977, 1980;
Giaume et al., 1980; Spray et al., 1981); the uncoupling is accompanied by

© 1985 by Elsevier Science Publishing Co., Inc.
Neurocircuitry of the Retina, A Cajal Memorial
A. Gallego and P. Gouras, Editors

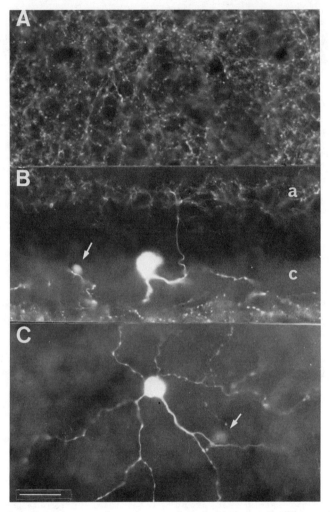

Fig. 1 Fluorescence photomicrographs of DA interplexiform cells taken from cryosections of the mullet (Mugil cephalus) retina. A and C, tangential; B, radial view; Scale, 40 µm. In B, small letters indicate the external horizontal cell layer (a) and the border (c) between the inner nuclear layer (INL) and the inner plexiform layer (IPL). In Band C, an intensely shining cell body with processes represents a DA interplexiform cell, while a weakly fluorescent cell body (arrow) belongs to a subclass of indoleamine-accumulating (IA) amacrine cells, which also took up noradrenaline intravitreally applied (see below). To enhance cellular fluorescence the retinas had been treated with intravitreal injection of noradrenaline (20 µg/10 µl saline/eye) 2 hours prior to enucleation. The retinas were fixed in a paraformaldehyde (4%) /glutaraldehyde (0.5%)/sucrose (30%) mixture in 0.1 M phosphate buffer at pH 7.4 (FGS solution) overnight, cryosectioned to 15 µm thickness, dried in a desiccator overnight, and examined under a fluorescence microscope (Nikon EF) after enclosing with Entellan (Merck). X400.

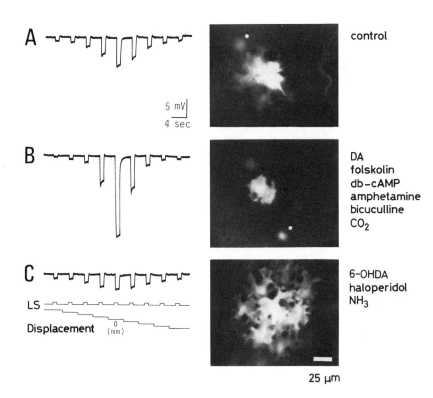

control

DA
folskolin
db-cAMP
amphetamine
bicuculline
CO_2

6-OHDA
haloperidol
NH_3

5 mV / 4 sec

LS

Displacement (mm) 0

25 μm

Fig. 2. Changes in S-potential amplitudes with spot displacement (left), and fluorescence photomicrographs of L-type horizontal cells intracellularly marked with Lucifer yellow (LY) in flatmounts (right). A, From a normal (control) retina; B, a retina in the presence of intravitreal dopamine (DA, 50 μM in the tissue); C, a retina deprived from DA cells with 6-hydroxydopamine intravitreally injected two weeks prior to the experiment. A star marks an endogenously DA-containing cell in A, and a DA-accumulated cell in B.

an increase in the gap-junctional resistance (Giaume et al., 1980; Spray et al., 1981). Recently we have found that CO_2 acts as an uncoupler like DA while NH_3 appears to act as a coupler like haloperidol on gap junctions between horizontal cells in the carp retina, presumably by changing the pH_i (Negishi et al., 1984).

The present paper summarizes our recent observations concerning the effects of DA, related compounds and of CO_2 and NH_3 on the spatial properties of horizontal cells in isolated carp retina (Teranishi et al., 1983; Negishi et al., 1983, 1984).

Morphology and neurotoxic destruction of DA interplexiform cells in the
fish retina

Fluorescence photomicrographs of cryosections (15μm thickness) of the
mullet retina are shown in Fig. 1. Typically a DA interplexiform cell
seen in a raidal section of the central region of the retina has a cell
body at the innermost level of the INL and sends processes towards both
the OPL and IPL. These processes form dense fiber networks in the distal
part of the INL surrounding the external horizontal cells (marked with a
in Fig. 1B) and in the IPL (c in Fig. 1B) as seen in tangential sections
through respective levels (Fig. 1A and C). This particular pattern of
dendritic distribution agrees well with that of DA interplexiform cells
described by earlier workers (Boycott et al., 1975; Ehinger, 1976; Dowling
and Ehinger, 1975).

When DA cells were examined in flatmounts of the carp retina, which
had been treated with intravitreal injection of noradrenaline (5 ug/10 ul)
plus 5,6-dihydroxytryptamine (5 μg) 2 hours before enucleation, DA and
indoleamine-accumulating (IA) cells (Ehinger and Floren, 1976, 1980) were
found to be distributed almost evenly over the entire retinal field,
except for the marginal region. The average density of both classes of
monoamine cell is approximately 40 cells/mm^2 in adult carp (body length,
30-35 cm in tip-to-tip (Negishi et al., 1981b). Although the population
of DA cells accounts for only 9.3% of the total number of cells located in
the amacrine cell layer (Negishi et al., 1981a), their dendritic network
heavily covers the entire retinal field (Fig.1). DA cells could be
destroyed by intravitreal injection of a neurotoxin, 6-hydroxydopamine
(6-OHDA) (Negishi et al., 1981b, 1982); these preparations, deprived of DA
cells, were useful for exploring the functional aspect of DA cells
(Teranishi et al., 1983, 1984; Negishi et al., 1983).

Effects of DA and related compounds on the lateral spread of S-potentials
and on dye diffusion between horizontal cells in the carp retina

During an intracellular recording of L-type S-potentials with a 4%-LY
filled glass-microelectrode, a spot of red (621 nm) light (0.5 mm
diameter) was displaced. Representative recordings of changes in
potential amplitude with spot displacement over various preparations are
illustrated in Fig. 2. When the spot stimulus was delivered to the
recording point (0 mm), the potential amplitude was maximal and gradually
decreased as the spot moved away from recording point in normal (control)
retinas (Fig. 2A, left). When LY was injected into a recording horizontal
cell, usually 5-6 cell bodies were seen in the flatmount (Fig. 2A, right).
The recordings of S-potentials from retinas treated with DA exhibited a
large center response while the amplitude shorply diminished as the spot
moved away, and the distant response (at 2 mm) was smaller than the
control one (Fig. 2B, left). In this case, a small amount (5 μl) of DA (2
mM)-containing Ringer's solution was applied to the residual vitreous
fluid beneath the isolated preparation 30 min before the recording. In
the retinas treated with DA, the injected LY was found to be restricted to
one cell (Fig. 2H, right), from which the recording was made. When the
same procedure was carried out with retinas deprived of DA cells, the
center response was small while the amplitude decay curve was gentle, and
the distant responce was larger than the control one (Fig. 2C, left).
Following intracellular LY-injection, many fluorescent horizontal cells
($>$ 10 cells) were consistently seen (Fig. 2C, right).

When DA was applied to retinas deprived of DA cells, high amplitude
S-potentials were recorded at 0 mm, but they were shaprly reduced in
amplitude with spot displacement. Correspondingly, the injected LY was
found restricted to single cells (Teranishi et al., 1983). The results

indicate that the postsynaptic membrane of horizontal cells is intact in retinas deprived of DA cells. It has been known that DA activates retinal adenylate cyclase, the enzyme that synthesizes cyclic AMP from ATP (Brown and Makman, 1972; Watling and Dowling, 1981). The effect of DA on horizontal cells, observed above in S-potentials and dye diffusion, might be mediated by the activation of DA-sensitive adenylate cyclase in the horizontal cell membrane. If this is the case, dibutyryl cyclic AMP could substitute for DA. A mixture of dibutyryl cyclic AMP (10 mM/5 μl) plus 3-isobutyl-1-methylxantine (1mM/5 μl) was applied to retinas deprived of DA cells. The amplitude of the center response was found to be larger than those seen in retinas deprived of DA cells and in normal retinas. The injected LY was restricted to single cells (Ternishi et al., 1983). A similar effect was produced by an adenylate cyclase activator, folskolin (Seamon et al., 1981).

A DAergic blocker, haloperidol (10 mM/5 μl) was similarly applied to normal retinas in combination with subsequent DA. In these cases, haloperidol was given 20-25 min prior to DA application, because the former appeared to slowly affect horizontal cells while the latter was rapidly effective. The blocker tended to prevent the appearance of DA effect on S-potentials and on dye diffusion (Teranishi et al., 1983; Negishi et al., 1984).

It was assumed that the effects of DA observed can be explained on the basis of an uncoupling action of DA, possibly by increasing of gap-junctional resistance between horizontal cells (Negishi and Drujan, 1978; Teranishi et al., 1983; Piccolino et al., 1983). This possibility was proved with a preliminary series of experiments with double and single mciroelectrodes, which were separated by about 70 um and inserted into different L-type horizontal cells in a center light spot (Takabayashi et al., 1984). Current pulses were applied into one cell through one of the double electrodes, and the voltage changes were recorded from both cells in response to the current pulses as well as to the center (0.5 mm dia.) and annular (1.0 mm i.d. and 4.0 mm o.d.) light stimuli. DA (100 μM) was breifly applied to the retina in the perfusate. Following the application the center response became larger while the surround response became smaller in amplitude, as already shown (Negishi and Drujan, 1978, 1979; Laufer et al., 1981). At the same time, the response to the injected currents was enhanced by about 3.2-fold, indicating that the input reistance was increased in the presence of DA. In only a few successful simultaneous recordings of S-potentials from 2 horizontal cells, it was estimated that the coupling ratio was reduced to one half, indicating that the gap-junctional resistance was increased by approximately 2-fold. These effects of DA briefly applied in the perfusate were reversible. Very recently, it has been shown that DA or cyclic AMP reduces the gap-junctional conductance between coupled horizontal cells in culture (Dowling, 1985).

Similar effects of DA were observed on L-type horizontal cells in the turtle retina (Neyton et al., 1982; Piccolino et al., 1983, 1985) although DA-containing cells belong to a subclass of amacrine cells (Ehinger, 1973; Witkovsky et al., 1984). In the turtle, DA was found to restrict the receptive field and dye diffusion of horizontal cells at the axon terminal level, also differing from our findings at the cell body level in the carp retina (Teranishi et al., 1983; Hida et al., 1984).

Effects of amphetamine and bicuculline on horizontal cells

Amphetamine is well known to facilitate monoamine release from monoamine neurons and also prevent uptake by monoamine neurons in the central nervous system. When amphetamine (2 mM/10 ul) was applied to normal retinas, it produced the same effects as those of DA. Amphetamine enlarged the center response and reduced the distant response as well as dye diffusion (Negishi et al., 1982). It is of interest to point out that if endogenous DA in interplexiform cells is fully mobilized by amphetamine, such marked effects of DA on horizontal cells can be induced. On the other hand, the GABA antagonists, bicuculline and picrotoxin, have been shown to produce effects similar to those of DA on L-type horizontal cells in the turtle retina (Piccolino et al., 1982; Neyton et al., 1982). In the carp retina, bicuculline (2 mM/10 μl) applied intravitreally produced effects similar to those of DA on horizontal cells (Negishi et al., 1983). The effects of both amphetamine and bicuculline were blocked by the preceding application of haloperidol and did not appear in carp retinas deprived of DA cells (Negishi et al., 1983).

Effects of ammonia and carbon dioxide on horizontal cells
    In this series of experiments, the isolated carp retina was placed receptor-side up in a specially designed air-tight chamber (80 ml; Negishi and Svaetichin, 1966), through which moist air was passed as the control gas medium. An alternating spot and annulus of red light stimuli, centered at the recording site, evoked respectively the center and surround responses of L-type horizontal cells. At the beginning of recording from each cell, the intensities of the spot and annular stimuli were adjusted by interposing neutral filters until the hyperpolarizing responses to both were approximately equal.

    While recording the horizontal cell membrane potential, a DA-containing Ringer's solution was briefly jetted from a nebulizer into the air flow so as to be applied over the entire retinal area (Fig. 3A). Following the application (arrow with DA), the membrane potential was depolarized by about 15mV, and the center response (c) was markedly enlarged while the surround response (s) was diminished in amplitude (c > s). This reciprocal effect of DA on both responses was comparable to that shown by intravitreal application of DA in Fig. 2B (left), and was the same as those seen after DA-application in the perfusate in our earlier reports (Negishi and Drujan, 1978, 1979; Laufer et al., 1981). The effect of DA on S-potentials was easily reversible, although Fig. 3A does not show it.

    When ammonia (NH_3) at a low concentration was introduced briefly (30-sec) into the chamber, the membrane potential of horizontal cells were initially slightly depolarized and subsequently hyperpolarized up to -60-70 mV (Fig. 3B). The amplitude of both center (c) and surround (s) responses was only slightly enlarged during the initial depolarization, while it was markedly reduced when the cells were being hyperpolarized. During the amplitude reduction, the center response was affected by NH_3 more than the surround response was, resulting in an amplitude smaller in the former than in the later (c < s). Since the effect of NH_3 was found to last for a long period (20-30 min) (Negishi, 1984), the isolated retina was renewed after such a recording was made. It should be noted that the photoreceptor remained responsive to light stimuli when horizontal cells were largely hyperpolarized by an exposure of the retina to NH_3 (Laufer et al., 1961; Negishi, 1984).

    When CO_2 (10% in air) was introduced into the chamber, the membrane potential was hyperpolarized by 10-20 mV, accompanied by a slight diminution of both responses. During the course of diminution, the surround response (s) was affected by CO_2 consistently more than the center response (c) was, producing an amplitude ratio of c > s (Fig. 3C). The effect of CO_2 was easily reversible.

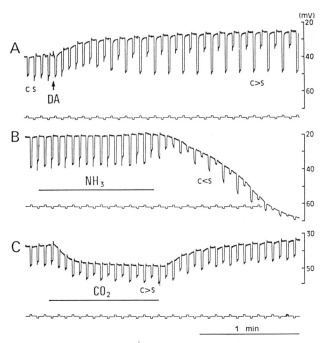

Fig. 3. Effects of DA, NH_3 and CO_2 on center and surround responses of
L-type horizontal cells. Hyperpolarizing shifts c and s represent the
center and surround response, respectively to a red (621 nm) light spot
(0.5 mm dia.) and a red (621 nm) annular light (1.8 mm i.d. and 4.0 mm
o.d) directed towards the recording site. At the beginning of recording,
the intensities of both light stimuli were adjusted by interposing neutral
filters to evoke almost equal sizes of the center and surround responses.
They were c/s=-0.5/-1.5 (A), -0.5/-0.5 (B) and 9.9/-0.5 log units (c),
respectively. Sign c s or c s implies that the amplitude is larger than
the other around the period of tiem. Normal retinas were used in A and C,
while a retina in the presence of amphetamine (100 uM) was used in B. In
A, a DA-containing (5 mM) Ringer's solution was briefly jetted from a
nebulizer into air-flow passing through an air-tight chamber (arrow), in
which the isolated retina was placed. In B and C., NH_3 (< 300 ppm) or CO_2
(10% in air) was applied over a period marked with underline. Scales are
indicated for the membrane potential (mV) and the recording speed (min).
Tracings B and C were from Negishi et al., (1985).

In the control condition under air flow, LY injected into horizontal
cells diffused to several neighboring cells (Fig. 4A), as already shown
(Fig. 2A, right). However, in the presence of CO_2 the injected LY was
found restricted to single cells (Fig. 4B). To examine firmly the effect
of NH_3 on dye diffusion, isolated retinas were kept under the influence
of DA or amphetamine. After several cells were marked singly with LY (see
Fig. 2B, right), the retinas were exposed to NH_3 (300-500 ppm) for 10-15
min, and then processed to fluorescent flatmounts. The injected LY was
found to have diffused to numerous neighboring cells (Fig. 4C).
Therefore, the effects of NH_3 and CO_2 appear to be also opposite on dye
diffusion.

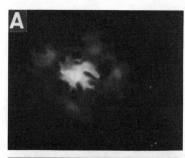
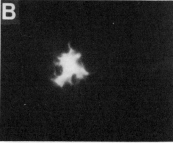
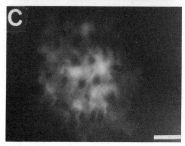

Fig. 4. Fluorescence photomicrographs showing effects of CO_2 and NH_3 on dye coupling between L-type horizontal cells in flatmounts. The dye LY was iontophoretically injected for 30 sec in these cases, and the retinas were fixed in a paraformaldehyde (4%) and sucrose (30%) mixture in 0.1 M phosphate buffer at pH 7.4 (FS solution). A: From a normal retina, which was placed in air for 20 min between dye injection and tissue fixation. B: From a retina, which was placed under 10% CO_2 in air. The dye was injected into the cell 10 min after exposure of the retina to CO_2, and the retina was kept in the presence of 15% CO_2 for a further 25 min before tissue fixation. C: From a retina, which was exposed to NH_3 (300-500 ppm). At first, a single cell was marked with LY in the presence of DA (50 μM) as shown in Fig. 2B, and then the preparation was exposed to NH_3 for 10 min before tissue fixation. Scale bar, 25 μm (magnification: x400) From data by Negishi et al., (1985).

There has been a general agreement that CO_2 reduces the pH_i (acidification), resulting in a decrease of the gap-junctional conductance (uncoupling) between cells (Turin and Warner, 1977, 1980; Giaume et al., (1980; Spray et al., 1981). In the present study on the carp retina, CO_2 appeared to interfere with the electrical coupling between horizontal cells, presumably by reducing the pH_i. On the other hand, the effect of NH_3 on horizontal cells is not consistent with earlier findings (Thomas, 1974; Giaume and Korn, 1980) in which ammonium sulfate was applied to electrically coupled pairs of invertebrate cells in the perfusate. In their experiments with the crayfish septate axon junction, Giaume and Korn (1980) noted that during an initial alkalinization following the application of ammonium sulfate the junctional resistance was not altered while the non-junctional resistance as well as the junctional conductance was decreased. A similar electrical decoupling could be induced when the external potassium concentration was increased. Therefore, they explained that the decoupling (reduced junctional conductance) resulted from a shunt of the gap junctions due to increased axonal membrane conductance; the junctional resistance proper was unaffected. Furthermore, a rebound phenomenon was found in the membrane potential, associated with intracellular acidification after the application of ammonium sulfate had been terminated (Giaume and Korn, 1980). During the rebound phase of intracellular acidification, uncoupling was caused due to a marked increase in the gap-junctional resistance; the non-junctional resistance was little affected in this case. In the horizontal cell membrane potential, such a rebound was not observed when NH_3 was eliminated from the chamber, and instead the effect of NH_3, diminishing the center response more than the surround response, was seen within 1 min after the termination of NH_3 application.

On the basis of the above view (Giaume and Korn, 1980), either intracellular alkalinization or acidification uncouples electrical gap junctions at the crayfish septate axon terminas, although the mechanisms underlying are different. In turn, our results show that NH_3 (applied in the gas form) appears to facilitate the lateral spread of S-potential as well as dye diffusion. Since we did not measure the intracellular pH and the membrane resistance, interpretation of the present findings would be so limited. Also, we could not detect under the fluorescence microscope when dye diffusion from one injected cell to its neighbors begins after an application of NH_3 to isolated retinas (Negishi et al., 1984). At present, it can not be ascertained whether or not factors other than intracellular alkalinization (such as changes in the concentration of external or internal ions) are involved in the NH_3-induced facilitation of coupling between horizontal cells. Futhermore, CO_2 and NH_3 certainly influence retinal cells other than horizontal cells. Among them, their effects on photoreceptor cells would be reflected to a considerable extent in the gas-induced changes in the horizontal cell membrane potential. CO_2 may rapidly act on cones, in which high carbonic anhydrase activity has been found (Parthe, 1981). It has also been assumed that the most sensitive site to NH_3 and anoxia is the synaptic region in the OPL. NH_3 readily interrupts synaptic transmission from photoreceptor to horizontal cells (Negishi and Svaetichin, 1966; Negishi, 1984), an action similar to that of L-glutamate, although the underlying mechanisms are completely different. The large hyperpolarization of horizontal cells after NH_3 application probably reflects the synaptic interruption, because cones remain responsive to light stimuli. Such general influences of CO_2 and NH_3 on retinal cells make it still more difficult to compare our results with other earlier data obtained with disected preparations of coupled cells (Thomas, 1973; Turin and Warner, 1977, 1980; Spray et al., 1981; Giaume and Korn, 1982).

The coupling and uncoupling phenomena observed between horizontal cells are assumed to be voltage-independent, because intravitreal application of L-glutamate (a depolarizing agent) or GABA (a hyperpolarizing agent) did not influence the restricted LY to single horizontal cells, which had been injected in the presence of DA or amphetamine (Netishi et al., 1984). Further, DA applied to paired horizontal cells in culture did not change the resting membrane potential while the coupling conductance was reduced (Dowling, 1985).

Comments in summary: Schematic circuitry related to the results obtained
The chemicals and agents used in the present experiments produced identical effects on all subclasses of cone-connected horizontal (L-, RG- and YRB-type) cells (Teranishi et al., 1984). They can be classified into 2 groups on the basis of their effects on the lateral spread of S-potentials and dye diffusion between horizontal cells. One group uncouples and the other couples horizontal cells in the fish retina. The former includes DA, folskolin, dibutyryl cyclic AMP, amphetamine, bicuculline and CO_2 while the latter includes 6-OHDA, haloperidol and possibly NH_3 (see Fig. 2).

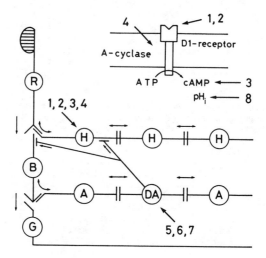

1, DA(+); 2, Haloperidol(-); 3, Dibutyryl cAMP
(analogue); 4, Folskolin(+); 5, Amphetamine
(+); 6, 6-OHDA(destruction); 7, Bcc
(desinhibition); 8, CO_2 & NH_3 (pH_i)

Fig. 5. Schematic circuitry of the carp retina related to the results
obtained. Symbols and signs: R, photoreceptor; H, horizontal cell; B,
bipolar cells; A, amacrine cells; DA, dopaminergic interplexiform cell; G,
ganglion cell; numbers 1-8, the reagents examined (see bottom); A-cyclase,
adenylate cyclase; pH_i, intracellular pH; thick arrows, acting sites of
the reagents; thin arrows (one and two ways), synaptic contacts (however,
two-way arrows between horizontal cells represent gap junctions).

The acting sites of the above reagents, however, are assumed to be
different. In a diagram of simplified circuitry of the fish retina, the
acting sites of respective reagents are indicated (Fig. 5). DA,
folskolin, dibutyryl cyclic AMP, haloperidol, CO_2 and NH_3 directly act on
horizontal cells, while 6-OHDA, amphetamine and bicuculline attack DA
interplexiform cells. For further details, DA and haloperidol bind with
D1-type receptors on the horizontal cell membrane, folskolin activates
adenylate cyclase and dibutyryl cyclic AMP is analogous to endogenous
cyclic AMP in the membrane. However, CO_2 and NH_3 may primarily change the
intracellular pH. The neurotoxin 6-OHDA destroys DA cells, amphetamine
releases endogenous DA from DA cells and bicuculline may let DA cells free
from GABAergic inhibition by amacrine cells (Yazulla, 1985). Since the
effect of externally applied or internally released DA simulates a
functional aspect of interplexiform cells, these cells appear to normally
regulate the spatial properties (gap junctions) of horizontal cells in the
fish retinas. At present, interrelation between the adenylate
cyclase-cyclic AMP system and intracellular pH, and also involvement of
intracellular calcium ions in the coupling phenomena between horizontal
cells remain unanswered.

Acknowledgements
     The authors thank Mrs. Tami Urano for her secretarial assistance. The series of experiments was supported in part by grants from the Ministry of Education of Japan, the Japan Society for the Promotion of Science, the Naito Foundation (82-128) and the Johnan Hospital in Takaoka. One of the authors (K.N.) expresses his gratitude to the Yamada Science Foundation for its partial support to his trip to Alicante, Spain.

References:
Boycott, B. B., J.E. Dowling, S.K. Fisher, H. Kolb, and A.M. Laties, Proc. R. Soc. Lond. Biol. B-191, 353-368 (1975).
Brown, J.H., and M.H. Makman, Proc. Natl. Acad. Aci. USA 69, 539-543 (1972).
Cohen, J.L., and J.E. Dlowling, Brain Res., 264, 307-310 (1983).
Dowling, J.E., E.M. Lasater and L. H. Young in: Circuitry in the Retina A. Gallego and P. Gouras eds. (Elsevier Press 1985) this volume.
Dowling, J.E., and B. Ehinger, Science 188, 270-273 (1975).
Dowling, J.E., and B. Ehinger, Proc. R. Soc. Lond. Biol. 201, 7-26 (1978).
Ehinger, B., in: Transmitters in the Visual Process S.L. Bonting, ed. (Pergamon Press 1976) pp 145-163.
Ehinger, B. and I. Floren, Cell Tiss. Res. 175, 38-48 (1976).
Ehinger, B. and I. Floren, Neurochem. Intenatl, 1, 209-229 (1980).
Galego, A., Vis. res. Suppl 3, 33-50 (1971).
Giaume, C. and H. Korn, Neurosci. 7, 1923-1930 (1982).
Giaume, C., M.E. Spira, and H. Korn, Neurosci. Lett. 17, 197-202 (1980).
Hida, E., K. Nehishi, and L.-I. Naka, J. Neurosci. Res. 11, 373-382 (1980).
Kaneko, A. J. Physiol (Lond) 213, 95-105 (1971).
Kaneko, A., and A.E. Stuart Neurosci. Lett. 47, 1-7 (1984).
Laufer, M. in: B. D. Drujan and M. Laufer eds. (Alan R. Liss 1982) pp. 257-279.
Laufer, M., K. Negishi, and B.D. Drujan Vis. Res. 21, 1657-1660 (1981).
Laufer, M., G. Svaetichin, G. Mitarai, R. Fatehand E. Vallecalle, and J. Villegas in: The Visual System: Neurophysiology and Psychophysics. R. Jung and H. Kornhuber eds. (Amsterdam: Elsevier 1961) pp. 457-463.
Naka, K.-I., and W.A.H. Rushton J. Physiol (Lond) 192, 437-461 (1967).
Negishi, K. J. Jūzen Med. Soc. 93, 341-351 (1984).
Negishi, K., and B.D. Drujan Sens. Processes 2, 388-395 (1978).
Negishi, K., and B.D. Drujan J. Neurosci. Res. 4, 311-334 (1979).
Negishi, K., S. Kato and T. Teranishi Acta Histochem. Cytochem. 14, 317-324 (1981a).
Negishi, K. and V. Sutija Vis. Res. 9, 881-893 (1969).
Negishi, K. and G. Svaetichin Pflugers Arch ges. Physiol. 292, 177-205 (1966).
Negishi, K., T. Teranishi and S. Kato, Acta Histochem. Cytochem. 14, 4490460 (1981b).
Negishi, K., T. Teranishi and S. Kato, Acta .Histochem. Cytochem. 15, 768-778 (1982).
Negishi, K., T. Teranishi and S. Kato, Neurosci. Lett. 37, 261-266 (1983).
Negishi, K., T. Teranishi and S. Kato, Brain Res. in press (1984).
Neyton, J., M. Piccolino and H. M. Gerschenfeld, Neurosci. Lett. Abstr. 8: 132 (1982).
Norton, Al., H. Spekreijse, M.L., Wolbarsht and H. G. Wagner, Science 160, 1021-1022 (1968).
Parthe, V, J. Neurosci. Res. 6, 119-131 (1981).
Piccolino, M., J. Neyton, P. Witkovsky and H.M. Gershenfeld, Proc. Natl. Acad. Aci. USA 79, 3671-3675 (1982).
Piccolino, M., J. Neyton, and H.M. Gershenfeld, J. Physiol (Paris) 78, 739-842 (1983).

88

Piccolino, M., J. Neyton, and H.M. Gershenfeld, J. Neurosci. 4, 2477-2488 (1984).

Seamon, K.B., W. Padgett and J.W. Daly, Natl. Acad. Sci. USA 78, 3363-3367 (1981).

Stewart, W., Cell 14, 741-759 (1978).

Spray, D.C., A.L. Harris and M.V.L. Bennett, Science 211, 712-715 (1981).

Takabayashi, A., G. Mitarai and K. Negishi, J. Physiol Soc. Jpn. Abstr. 46, 437 (1984).

Teranishi, T., Jpn. J. Physiol. 33, 417-428 (1983).

Teranishi, T., K. Negishi and S. Kato, Nature 301, 243-246 (1983).

Teranishi, T., K. Negishi and S. Kato, J. Neurosci. 4, 1271-1280 (1984).

Thomas, R.C., J. Physiol (Lond) 238, 159-180 (1974).

Tomita, T., T. Tosaka, K. Watanabe, Y. Saito, Jpn. J. Physiol. 8, 41-50 (1958).

Tonosaki, A., H. Washioka, H. Nakamura K. Negishi, J. Elet. Micr. Tech. in press (1984).

Turin, L., A.E. Warner Nature 270, 56-57 (1977).

Watling, K.T. and J.E. Dowling, J. Neurochem. 36, 559-568 (1981).

Witkovsky, P., W. Eldred and H.J. Karten, J. Comp. Neurol. 228, 217-225 (1984).

Yamada, E. and T. Ishikawa, Cold Spring Harbor Symp. Quant. Biol. 303, 383-392 (1965).

Yazulla, S. in: Neurocircuitry of the Retina (this volume) (1985).

GABA sensitivity in solitary turtle cones: Evidence for the
feedback pathway from horizontal cells to cones

A. Kaneko, T. Ohtsuka, M. Tachibana
National Institute for Physiological Sciences
Okazaki, Japan

The vertebrate retina receives chromatic information by three sets of cones having different spectral sensitivity and processes it into opponent responses at an early stage of the neural network. The underlying mechanism responsible for the color opponent responses of biphasic and triphasic horizontal cells has been studied extensively in the past decades. The model proposed by Fuortes and Simon (1974) on the turtle retina has been widely adopted as the most likely interpretation. Their model involves subtype-specific feedforward and negative feedback connections between cones and horizontal cells (Fig. 1). Similar model has been suggested also in the fish retina based on the subtype-specific synaptic morphology of cone terminals (Stell and Lightfoot, 1975; Stell et al., 1975). The feedback circuit attracted many investigators, and has been used to explain not only color opponency (Fuortes et al., 1973; Fuortes and Simon, 1974; Murakami et al., 1982; Toyoda and Fujimoto, 1983), but also the center-surround antagonism of the receptive field (Baylor et al., 1971; O'Bryan, 1973; Piccolino and Gerschenfeld, 1980; Gerschenfeld and Piccolino, 1980; Gerschenfeld et al., 1980). The feedback effect from horizontal cells to cones was first demonstrated by Baylor et al (1971), who showed that polarization of horizontal cell by injection of an extrinsic current caused polarization of opposite polarity in nearby cones. In spite of popularity of the feedback syanpse, supporting evidence is still limited.

γ-Aminobutyric acid (GABA) has been suggested as a candidate of the neurotransmitter of a subtype of horizontal cells, the monophasic horizontal cell. This type of horizontal cell is characterized by its hyperpolarizing responses to monochromatic light flashes of all visible wavelengths (Simon, 1973; Saito et al., 1974). It has been shown in fish and toad that monophasic horizontal cells synthesize GABA (Lam, 1972; Lam et al., 1979), accumulate extrinsic GABA by a high affinity uptake mechanism (Lam and Steinman, 1971; Marc et al., 1978; Schwartz, 1982) and release stored GABA when exposed to high $[K^+]_o$ (Schwartz, 1982) or to L-glutamate (Miller and Schwartz, 1983). Application of GABA agonists or antagonists affects chromatic responses of biphasic and triphasic horizontal cells (Murakami et al., 1982; Toyoda and Fujimoto, 1983).

Difficulty in analyzing the retinal circuitry arises partly from the complicated network of closely packed retinal neurons. Solitary retinal cells dissociated from the network provide an ideal preparation to get out of such complexity. They are particularly suitable for examining the chemosensitivity, not only because they are independent of interaction with other cells, but also because they are free from the diffusion barrier, or from a population of surrounding cells which sequester the applied chemical compounds such as amino acids from the extracellular space by an active uptake (cf. Ishida and Fain, 1982).

Another advantage of solitary cells is that they can be recorded by using "Giga-seal" suction electrodes either under voltage-clamp or under current-clamp conditions (Hamill et al., 1981). The plasma membrane of dissociated cells is cleaned by an exposure to proteolytic enzymes, which is one of the prerequisite for recording with the suction electrode. Small size of retinal cells, which had set the technical limitation for intracellular penetration with microelectrode, is now advantageous to achieve perfect space clamp.

Neurocircuitry of the Retina, A Cajal Memorial
A. Gallego and P. Gouras, Editors

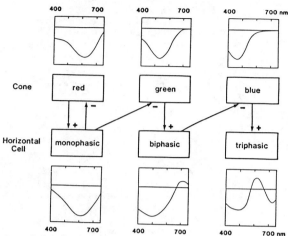

Fig. 1. A model of the outer plexiform layer of the turtle retina. Modified from Fuortes and Simon (1974). Arrows indicate synapses and the direction of signal transmission. Positive sign represents the sign-conserving synapse at which the response polarities of presynaptic and postsynaptic cells are identical. Negative sign represents the sign-inverting synapse at which the response polarity of presyanptic cells is reversed in the postsyanptic cell. Curves in boxes illustrated above each type of cones or below each type of horizontal cells represent the envelop of response amplitudes of each cell to monochromatic light flashes of various wavelengths (in the spectral range of approximately between 400 nm and 750 nm). Horizontal straight lines in the boxes indicate the dark membrane potential level: deflections above this level indicate depolarizing responses, while deflections below this level indicate hyperpolarizing responses.

This chapter will summarize our recent studies (Tachibana and Kaneko, 1984; Ohtsuka, 1984, 1985) of measuring GABA sensitivity in various types of solitary photoreceptors dissociated from the fresh-water turtle (Geoclemys reevesii) retina. Our results may provide a new piece of supporting evidence for the GABA-operated negative feedback connection from monophasic horizontal cells to red-sensitive and green-sensitive cones.

Morphological identification of turtle photoreceptors

Turtle photoreceptors are classified morphologically into seven types (Ohtsuka, 1985) by their unique cell shape and by various colors of the oil droplets located at the distal end of the inner segments; four types of single cones, one type of double cone consisting of the principal and accessory members, and one type of rod. These morphological features were correlated with the results of microspectrophotometric (MSP) measurements of spectral absorption of photopigments contained in the outer segments (Liebman and Granda, 1971; Liebman, 1972; Granda and Dvorak, 1977). Their results have provided the basis of identification of cell types in physiological experiments (Baylor and Hodgkin 1973; Richter and Simon 1974). According to their identification of cell types in physiological experiments (Baylor and Hodgkin, 1973; Richter and Simon 1974). According to their identification single cones containing red oil droplet were red-sensitive, those containing orange oil droplet were green-sensitive, and those containing clear (or colorless) oil droplet were blue-sensitive: double cones were described as consisting of red-sensitive principal member and green-sensitive accessory member.

Recently, however, one of the authors reexamined the correlation between the spectral sensitivity and the type of oil droplets both in Geoclemys (Ohtsuka, 1985) and in Pseudemys (in preparation) by intracellular recording and subsequent staining with Lucifer yellow with identical results in both species. The fore-mentioned morphological and physiological correlation was confirmed on single cones containing either red or orange oil droplet, on the principal member of double cones, and on rods. However, surprising results were obtained that the previous identification on the accessory member of double cones and on single cones containing clear oil droplet need corrections.[*]

In the past, the accessory member of a double cone was thought to be green-sensitive, but the present study revealed that it is red-sensitive. The previous identification was based on MSP made on the outer segment of a presumably "detached accessory member of a double cone" (Liebman and Granda, 1971). Since the accessory member of a double cone closely resembles to the rod, a careful observation is needed to identify it morphologically, if detached from its counterpart. A reliable criterion of the identification is the diameter of the axon which connect the cell body with the terminal. Rods have a stout (> 4 µm) axon, while the accessory member of double cones has a thin (< 1 µm) axon. Consistent with the present electrophysiological study, recent MSP measurements on a large sample (Lipetz and MacNichol, 1982; Lipetz, 1984) revealed that, without exception, both members of double cones contained red-absorbing visual pigments.

When the flat mount preparation of the turtle retina is observed under a fluorescence microscope, about two-thirds of colorless oil droplets emitted a strong autofluorescence, while remaining one-third did not (Ohtsuka, 1984). Fluorescent colorless oil droplets were localized to red-sensitive cones, while nonfluorescent colorless oil droplets to blue-sensitive cones (Ohtsuka, 1984). In 1957, Fujimoto et al., reported two types of colorless oil droplets, "pale-green" and "transparent", which seem to correspond to the two types of colorless oil droplets found in the present study. Under the ordinary light microscope, pale-green oil droplets are lightly tinted and are slightly larger in size, while transparent oil droplets has no tint and are smaller. Since the morphological difference between these two types of oil droplets was smaller than the difference between those and the other brilliantly colored oil droplets, they were treated as homogeneous group in later papers under the name of "colorless" or "clear" oil droplet (e.g., Liebman, 1972). Recently, two types of "clear" oil droplets were reconfirmed by MSP in the Pseudemys retina, and they were localized to red-sensitive (fluorescent, pale-green oil droplet) and to blue-sensitive (non-fluorescent) cones (Lipetz and MacNichol, 1982; Lipetz, 1984).

Spectral sensitivity of each type of photoreceptors is summarized in Table 1.

GABA sensitivity of solitary cones
Solitary photoreceptors (an example in Fig. 2) were obtained from the retina of the dark-adapted turtle by incubating the retina in a solution containing 6 U/ml papain and 5 mg/ml collagenase (Tachibana and Kaneko, 1984). Cells were plated in a culture dish and incubated until they attached to the bottom of the dish made of a concanavalin A-coated cover

92

T A B L E   1

Morphological Features and Spectral Sensitivity
of Turtle (Geoclemys) Photoreceptors

	Color of the oil droplet	Spectral sensitivity
Single cones	red	red-sensitive
	orange*	green-sensitive
	colorless (fluorescent)	red-sensitive
	colorless (non-fluorescent)	blue-sensitive
Double cones		
principal	yellow*	red-sensitive
accessory	no oil droplet	red-sensitive
Rods	no oil droplet	scotopic spectral sensitivity

*color of the oil droplets contained in the principal member of double
cones and those in green-sensitive single cones appears different in the
two species of turtle, Geoclemys and Pseudemys.   In this Table the colors
of Geoclemys photoreceptors are listed.

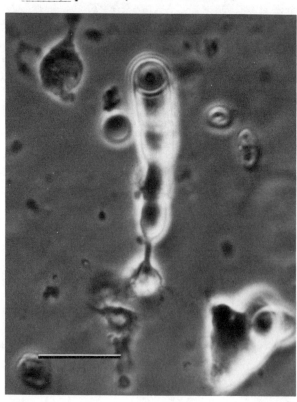

Fig. 2.   Photo-
micrograph of a single
cone containing red
oil droplet dissociat-
ed from Geoclemys
reevesii. Calibra-
tion 20 μm.

glass. During recording, cells were superfused by a solution whose composition was similar to physiological saline; (in mM) NaCl 79, KCl 10, $CaCl_2$ 2.5, $MgCl_2$ 1, glucose 16, HEPES 2, choline Cl 37 (maintained 15°C, pH 7.4). Since the outer segments had been lost during dissociation, no light responses were obtained from solitary photoreceptors. Nevertheless, the type of photoreceptors was unequivocally identified by the fore-mentioned morphological criteria, since their morphology was well maintained even after dissociation.

Since photoreceptors are small (Fig. 2), approximately 5 to 7 μm in diameter, it was difficult to obtain stable recordings by the conventional intracellular recording technique. Thus, we used suction pipettes (ca. 3 μm o.d. and 1 μm i.d.) filled with 120 mM KCl, 5 mM EGTA and 10 mM HEPES (pH 7.4) in the whole-cell clamp configuration (Hamill et al., 1981). After the giga-seal was established between the pipette tip and the cell membrane, the patch membrane at the pipette tip was ruptured by a brief strong suction. The giga-seal remained intact, and a low resistance communication was formed between the intracellular solution and the pipette. We measured membrane voltages by connecting the pipette to a voltage follower, or the membrane current by switching the preamplifier to a current-voltage converter. The resting membrane potential of all types of solitary photoreceptors was usually between -30 mV and -40 mV. GABA was applied either ionophoretically from a fine-tipped glass pipette by passing brief current pulses (1 - 50 msec, 1 50 nA) or by pressure ejection (Ishida et al., 1984) from a 20 μm-tip pipette filled with 0.1 - 10 μM GABA.

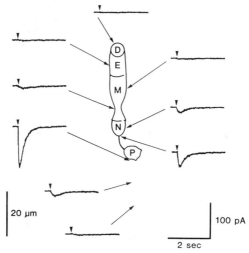

Fig. 3. Responses of a single cone containing red oil droplet to GABA applied ionophoretically at various positions on the cell surface. The recording suction pipette was positioned at the cell body. Holding potential (V_h) was -60 mV. GABA was applied ionophoretically by passing brief current pulses (5 msec, 25 nA; timing indicated by arrow heads) through a fine-tip glass micropipette. At the pedicle this dose of GABA evoked a response whose amplitude was about 1/3 of the maximum. Braking current -5 nA. Responses to GABA applied 10 and 20 μm away from the pedicle are also illustrated to demonstrate a limited distance of GABA diffusion. D, oil droplet; E, ellipsoid; M, myoid; N, cell body containing the nucleus; P, cone pedicle.

Localization of GABA sensitivity
    When GABA was applied ionophoretically to a cone containing red oil
droplet (holding potential, -60 mV), an inward current was evoked (Fig.
3). There was a large regional difference in GABA sensitivity. As seen
in Fig. 3, the amplitude of the GABA-evoked current was maximum (> 100 pA)
when GABA was applied at the cone pedicle, and sharply declined when the
site of GABA application was moved away from the cone pedicle; to about
13% of the maximum at the cell body, and to less than 2% at the myoid and
ellipsoid. Localized sensitivity at the pedicle was further confirmed by
the observation that GABA sensitivity was extremely low in single cones
(containing red oil droplet) whose pedicles were lost during dissociation.

Difference in GABA sensitivity among cell types
    The amplitude of the GABA response was dose-dependent (Fig. 4). In
this figure, the dose (unit, nC) is expressed as the electric charge which
carried ionophoretic current (the product of the current intensity and
duration). The dose-response curve had a sigmoid shape covering a range
of about 1 log unit. Fig. 4 also illustrates that the single cone
containing red oil droplet (red-sensitive cone) and the single cone
containing orange oil droplet (green-sensitive cone) showed nearly equal
maximal response amplitudes, and that both of them showed larger maximal
amplitude than the single cone containing non-fluorescent colorless oil
droplet (blue-sensitive cone). However, the threshold dose (50 to 100 pC)
and the dose at which the response saturates were similar in all types of
cells. The least effective dose determined by a pressure application of
known concentration of GABA was approximately 100 nM.

    Figure 5 illustrates the GABA sensitivity histograms for each cell
type. The sensitivity was defined by the maximum response amplitude to
the saturating dose of GABA. Single cones with red oil droplet
(red-sensitive cones) and single cones with orange oil droplet
(green-sensitive cones) were categorized in the high sensitivity group.
Single cones with fluorescent colorless oil droplet (red-sensitive cone)
showed a large saturating response, while cells with non-fluorescent
colorless oil droplet (blue-sensitive cones) showed a low GABA
sensitivity. The principal member of double cones belonged to the high
GABA sensitivity group, while the accessory member belonged to the low
GABA sensitivity group, although both members are red-sensitive. Rods
were very low in GABA sensitivity.

Ionic mechanisms of GABA-induced currents
    The polarity of GABA-induced current may appear contradictory to what
is expected from the inhibitory effect of GABA, because the inward current
depolarizes the cell membrane. We first determined the ionic species
which carry the GABA-induced current to answer this puzzle, by measuring
the reversal potential. GABA-induced current was inward at the holding
potential (V_h) of -60 mV (Fig. 3), but its polarity was reversed to
outward at $V_h > 0$ mV. The reversal potential of GABA-induced current was
estimated to be 6.1 ± 4.5 mV (mean ± SD), which was very close to the
estimated equilibrium potential of 1^- (E_{Cl}). The reversal potential was
shifted to -17.2 ± 3.9 mV when 70% of Cl^- in the pipette solution were
replaced with non-permeant glutamate ions. The amount of shift of the
reversal potential was close to the value estimated by the Nernst equation
for Cl^-. No appreciable shift in the reversal potential nor change in
response amplitude was seen when either the concentration of Na^+ or the
concentration of K^+ of the superfusing solution was changed. These
observations strongly suggest that the current induced by GABA is carried
by Cl^- almost exclusively. Reversal potentials examined in other types of
cells were all similar to the above value.

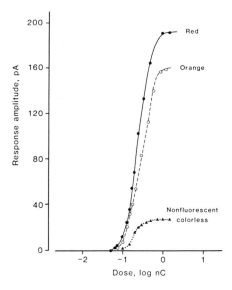

Fig. 4. Dose-response curves of GABA examined in a single cone with red oil droplet (red-sensitive cone; filled circles connected with an uninterrupted line labeled "Red"), a single cone with orange oil droplet (green-sensitive cone; open circles connected with a broken line labeled "Orange"), and a single cone with non-fluorescent colorless oil droplet (blue-sensitive cone; filled triangles connected with a dotted line labeled "nonfluorescent colorless"). GABA was applied to pedicles in all cells. The dose (nC) is the product of the intensity (varied from 5 to 50 nA) and duration (varied from 5 to 50 msec) of ionophoretic current. Braking current −5 nA in red, −10na in orange, and -11 nA in colorless.

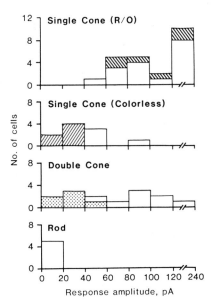

Fig. 5. GABA-sensitivity histogram for each morphological type of cells. The sensitivity in this Figure was defined by the maximum response amplitude to the saturating dose of GABA. The right-most column includes cells showing response amplitudes exceeding 120 pA. Top row; single cones with either red (non-shaded) or orange (shaded) oil droplet. Second row; single cones with either fluorescent (non-shaded) or non-fluorescent (shaded) colorless oil droplet. Third row; principal (non-shaded) and accessory (shaded with dots) members of double cones. Bottom row; rods.

E_{Cl} in in situ photoreceptors is presumably at more negative value than what we have seen in solitary cells under the whole-cell clamp. Diffusion of Cl^- from the suction pipette to the cell interior seems to be quite rapid and must have raised the intracellular Cl^- concentration Cl^- soon after the rupture of the patch membrane. To observe the effect of GABA on cells before Cl^-_i increase, we recorded voltage responses of solitary cones immediately after rupture of the patch membrane. Within a few seconds after the rupture, GABA caused a hyperpolarization in a cell whose resting potential was -37 mV. About 10 sec after the rupture, the polarity of the GABA response reversed to depolarizinging, suggesting $[Cl^-]_i$ has increased. This observation strongly suggests that GABA induces a membrane hyperpolarization in in situ cones.

Physiological role of GABA-operated feedback circuit

The present study has demonstrated that turtle cones are sensitive to GABA and that the sensitivity varies among subtypes. It is inferred that both red-sensitive (except for the accessory member of double cones) and green-sensitive cones have high sensitivity to GABA, while blue-sensitive cones and rods have very low sensitivity. It is tempting to believe that GABA is the transmitter substance used in the interaction between the monophasic horizontal cell and red-sensitive and green-sensitive cones, since GABA was effective at a concentration as low as 100 nM, and the GABA sensitivity was clearly localized to the cone pedicle where they make contacts with horizontal cells.

Finally we wish to speculate the functional aspects of the GABAergic negative feedback synapse from monophasic horizontal cells to red-sensitive and green-sensitive cones. In the dark, cones release their transmitter tonically. There are a number of reports that transmitter substance of cone photoreceptors depolarize horizontal cells (Trifonov, 1968; Dowling and Ripps, 1973; Cervetto and Piccolino, 1974; Kaneko and Shimazaki, 1975). Depolarization triggers release of GABA from monophasic horizontal cells (Schwartz, 1982; Miller and Schwartz, 1983), which, in turn, causes membrane hyperpolarization in both red-sensitive and green-sensitive cones. Illumination of light hyperpolarizes photoreceptors, and sequence of events of the opposite polarity is expected to occur during light flashes.

It seems possible that the negative feedback interaction (Fig. 1) plays three important roles in the function of the retina; color opponent responses of biphasic horizontal cells, center-surround antagonism, and the gain control of cone output. If the fore-mentioned sequence of events in the neural chain starts from the red-sensitive cone, and is relayed by the monophasic horizontal cell to green-sensitive cones, biphasic horizontal cells respond with depolarization to red light. If and when the negative feedback operates between red-sensitive cones and monophasic horizontal cells bidirectionally, such interaction would result in surround antagonism in red-sensitive cones, since the spatial summation in monophasic horizontal cells is much larger than in red-sensitive cones. This circuit may also contribute in compressing the light-evoked voltage responses of both red-sensitive cones and horizontal cells.

Morphological studies have shown that biphasic =, and triphasic horizontal cells also have subtype-specific connections (Leeper, 1978); biphasic cells with green-sensitive and blue-sensitive cones, and triphasic cells with blue-sensitive cones. It is also shown that these types of horizontal cells neither accumulate GABA nor have a machinery to synthesize GABA (Lam, 1972; Lam and Steinman, 1971; Marc et al., 1978; Lam et al., 1979). Low GABA sensitivity in blue-sensitive cones agree with those reports, but the question how these types of horizontal cells communicate with photoreceptors still remains open.

Acknowledgements
We thank Miss Michi Hosono for her excellent technical assistance of preparing solitary photoreceptors. This research was supported in part by the Grants in Aid for Scientific Research from the Ministry of Education, Science and Culture (Nos. 58480117, 58870015 AK, principal investigator; 58770085, 59770116 to MT), and by Prof. Kato Memorial Research Fund for Physiology and Medicine to MT.

References
Baylor, D.A., M.G.F. Fuortes and P.M. O'Bryan J. Physiol (Lond) 214, 265-294 (1971).
Baylor, D.A. and A.L. Hodgkin J. Physiol (Lond) 234, 163-198 (1973).
Cervetto, L. and M. Piccolino, Science, 183, 417-419 (1974).
Dowling, J.E. and H. Ripps, Nature, 242, 101-103 (1973).
Fujimoto, K., T. Yanase and T. Hanaoka, Jpn. J. Physiol. 7 339-346 (1957).
Fuortes, M.G.F., E.A. Schwartz and E.J. Simon, J. Physiol (Lond) 234, 199-216 (1973).
Fuortes, M.G.F. and E.J. Simon, J. Physiol (Lond) 240, 177-198 (1974).
Gerschenfeld, H., M. Piccolino, Proc. Roy. Soc. Lond. B 206, 465-480 (1980).
Gerschenfeld, H., M. Piccolino and J. Neyton, J. Exp. Biol. 89, 177-192 (1980).
Granda, A.M. and C.A. Dvorak in: Handbook of Sensory Physiology F. Crescitelli (ed) (Springer-Verlag Berlin 1977)pp. 451-495.
Hamill, O.P., A. Marty, E. Neher, B. Sakmann and F.J. Sigworth, Pflugers Archiv 391, 85-100 (1981).
Ishida, A.T. and G. Fain, Proc. Natl. Acad. Sci. USA 78, 5890-5894 (1982).
Ishida, A.T., A. Kaneko and M. Tachibana, J. Phsyiol. (Lond) 348, 255-270 (1984).
Kaneko, A. and H. Shimazaki, J. Physiol (Lond) 252, 509-522 (1975).
Lam, D.M.K., J. Cell Biol. 54, 225-231 (1972).
Lam, D.M.K. and L. Steinman, Proc. Natl. Acad. Sci. USA 68, 2777-2781 (1971).
Lam, D.M.K., Y.Y.T. Su, L. Swain, R.E. Marc, C. Brandon and J.Y. Wu, Nature 278, 565-567 (1979).
Leeper, H.F., J. Comp. Neurol. 182, 795-810 (1978).
Liebman, P.A. in: Handbook of Sensory Physioloy H.J.A. Dartnall ed. (Springer-Verlag Berlin 1972) pp. 507-509.
Liebman, P.A. and A.M. Granda, Vis. Res. 11, 105-114 (1971).
Lipetz, L.E. in: The Visual System A. Fein (ed) (Alan R. Liss New York 1984) in press.
Lipetz, L.E. and E.F. MacNichol, Jr., Biol. Bull. 163, 396 (1982).
Marc, R.E., W.K. Stell, D. Bok, and D.M.K. Lam, J. Comp. Neurol. 182, 221-246 (1978).
Miller, A.M. and E.A. Schwartz, J. Physiol. (Lond) 334, 325-349 (1983).
Murakami, M., Y. Shimoda, K. Nakatani, E., Miyachi and S. Watanabe, Jpn. J. Physiol 32, 927-935 (1982).
O'Bryan, P.M., J. Physiol (Lond) 235, 207-223 (1973).
Ohtsuka, T., Neurosci Lett. in press (1985).
Ohtsuka, T., J. Comp. Neurol. 52, 241-245 (1985).
Piccolino, M. and H.M. Gerschenfeld, Proc. R. Soc. Lond B. 206, 439-463 (1980).
Richter, A. and E.J. Simon, J. Physiol (Lond) 242, 673-683 (1974).
Saito, T., W.H. Miller and T. Tomita Vis. Res. 14, 119-123 (1974).
Schwartz, E.A., J. Physiol. (Lond) 323, 211-227 (1982).
Simon, E.J., J. Physiol. (Lond) 230, 199-211 (1973).
Stell, W.K. and D.O. Lightfoot J. Comp. Neurol. 159, 473-502 (1975).

Stell, W.K., D.O. Lightfoot, T.G. Wheeler and H.F. Leeper, Science 190, 989-990 (1975).

Tachibana, M., J. Physiol (Lond) 345, 329-351 (1983).

Tachibana, M. and A. Kaneko Proc. Natl. Acad. Sci. USA 81, 7961-7964 (1984).

Toyoda, J. and M. Fujimoto Vis. Res. 23, 1143-1150 (1983).

Trifonov, Yu.A., Biofizika 13, 809-817 (1968).

Properties of Amino Acid Binding Sites on Horizontal Cells
Determined by Electrophysiological Studies on the Isolated Roach Retina

M. W. Hankins,[1] J. S. Rowe,[2] K. H. Ruddock[1]
Imperial College[1]
London, England

McMaster University[2]
Hamilton, Ontario Canada

Neurotransmission between photoreceptors and second order retinal neurones has been subject to considerable research and several independent lines of investigation indicate that the transmitter acting at these synapses is an analogue of L-glutamate (Ishida and Fain, 1981; Rowe and Ruddock, 1982a; Dowling et al, 1983; Ishida et al, 1984). In this paper, we present data relating to the neurotransmission between photoreceptors and horizontal cells obtained by electrophysiological recording from the isolated, superfused retina of a cyprinid fish, the roach (Rutilus rutilus). Intracellular recordings from retinal neurones were first obtained from isolated retinae of cyprinid fish (Svaetichin, 1953) and subsequently, perfusion studies were performed with this preparation (Kaneko and Shimazaki, 1975). None-the-less, rather few workers have persevered with the perfused fish retina for the purpose of studying retinal neurotransmission. We consider three aspects of our experimental results, which extend the previous reports by Rowe and Ruddock (1982a,b) and Hankins and Ruddock (1984a,b,c). Firstly we examine the suppression of retinal responses by extracellular calcium, which unexpected phenomenon may have contributed to the relative neglect of the cyprinid retinal preparation. We then present perfusion data for a variety of neuro-active substances, which provide a pharmacological profile of the excitatory binding sites on the horizontal cells. Finally, we describe the actions of certain excitatory amino acids dissolved in perfusates of various ionic compositions.

Methods:
Intracellular responses were recorded from all classes of retinal neurones, except photoreceptors, by conventional micropipette electrodes containing 2.5mM KCl (D.C. tip resistance 60 to 120 MΩ). Retinae were removed from the eyes of freshly killed, fully dark adapted fish, except for experiments which specifically required light adapted retinae. The isolated retina was clamped receptor side up in a circular chamber by a metal ring covered by a coarse mesh net, which arrangement provided great stability for intracellular recording during perfusion. Pharmacological substances were dissolved in Ringer solution, bubbled continuously with a mixture of 95% O_2 and 5% CO_2 and adjusted to pH 7.7. Unless otherwise specified, the ionic composition of the Ringer was 110mM NaCl; 2.5mM KCl; 20mM $NaHCO_2$; 20mM glucose; 20 μM $CaCl_2$.

Results:
1. Effects of Calcium on Retinal Electrophysiological Responses
During development of the perfusion system, we included 2mM calcium in the perfusate, and found that all horizontal cells were hyperpolarized and their light evoked S-potentials suppressed, despite the fact that immediately prior to perfusion, the isolated retinae functioned normally. Recordings made with a number of perfusates, each of different ionic composition, established unequivocally that in solutions without added calcium, retinae functioned as in the unperfused state, whereas addition of 1 to 2mM calcium suppressed all light evoked activity. The effects of calcium on cone and rod-driven horizontal cells and on amacrine cell

© 1985 by Elsevier Science Publishing Co., Inc.
Neurocircuitry of the Retina, A Cajal Memorial
A. Gallego and P. Gouras, Editors

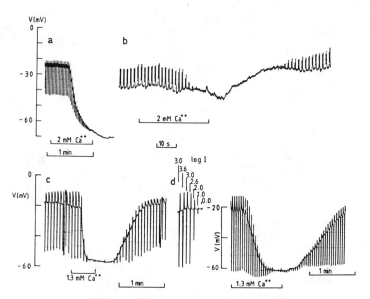

Fig. 1. Effects of Ca^{++} on electrophysiological responses of neurones of the isolated roach retina. Ca^{++} was added to the perfusate, applied to the photoreceptor surface, as indicated by the horizontal bars. Light responses were elicited by periodic light flashes of 300 m sec duration. Membrane voltage V,(mV), is displayed against time, with depolarizing responses corresponding to upward displacement. (a) Cone-driven horizontal cell (b) and amacrine cell. The light stimulus was of wavelength 650 nm, giving retinal flux of 10μW, and in the form of a circular spot of diameter 3mm. (c) and (d) Rod-driven horizontal cells. Stimulus wavelength 495 nm; spot diameter 3mm. To the left of Fig. 1d are shown the responses of the cell to flashes of different illuminations, I, defined as log$_{10}$ I. On this scale of illumination, threshold for the dark adapted human eye, with the stimulus located 10° eccentrically, was about 1 log unit.

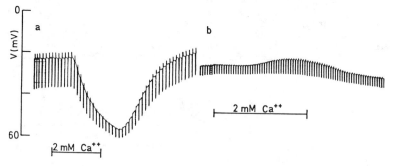

Fig. 2. Effects on horizontal cell responses of Ca^{++} applied a) to the photoreceptor surface and b) to the vitreal surface of the same retina. Stimulus conditions as for Fig. 1a.

responses are illustrated in Fig. 1. Measurements made for 65 cone-driven horizontal cells taken from 27 retinae gave a mean dark membrane potential of -21 mV during perfusion with low calcium perfusate, and -62 mV during perfusion with 2mM calcium perfusate. For comparison, corresponding values were -20 mV for low calcium perfusate and -58 mV when 2mM cobalt chloride was included in the perfusate (35 cells from 25 retinae). Calcium at mM concentrations also strongly hyperpolarised horizontal cells in retinae taken from light adapted fish, the receptor surfaces of which were covered with the pigment epithelium. Application of 2mM calcium to the vitreal surface of the retina does not, however, have the same effects as those observed when it is applied to the photoreceptor surface (Fig. 2).

II. Action of Amino Acids on Horizontal Cell Responses

Rowe and Ruddock (1982a) demonstrated that kainate (KA) and quisqualate (QA) depolarize horizontal cells of the isolated cyprinid retina, whereas N-methyl-D-aspartate (NMDA) does not, from which observation they concluded that the neurotransmitter at the photoreceptor - horizontal cell synapse is an analogue of L-glutamate rather than of L-aspartate. In Table 1, data are given for a number of other excitatory substances which are classified as agonists either for NMDA or for KA/QA binding sites. The classification is based on binding studies (Coyle, 1981; Redburn, 1981) and electrophysiological data (McLennan and Lodge, 1979; Perkins and Stone, 1983). It is apparent that those substances classified as KA/QA agonists depolarize the horizontal cells and suppress the light-evoked S-potentials, whereas those classified as NMDA agonists do not. Unexpected variability was observed both with NMDA and with the endogenous substance quinolinic acid, both of which usually hyperpolarize horizontal cells, but on some occasions were either ineffective, or even depolarized the cells with relatively little change in the S-potential amplitude. These effects are illustrated for quinolinic acid in Fig. 3a,b.

A number of proposed antagonists of L-glutamate, KA and QA were ineffective in blocking depolarization of horizontal cells by these excitatory amino acids, although glutamate diethyl ester (GDEE) and γ-D-glutamyl glycine (DGG) on occasion selectively suppressed the depolarizing effects of, respectively, QA and KA. Folic acid (5mM), which simulates the neurotoxic effects of glutamate in the rat amygdala (Olney et al, 1981) proved an effective antagonist of $50\mu M$ KA and $50\mu M$ QA, but was less reliable in antagonising the depolarizing effects of $50\mu M$ L-glutamate potentiated by 3mM D-aspartate (Ishida and Fain, 1981). Kynurenic acid, which acts as a non-specific antagonist of excitatory responses in the rat cortex (Perkins and Stone, 1982), hyperpolarizes horizontal cells and abolishes their S-potentials when applied at 1mM concentration (Fig. 3c). It proved a potent antagonist of $50\mu M$ KA, 50 μM QA and 25 to $50\mu M$ L-glutamate potentiated by 3mM D-aspartate (Fig. 3d,e); but, like folic acid, it fails to antagonise the depolarizing effects of 5mM L-glutamate (Table 1). Kynurenic acid also fails to block depolarization of horizontal cells by $20\mu M$ dopamine.

III The Ionic Composition of the Perfusate

The extracellular concentrations of the principal ions, namely $(Na^+)_o$, $(K^+)_o$ and $(Cl^-)_o$ were varied independently in order to examine their separate contributions to the depolarization of horizontal cells by excitatory amino acids. Increase of $(K^+)_o$ to 12.5mM depolarizes the horizontal cells, but addition of $50\mu M$ KA further depolarizes them to a level similar to that found in solutions with normal (2.5mM) $(K^+)_o$ concentration (Fig. 4a). Even with $(K^+)_o$ raised to 110mM, addition of $50\mu M$ KA still produces further depolarization of the horizontal cell

T A B L E   1

Substance	Threshold Concentration for Depolarization	Antagonistic response to:	
		Kynurenic Acid	Folic Acid
A			
Kainate	7 uM	Yes	Yes
Quisqualate	7 uM	Yes	Yes
L-Glutamate	1 mM	No	No
L-Glutamate + D-Aspartate	25 uM	Yes	Yes[a]
L-Cysteate	5 mM	No	No
L-Cysteate + D-Aspartate	hyperpolarize at 100 uM	-	-
L-Cysteine Sulf	1mM[b]	No	No
L-Cysteine Sulf + D-Aspartate	hyperpolarize at 100 uM	-	-
B			
NMDA[c]	hyperpolarizes up to 10 mM	-	-
Homo-cysteate	hyperpolarizes up to 1 mM	-	-
Ibotenate	hyperpolarizes up to 250 uM	-	-
Quinolinate[c]	hyperpolarizes up to 10 mM	-	-
Kynurinate	hyperpolarizes up to 5 mM	-	-
D-Aspartate	hyperpolarizes up to 3 mM	-	-

a) Antagonism observed on about 50%
b) Observed only after several ineffective applications
c) On some occasions slight depolarization without change in the S-potential amplitude is observed.

Responses of retinal horizontal cells to a number of neuro-active substances.
A. Those which bind selectively to QA/KA sites.
B. Those which bind selectively to NMDA sites.

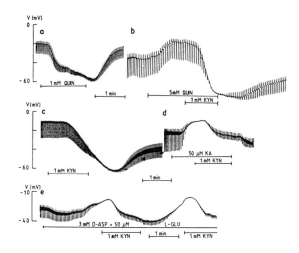

Fig. 3. Responses of retinal horizontal cells. Stimulus conditions as for Fig. 1a. (a) Hyperpolarizing effect of quinolinic acid (QUIN); (b) Depolarizing effect of quinolinic acid, reversed by kynurenic acid (KYN); (c) Hyperpolarizing effect of kynurenic acid; (d) Reversal of depolarizing effect of kainic acid (KA) by kynurenic acid; (e) Reversal by kynurenic acid of the depolarizing effect of L-glutamate potentiated by 3mM D-aspartate.

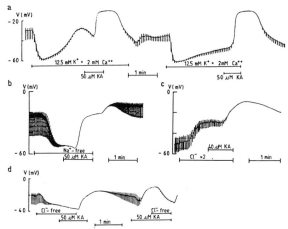

Fig. 4. Responses of retinal horizontal cells to KA in perfusates of different ionic compositions. Stimulus conditions as for Fig. 1a. a) with $(K+)_o$ increased to 12.5 mM, and with addition of 2mM Ca^{++} to suppress the endogenous transmitter. b) Na^+-free perfusate, with NaCl replaced by choline chloride. c) With $(Cl^-)_o$ doubled by the addition of 110 mM choline chloride. d) Cl^--free perfusate, with NaCl replaced by 110 mM Na_2SO_4.

membrane (Table 2). Substitution of choline chloride for sodium chloride partially blocks the depolarization induced by KA and QA, although the latter effect is still significant (Fig. 4b and Table 2). $(Cl^-)_o$ was both increased, by addition of choline chloride, and decreased, by substitution of various anions for Cl^-. In the former case, doubling $(Cl^-)_o$ depolarizes the horizontal cells, and addition of 50μM KA further depolarizes them to -5 mV, i.e. the level found in normal Ringer (Fig. 4c). Substitution of $(Cl^-)_o$ by 55mM SO_4 hyperpolarizes the membrane potential to about -45 mV and partially blocks the depolarizing effects of KA and QA, addition of which raises the membrane potential to -31 mV, compared with -5 mV for normal $(Cl^-)_o$. Similar effects are observed for other anion substitutions. In a hypertonic Cl^--free perfusate containing 110mM Na_2SO_4, however, KA and QA fail to induce membrane depolarization significantly above the level found for the Cl^--free perfusate itself (Fig. 4d, Table 2).

T A B L E   2

Ion	Modified Conc.	Dark Membrane Potential (mV)				Cells/ Retinas
		Normal	Modified	Modified +Ka	Normal +KA	
K^+	110	-35±6	-16±2	-5±2	-5±1	7:3
Na^+	0	-19±2	-44±2	-19±1	-5±1	6:3
Cl^- (55mM SO_4^-)	0	-31±2	-41±1	-16±2	-5±1	8:3
Cl^- (110mM SO_4^-)	0	-27±4	-23±3	-21±2	-6±1	6:2
Cl^- (110mM SO_4- +2mM Co^{++})	0	-30±3	-	-46±5	-7±1	3:1
Cl^- (110mM SO_4- +2mM Ca^{++})	0	-18±4	-50±8	-35±1	-6±1	4:2
				+QA	+QA	
Cl^- (110mM SO_4^-)	0	-21±4	-57±1	-37±1	-5±1	5:2
Cl^- (110mM SO_4- +2mM Co^{++})	0	-20±2	-58±1	-38±2	-5±1	3:2
				+3mM D-asp +50uM L-glu	+3mM D-asp +50uM L-glu	
Cl^- (110mM SO_4^-)	0	-20±4	-25±2	-30±2	-12±1	3:2

Data for retinal horizontal cells recorded in ionic solutions of various concentrations. The first column defines the ion which is changed in the modified Ringer and the second, the mM concentration of the ion. Species roach (Rutilus rutilus)

Discussion:
1 to 2mM $(Ca^{++})_o$ applied to the photoreceptors but not to the vitreal surface of the retina (Fig. 2) is as effective in hyperpolarizing the horizontal cells and abolishing their S-potentials as is 2mM cobalt. Thus, according to Trifonov's (1968) hypothesis, mM $(Ca^{++})_o$ blocks neurotransmission between photoreceptors and horizontal cells as efficiently as mM $(Co^{++})_o$. (Co^{++}) also hyperpolarizes goldfish cones and suppresses their responses to light (Rowe, unpublished observation), and abolishes the photoreceptor component of the roach ERG isolated by 5mM glutamate (Rowe and Ruddock, 1982a). In contrast, (Co^{++}) affects neither of these receptoral response functions (see also Cervetto and Piccolino, 1974). Extracellular Ca^{++} significantly reduces the trans-membrane current of rod photoreceptors (Yau et al, 1981), and it seems likely that such an effect is occurring when we apply 1 to 2mM calcium to the photoreceptor surface of the roach retina. The unexpected aspect of the present results is that retinal responses recorded in low levels of $(Ca^{++})_o$ are closely similar to those recorded from the non-perfused, isolated retina and from the eyecup (Hankinson and Rowe, 1983), whereas in 1 to 2mM $(Ca^{++})_o$, responses are effectively suppressed. We have considered a number of possible objections to our experimental procedure and we review these briefly:

a) The Photoreceptors of the Isolated Retinae are Damaged Except on those occasions when we wished to examine the effects of the pigment epithelium on retinal responses, retinae were removed from dark adapted eyes, under dim red ($\lambda > 640nm$) light. Under these conditions, the retina is mechanically separated from the pigment epithelium and it is necessary only to sever the optic nerve in order to peel it from the eyecup. Scanning and transmission electron microscopy established that both rod and cone photoreceptors of retinae isolated in this way are structurally intact (Djamgoz and Ruddock, 1978; Downing, 1983) and it is difficult to envisage how severance of the optic nerve could damage all retinal photoreceptors in such a way that they function normally in low calcium, but are completely suppressed by 1 to 2mM calcium. The possibility that removal of pigment epithelium causes the observed effects of extracellular calcium appears to be eliminated by the observation that they persist in retinae, taken from light adapted fish, extensively covered by the pigment epithelium.
b) The Retinae are Light Adapted during their Isolation from the Eyecup The retinae isolated from dark adapted fish were free of pigment epithelium, thus establishing that dark adaptation of the fish proceeded normally. The responses recorded from the isolated retinae superfused with low calcium Ringer are closely similar to those recorded from the same retinae immediately prior to superfusion, and no change in adaptation occurred between the two recordings. On several occasions, we recorded continuously from the same cell both before and following the onset of perfusion with low calcium Ringer, and no significant shift in dark resting potential or S-potential amplitude occurred as a result of per-fusion. The experiments with the rod-driven horizontal cells (Fig. 1) show that the light sensitivity of the dark-adapted fish retina is comparable to that of the dark-adapted human eye, thus providing further evidence that the isolated retina cannot be significantly light adapted.

c) Low Calcium Perfusate leads to Abnormal Neurotransmission and/or Abnormal Membrane Properties of the Horizontal Cells. This proposition can be immediately rejected on the evidence that horizontal (and amacrine) cell responses recorded in low calcium are similar to those recorded from the unperfused retina and depolarization responses to excitatory amino acids are identical in low calcium Ringer and in 2mM Ca^{++} Ringer. Further, the neuropharmacological data obtained with low calcium Ringer applied to the isolated retina have been largely supported by observations on isolated horizontal cells maintained in 2mM Ca^{++} Ringer (e.g. Dowling et al, 1983; Ishida et al, 1984).

We interpret our data as evidence that in the dark adapted roach retina, calcium levels around the photoreceptors are maintained at a low value, perhaps by the active pumping mechanism revealed in diffusion measurements made with $^{45}Ca^{++}$ (Galley et al, 1982). We have observed similar effects of calcium in other cyprinid fish including rudd (Scardinius erythrophthalmus), bream (Abramis brama), goldfish (Carassius auratus) and tench (Tinca tinca), and they also occur in carp (Cyprinus carpio) (J.E. Dowling, personal communication). Low $(Ca^{++})_o$ around the photoreceptors appears to be a requirement for the elongation of the cone myoids which characterises the dark adapted teleost retina (Dearry and Burnside, 1984). Low $(Ca^{++})_o$ in the dark adapted retina is also consistent with the periodicity of disc shedding in amphibian retinae (Greenburger and Besharse, 1983; Hoffmann and Matthes, 1976). Finally, we note that low $(Ca^{++})_o$ has been used previously in studies involving the isolated retina (e.g. Borchard and Erasmi, 1974).

The experiments with different pharmacological agents, summarised on Table 1 and Fig. 3, establish that those classified as KA/QA agonists depolarize retinal horizontal cells and abolish their S-potentials, whereas those classified as NMDA agonists usually hyperpolarize the cells and when they cause depolarization, this is not accompanied by significant reduction of the S-potential amplitude (Fig. 3b). L-glutamate, potentiated by the uptake blocker D-aspartate, is active at $25\mu m$, whereas none of the other endogenous putative neurotransmitters (L-aspartate, L-cysteate and L-cysteine sulfinate) are so potentiated. The variable response pattern observed for NMDA and quinolinic acid (Fig. 3a,b) is not readily explained, but implies that the horizontal cells are controlled by more than one pharmacological pathway influenced by NMDA agonists. In contrast to KA and QA, NMDA and quinolinic acid fail to depolarize horizontal cells in the presence of 2mM Co^{++} or Ca^{++} which implies that they do not exert a direct polarizing effect on the horizontal cell membrane. The most interesting new finding is that kynurenic acid is an effective blocker of exogenously applied KA, QA and potentiated L-glutamate (Fig. 3d,e), as well as of the endogenous neurotransmitter acting at the photoreceptor-horizontal cell synapse (Fig. 3c0. It does not, however, lock depolarization by 5mM glutamate, even though this is only about x5 threshold concentration (Table 2), whereas it blocks depolarization by $50\mu M$ KA, which is about x7 threshold concentration. The depolarization of horizontal cells by high concentrations of L-glutamate appears, therefore, to be mediated by sites different from those sensitive to the endogenous transmitter and to low concentrations of excitatory amino acids, and these sites may correspond to the extra-junctional glutamate binding sites described by Ishida et al (1984). The slight recovery of S-potential responses which occurs e.g. when kynurenic acid reverses the depolarization caused by $50\mu M$ KA, suggests, however, that there is a sub-population of junctional sites sensitive to the endogenous transmitter which is blocked neither by kynurenic acid nor by KA. Folic acid at 5mM concentration also acts as an antagonist of excitatory amino acid effects on horizontal cells.

The experiments with high $(K^+)_o$ perfusates establish that the depolarization exerted by excitatory amino acids is not influenced by the value of $(K+)_o$ (Fig. 4a; Table 2). Thus, the increase in $(K+)_o$ to about 10mM, which accompanies application of L-glutamate to the retina (Djamgoz, 1985) makes no significant contribution, either direct or indirect, to the observed level of depolarization. Removal of Na^+ from the perfusate only partially blocks the depolarization of horizontal cells by 50μM QA and KA (Fig. 4b; Table 2), which implies that ions other than Na^+ are involved in the depolarizing response. The experiment with hypertonic Ringer, containing 110mM Na_2SO_4, confirms the conclusion, as in this case $(Na^+)_o$ is at double the normal concentration, yet the depolarization effects are abolished (Fig. 4d, Table 2). Other studies on both perfused retinae and isolated horizontal cells have demonstrated that $(Na^+)_o$ contributes to the depolarization of horizontal cells by excitatory amino acids (Kaneko and Shimazaki, 1975; Waloga and Pak, 1976; Ishida et al, 1984,) and the photoreceptor dark current is probably also carried by Na^+ (Yau et al, 1981). Thus in Na^+-free Ringer, both photoreceptors and horizontal cells should be subject to hyperpolarization. Even so, roach horizontal cells hyperpolarize only to some -45mV in Na^+-free Ringer, compared with a level around -60mV in Ringer containing mM Co^{++} or Ca^{++} (Table 2). Na^+-free conditions do not, therefore, produce full hyperpolarization of the horizontal cells, which is again consistent with the view that depolarization by synaptic binding, in this case of the endogenous neurotransmitter, cannot be mediated solely by Na^+. In Cl^--free solution containing SO_4^-, the horizontal cells of the roach depolarize and then hyperpolarize, a response pattern which has been reported previously for the retina eyecup preparation of the mudpuppy by Miller and Dacheux (1983). They interpret this response in terms of a reduction during light stimulation of chloride conduction at the synapse, resulting in a movement of Cl^- out of the cell. In the steady state, roach horizontal cell hyperpolarize in Cl^--free perfusate to about -40mV, and are depoalrized by addtion of 50μM KA to about -16mV, compared to a level of -5mV in normal Ringer containing 112.5mM $(Cl^-)_o$ This reduction in KA effectiveness may indicate that its action involves a Cl^- mechanism similar to that proposed by Miller and Dacheux, but some excitatory amino acid binding is dependent on $(Cl^-)_o$ (Monaghan et al, 1983). The almost complete suppression of KA and QA induced depolarization in Cl^--free solution containing 110 mM Na_2SO_4 however, militates against the latter explanation, as the binding conditions should be the same in all Cl^--free solutions.

Conclusions:

Perfusion of the isolated fish retina yields pharmacological data for horizontal cells broadly similar to those found by other techniques, with responses to a range of excitatory amino acids consistent with identification of the binding sites as glutamate-like.

References:

Borchard, U. and Erasmi, W. Vis. Res. 14, 17-22 (1974).
Cervetto, L and Piccolino, M. Science 183, 417-419 (1974).
Coyle, J.T. in: Neurosci. Res. Prog. Bull. 19 (4) J.T. Coyle, ed. 354-359 (1981).
Dearry, A. and Burnside, B. J. Gen. Physiol. 83, 589-611 (1984).
Djamgoz, M.B.A. J. Physiol. (Lond) 358, 11P (1985).
Djamgoz, M.B.A. and Ruddock, K.H. Neurosci. Letters 7, 251-256 (1978).
Dowling, J.E., Lasater, E.M., Buskirk, R. van and Watling, K.J. Vis. Res. 23, 421-432 (1983).
Downing, J.E.G. Ph.D. thesis, University of London (1983).
Galley, J.E., Hankins, M.W., Rowe, J.S. and Ruddock, K.H. J. Physiol. (Lond) 332, 15-16 P (1982).
Greenberger, L.M. and Besharse, J.C. Vis. Res. 24, 1456-1464 (1983).
Hankins, M.W. and Ruddock, K.H. Nature (Lond) 308, 360-362 (1984a).
Hankins, M.W. and Ruddock, K.H. Neurosci. Letters 44, 1-6 (1984b).
Hankins, M.W. and Ruddock, K.H. J. Physiol (Lond) 348, 18 P (1984c).
Hankinson, K.C. and Rowe, J.S. J. Physiol. (Lond) 345, 68 P (1983).
Hoffmann, R. and Matthes, M. Science 194, 1074-1076 (1976).
Ishida, A.T. and Fain, G.L. Proc. Nat. Acad. Sci. USA 78, 5890-5894 (1981).

Ishida, A.T., Kaneko, A. and Tachibana, M. J. Physiol. (Lond) 348, 255-270 (1984).

Kaneko, A. and Shimazaki, H. J. Physiol. (Lond) 252, 509-522 (1975).

Monaghan, D.T., Holets, V.R., Toy, D.W. and Cotman, C.W. Nature 306, 176-179 (1983).

McLennan, H. and Lodge, D. Brain Res. 169, 83-90 (1979).

Miller, R.F. and Dacheux, R.F. Vis. Res. 23, 399-411 (1983).

Olney, J.W., Fuller, T.A. and de Gubareff, T. Nature (Lond) 292, 165-167 (1981).

Perkins, M.N. and Stone, T.W. Brain Res. 247, 184-187 (1982).

Perkins, M.N. and Stone, T.W., J. Pharmacol. and Exptl. Therapeuc. 226, 551-557 (1983).

Redburn, D.A. in: Glutamate as a Neurotransmitter G. diChiara and G.L. Gessa eds (Raven New York 1981) pp. 79-89.

Rowe, J.S. and Ruddock, K. H. Neurosci. Letters 30, 257-262 (1982a).

Rowe, J.S. and Ruddock, K. H. Neurosci. Letters 30, 251-256 (1982b).

Svaetichin, G. Acta Physiol. Scand. 106, 565-600 (1953).

Trifonov, Yu A Biofizika 13, 809-817 (1968).

Waloga, G. and Pak, W.L. Science 191, 964-967 (19)

Yau, K.W., McNaughton, P.A. and Hodgkin, A.L. Nature (Lond). 292, 502-505 (1981).

Spectral Mechanisms in Cat Horizontal Cells

R. Nelson, T. Lynn, A. Dickinson-Nelson, H. Kolb[*]

Laboratory of Neurophysiology
National Institute of Neurological and
Communicative Disorders and Stroke
Bethesda, Maryland 20205
Department of Physiology[*]
University of Utah
Salt Lake City, Utah   84112

A- and B-type horizontal cells: Morphology and connectivity.

Since the time Cajal (1933) first observed Golgi-stained vertebrate retinas and described their neurons, retinal horizontal cells have attracted the attention of many excellent neuroanatomists, including our symposium organizer, Antonio Gallego. In Figure 1 is a camera lucida drawing of the two sorts of horizontal cells of the cat retina, here revealed by the more modern technology of intracellular injection of horseradish peroxidase (HRP). These are the A- and B-type cells. The A-type cell is the larger and coarser of the two: at a given retinal eccentricity, or distance from the optic axis, its dendritic extent is about 50% greater than that of the dendrites immediately surrounding the B-type cell body (Gallego, 1971, 1976; Kolb, 1974; Boycott and Wassle, 1978). In peripheral retina the A-type cell attains a diameter of 200 or more um. The B-type horizontal cell is particularly striking visually, possessing an axon-like process several hundreds of um long, which arborizes profusely at the end into a large axon terminal (at, Fig. 1).

All these three horizontal cell structures, the A-type cell, the B-type cell body region, and the B-type axon terminal have been examined in cat retina by the technique of Golgi-electron-microscopy to determine their connections with photoreceptors (Kolb, 1974). Dendrites from the perikaryal regions of both A- and B-type cells terminate as lateral elements in the synaptic triads of cone pedicles. The axon terminal of the B-type cell contains several thousands of little lollipop-like terminals which contact rod spherules as lateral elements. Thus the A- and B-type cell body regions contact only cones, while the B-type axon terminal contacts only rods.

Role of the B-type axon

The B-type cell has raised questions for the electrophysiologist. Although no horizontal cell has ever been seen to fire an action potential in the retina, nonetheless this horizontal cell, as well as certain types of horizontal cells in most other vertebrate species, possess an axon. What is the role of this axon? If it acts simply as a passive cable, one can calculate how much of a signal generated at one end of the cell might reach the other. This turns out to be less than 1% for signals propagating from cell body to terminal, and about 1% for signals propagating in the reverse direction. This result (Nelson et al., 1975) is due not so much to the electrotonic length of the axon, but to the large electrical loads placed on either end of it by the huge surface areas of either the terminal or the cell body (see appendix). Because the beauty of the anatomical features of the B-type cell suggest that it would be ideal to mediate some sort of interaction between rods and cones, the modeling result is hard to accept. Therefore the analytical considerations are presented in detail in the appendix. The calculation above is based on a specific membrane resistance of 2000 ohm cm^2 measured by Barrett and Crill (1974) in cat spinal motor neurons. However even a

Published 1985 by Elsevier Science Publishing Co., Inc.
Neurocircuitry of the Retina, A Cajal Memorial
A. Gallego and P. Gouras, Editors

110

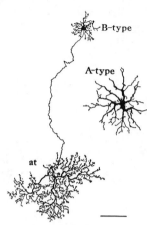

Fig. 1. Camera lucida drawings of horizontal cells stained by intracellular injection of horseradish peroxidase (HRP) as seen in wholemount of cat retina. The A-type horizontal cell is a stellate, axonless cell with thick dendrites covering a 125 μm dendritic field. The cell body is contiguous with the main dendrites and not obvious. Find dendritic terminals make synaptic contact with cone pedicles. The B-type horizontal cell has a small bushy dendritic tree and a distinct cell body. The dendritic terminals also contact cones. The axon terminal (at) is strikingly larger in extent than the cell body and bears thousands of tiny button-like terminals contacting rod spherules. The fine axon connects the axonal arborization to the cell body, 300 μm away. The cell body, in this case filled by retrograde transport from the axon terminal, is relatively poorly stained in comparison to the axon terminal and the full number of dendrites and terminals may not be represented. Scale bar 50 μm.

specific resistivity of 20,000 ohm cm^2 for the cell under consideration yields an attentuation of more than 20 between cell body and terminal. The relatively rapid risetimes of the cellular response to light tend to exclude resistivities greater than this.

So calculations based on passive electrical spread indicate that the two ends of the B-type horizontal cell should be physiologically isolated, and from an electrical standpoint the A- and B-type cell body regions and the B-type axon terminal are three distinct horizontal cell entities. The first two entities are devoted to cones, and the last to rods. One might ask how the cones got two cells and the rods only one. Based on investigations in fish retinas (Stell, 1975) one might suppose that different spectral types of cones each deserved special attention from a horizontal cell type. In cat, however, there is neither anatomical nor physiological evidence in favor of this notion.

Intracellular stains

We have obtained intracellular recordings from each of these horizontal cell entities, characterized them physiologically, and injected them with a variety of stains for morphological identification. In Fig. 2a is a wholemount view of an A-type or axonless horizontal cell, stained by intracellular injection of HRP and subsequent histochemical techniques. The cell, drawn in Fig. 1, has a typical radiating pattern of wavy dendrites, and cell body confluent with major branches. In Fig. 2b is another A-type cell, this time seen in vertical section and at higher magnification. The resolution of fine processes with the HRP staining method is superb. One can see dendritic stalks carrying terminals (arrows), arising from a main dendrite, and innervating a cone pedical, one can imagine, with a lateral element.

In Fig. 2c is a B-type horizontal cell injected with HRP. On the right is the axon terminal end with its large floral appearance and multitude of tiny projections contacting rods. The dark spot comes from Muller cell staining and marks the site of injection. There is an axon (not visible in the mircograph) traveling to the left and ending in a stained B-type cell body with a much smaller arborization than the terminal. An example of another axon terminal is seen in Fig. 2d, and

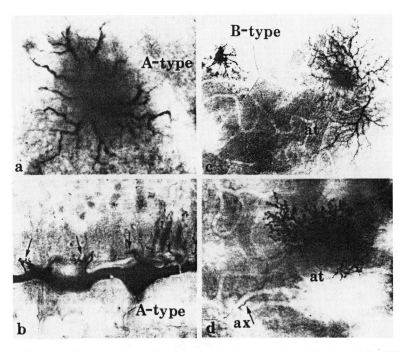

Fig. 2. a) Light micrograph of an A-type horizontal cell stained by HRP and viewed in whole-mount. The stellate, radiate dendritic tree of thick dendrites has been drawn in Fig. 1. The cell body is particularly dark because it was the site of the electrode penetration. x425. b) HRP stained A-type horizontal cell as seen in vertical section. The large cell body thinning into the major dendrites can be seen. Fine dendritic branches project to the cone pedicles and bear clusters of terminals (arrows) that become lateral elements in cone synaptic triads. x940. c) Complete B-type horizontal cell stained by HRP and viewed in whole mount. The injection site was in a branch of the axon terminal (black mark), which is well stained, leaving the cell body (210 um distant) relatively faintly stained. The fine axon is not visible in the plane of the micrograph. Note the background capillary bed of the retina. x240. d) HRP stained axon terminal of a B-type horizontal cell. The injection site again was a branch of the axon terminal arborization, as shown by the dense mark. The fine terminals are extraordinarily well stained as is the fine axon running to the left (arrow). The entire cell can be seen drawn in Fig. 1 x240.

here the axon is also visible. Although not illustrated in Fig. 2d, the cell body was stained, and a camera lucida drawing of the complete cell appears in Fig. 1 (B- type). In this case fixation occurred less than 20 minutes after injection, demonstrating transport of proteins between terminal and cell body within this time frame. Conceivably chemical messages of neurophysiological importance could be similarly transported. Intracellularly injected HRP appears to move more readily through the horizontal cell axon in the retrograde than the orthograde direction, both in cat, and in rabbit (Bloomfield and Miller, 1982).

In the backgrounds of Figs. 2c and d, a network of bright channels can be seen. This is a retinal capillary bed running in the plane of the outer plexiform layer. The red cells, which would otherwise stain darkly in the histochemical reactions for HRP, have been washed out because the preparation is an arterially perfused cat eyecup (Nelson, 1977), similar to perfused eye preparations described by Gouras and Hoff (1970) and Niemeyer (1980).

Properties of intracellular responses to light

Physiological responses to light of A- and B-type horizontal cell bodies and the b-type axon terminal are illustrated in Fig. 3. All units responded with the slow graded hyperpolarizations typical of horizontal cells. An assay for the rod and cone contributions to these responses is the dynamics of the rod off-response. It is a general property of rods that with very bright, supersaturating stimuli, they remain hyperpolarized for extended periods after the stimulus is turned off. This "rod after-effect" was first appreciated by Steinberg (1969). The response of the axon terminal (Fig. 3, B at) exhibits rod after-effects lasting many seconds after the termination of the stimulus. Here, as with other elements of Fig. 3, three responses to increasing intensities of stimulation in a range beyond rod saturation have been superimposed. The longer after-effects correspond to the brighter stimuli. Cones, exposed to the same stimulus levels, repolarize rapidly at stimulus-off. Furthermore the dynamic range of the cones is displaced towards brighter stimuli by some two to three log units, so even at these levels, they are able to modulate with increases in response amplitude to increased stimulation (Nelson, 1977). In the responses of the A- and B-type cell bodies (Fig. 3; A cb, B cb) there are both increases in response amplitude with brighter stimuli, and a component which repolarizes rapidly at stimulus off. This is the cone signal, present in both the A- and B-type cell bodies, as predicted from the anatomy. Such signals are hardly seen in the responses of the axon terminal, which is dominated by lengthy rod after-effects (Fig. 3, B at). As calculations based on cellular morphology suggested, the two ends of the B-type cell are physiologically separate and distinguishable. The axon terminal is rod dominated while the cell body region is dominated by cones.

One also notices rod after-effects in the A and B-type cell bodies (Fig. 3). Where have these signals come from? The rod signals in the A-type cell are particularly puzzling since this cell has no known contacts with rods.

Spectral sensitivities under selective chromatic adaptation

Consistent with the rod after-effects observed in Fig. 3, threshold spectral sensitivities of horizontal cell bodies resemble those of rods (Steinberg, 1969; Neimeyer and Gouras, 1973). But spectral sensitivity curves obtainable from dark adapted horizontal cell bodies depend on the criterion level chosen: Low levels give rod-like spectra, while high levels give red-shifted, cone-like spectra (Niemeyer and Gouras, 1973). This shifting of spectral curves with criterion level is thought to arise from rod saturation at higher levels. We have used this same approach to identify different spectral classes of cone input into horizontal cell bodies as examined under conditions of selective chromatic adaptation of cones, sufficient to eliminate the rod signal through light adaptation. At least two different patterns of cone input are seen. The pattern observed in Fig. 4 is perhaps the easiest to interpret. With a blue background (lower, solid set of curves) only a single spectral sensitivity function is seen, peaking at 562 nm, for all criteria between 4 and 18 mV. With the red background, upper, dashed set of curves (Fig. 4), this is not the case. Lower criteria reveal a definite increment in sensitivity

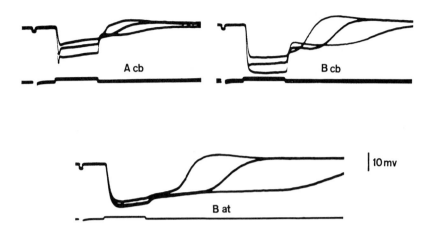

Fig. 3. Intracellular responses of A- and B-type horizontal cell bodies
(A cb, B cb) and the B-type horizontal cell axon terminal (B at) to rod
saturating blue stimuli. Three responses to different levels of
stimulation are superimposed with the larger peak deflections and the
longer rod after effects being associated with the brighter stimuli.
Stimuli, 520 msec in duration (illustrated below responses), are in the
range of 10 to 50 times brighter than rod semisaturation. Stimulus
irradiances (400 nm) in log quanta um^{-2}s^{-1}: A hc= 4.5, 5.3, 5.9; B hc=
4.5, 5.3, 5.9; B at= 4.2, 4.8, 5.6.

between 400 and 500 nm. At longer wavelengths, the curves converge to the
dominant red mechanism peaking at 563 nm. The spectral behavior on red
backgrounds is readily interpreted as an admixture of blue and
long-wavelength cone input. With red backgrounds (Fig. 4) the sensitivity
in the 400-500 nm region decreases with increasing criterion level. By
analogy with rod behavior, the loss of blue sensitivity at high criteria
may be a blue cone saturation effect. Both A- and B-type cells exhibit
blue as well as red cone input of this kind.

In Figs. 4 and 5 we have used a regression to fit the best fifth
order polynominal to the points. To eliminate the clutter, only the
curves are shown and not the actual data points. All curves have been
normalized to 650 nm, since at this wavelength there is likely to be only
one, long-wavelength cone mechanism observable, and a region of
superimposable curves in this spectral region is thus expected. In these
figures backgrounds are beyond 90% saturation for the rods so that rod
spectral contributions are not observed.

In Fig. 5 a more complex spectral pattern is seen. In the red adapted
spectra (upper, dashed curves), the 1 mV criterion reveals a spectral peak
in the blue at 440 nm. With increases in level, the spectral peak shifts
to an intermediate value at 543 nm, and at the highest criteria, the
typical red cone peak at 559 nm is revealed. The blue background (lower,
solid curves) suppresses most of the short wavelength activity, however
evidence of blue cones can still be seen between 400 and 500 nm. It is
hard to explain the lower curves on the basis of just two spectral mechanisms. These curves don't converge to one spectral mechanism until about
620 nm. No one supposes that blue cone responses are detectable here. As
seen in Fig. 4, blue and red cone sensitivities become equal near 500 nm.

114

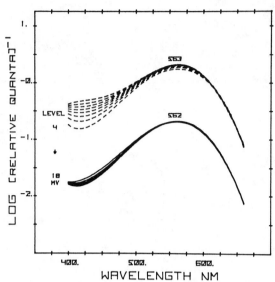

Fig. 4. Spectral sensitivity of a horizontal cell body with selective chromatic adaptation. This class of cell exhibited synergism between red and blue cones. Upper, dashed curves were obtained with a broadband red background (cutoff about 620 nm) and lower solid curves, with a broadband blue background (cutoff about 440 nm), both backgrounds beyond 90% saturation for rods. In each case spectral sensitivities were generated at 8 criterion levels spanning the dynamic range of the cell 4-18 mV, 2mV steps), fit with a 5th order polynominal (11 wavelengths), and adjusted to be equal at 650 nm. On the blue background spectral curves were nearly invariant with criterion level, revealing a single 562 peaking (red) mechanism. With the red background spectral curves were invariant in the 500-650 nm region, but diverged in the 400-500 nm region, indicative of blue input. Greatest relative sensitivities in this region occurred with low criteria (including small departures with blue backgrounds). Wavelengths: 400, 441, 462, 485, 498, 521, 542, 575, 617, 647 658 nm.

The red adapted curves thus reveal a third, midspectral or green cone mechanism, though they do not precisely define its spectral peak.

What is surprising is that blue light selectively adapts the midspectral mechanism. In Fig. 5 blue and red backgrounds are matched for rods so as to adapt them equally. Therefore the midspectral cones should not be selectively adapted by either background. Nonetheless they appear more sensitive to blue adaptation than do the blue cones themselves. In this an example of a chromatic interaction or opponency? Do blue cones inhibit green? And if so, what outer plexiform layer circuits underlie such an interaction?

Contacts between photorecpptors
    The presence of rod signals in cat horizontal cell bodies, particularly the A-type cell in which no direct contacts with rods are observed, were better understood after recordings were obtained from cat cones. In Fig. 6 appear responses of a cat cone to rod-saturating stimuli. These responses exhibit rod after-effects! They are just like

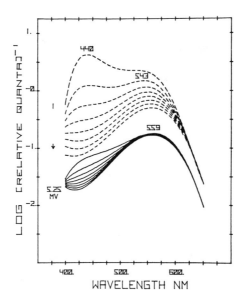

WAVELENGTH NM

Fig. 5. Spectral sensitivity of a horizontal cell body with selective chromatic adaptation. This cell exhibits synergism between red, green and blue cone mechanisms. The format of this figure is similar to Fig. 4 except that the backgrounds are monochromatic (red = 627nm, blue = 418 nm) and matched in energy (about 90% saturating) for the rods. For the lowest criteria (2 mV) the sensitivity with the red background (upper, dashed curves) peaked at 440 nm (blue cone peak) with intermediate criteria, a midspectral peak (543 nm) was observed, reflecting a mixture of red and green cone mechanisms. With the highest criteria available, the peak shifted to 559 nm, and the spectral shape resembled that of the red cones alone. The blue background (lower curves) depressed sensitivity in both the midspectral and short wavelength regions revealing an invariant region between 500 and 650 nm and a 559 nm peak (red cones). Blue cones were incompletely suppressed as seen by the divergence of curves in the 400-500 nm region. In all spectral regions sensitivity relative to 650 nm was reduced with increasing criterion level. The 5th order polynomials were fit to sensitivities at 15 wavelengths: 400, 420, 441, 462, 485, 498, 521, 542, 550, 575, 600, 617, 636, 647, 658 nm.

the responses of horizontal cell bodies. Apparently the synergistic mixing of rod and cone signals arises at the level of the photoreceptors themselves.

An anatomical network has been discovered which may explain this cone physiology. In Fig. 7a is an electron micrograph of a process projecting from a cone pedicle to form a punctate gap junction with a neighboring rod spherule. Further investigation of rod spherules in cat (Kolb, 1977) reveals that they may be surrounded by a basket of such cone telodendria, making gap junctions. Another outer plexiform layer gap junction is revealed in Fig. 7b. This is between basal processes of two adjacent cone pedicles. Analogous interreceptor junctions have been observed in primate

116

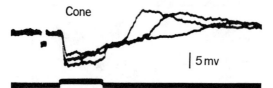

Cone

| 5 mv

Fig. 6. Intracellular responses of a cat cone to rod saturating blue stimuli. Traces are superimposed as in Fig. 3. Cat cones exhibit rod after-effects similar to those seen in the cone-connected A- and B-type horizontal cell bodies. Intermixing of rod, and perhaps different spectral classes of cone, signals may occur in the cones themselves. Stimulus conditions: 441 nm; log quanta $\mu m^{-2} s^{-1}$=4.0, 4.6 and 5.2. The larger responses and longer after-effects correspond to the brighter stimuli. The flash length is 540 msec and the calibration pulse preceding the responses (downward impulse) is 4.1 mV.

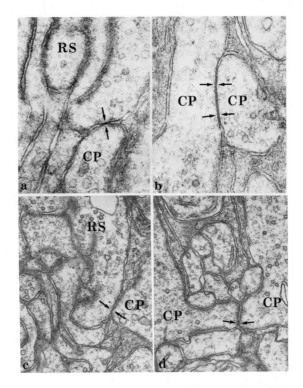

Fig. 7. a) Electron micrograph of a small punctate gap junction (arrows) made between a cone pedicle (CP) basal process and a neighboring rod spherule (RS) in the cat retina. x60,000. b) Larger gap junction (arrows) between two cone pedicle (CP) basal processes where they touch each other in the neuropil of the OPL. Cat retina. x60,000. c) Punctate gap junction (arrows) between a cone pedicle base (CP) and a neighboring rod spherule (RS) in the monkey retina. x47,000. d) Small gap junction (arrows) between neighboring cone pedicles (C)) at basal projections in the monkey retina. x47,000.

retina. In Fig. 7c a gap junction interconnects a cone pedicle and a rod spherule to the rhesus monkey too. Here the connection does not involve a directed cone process, but is effected by direct apposition of the membranes of a cone pedicle and a rod spherule. This difference between cat and monkey may relate to the lesser density of rods in monkeys, allowing a greater proportion of rod spherules to directly touch cone pedicles. In Fig. 7d a punctate junction is observed between basal processes of two adjacent cone pedicles of rhesus foveal slope. Cone to cone junctions as long and pronounced as seen in cat (Fig. 7b) are rarely seen in monkey.

Discussion

We argue that the rod input seen in cones and horizontal cell bodies in the cat retina comes about as a result of such interreceptor contacts between rods and cones. It is tempting to argue that some of the mixing of different cone signals seen at the horizontal cell level in cat also arises through interreceptor junctions, and might be manifest in cones themselves. Turtle cones mix signals from red and green cone pigments (Normann et al., 1984). In cat the ubiquitous blue cone signal may arrive through such a path, analogous to the rod signal. We do not know the extent to which horizontal cell dendrites specifically innervate a particular spectral class of cone in cat retina. In the case of A- and B-type cells, about 60% of cones might be connected in common (red cones?), while the remainder might not (Wassle et al, 1978). Furthermore, although juxtaposition of lateral elements directly beneath synaptic ribbons argues in favor of a direct, photoreceptor to horizontal cell input, shown physiologically to be excitatory, the site of inhibitory or other output of horizontal cells, particularly onto photoreceptors is poorly defined anatomically and might yet prove specific. Thus the possibilities of partial specificity of horizontal cells for particular spectral classes of cone, and of horizontal cell mediated interactions among cone mechanisms in the mammalian outer plexiform layer, remain as intriguing as they are unresolved. Physiologically it is clear that, as reported above, there are at least two spectral classes of horizontal cell in the cat retina: One mixing red and blue signals, and the other red green and blue.

The findings reported here of a common intermixing of two or three spectral classes of cone signal at the horizontal cell level confirms in a general way views first promulgated by Ringo et al (1977) and Crocker et al (1980), analyzing spectral properties of cat ganglion cells. Although on neutral backgrounds there is a rare, overt opponency between red and blue cone signals at the ganglion cell level, (Pearlman and Daw, 1970), appropriate selective chromatic adaptation commonly revealed admixtures of blue as well as green cone input with the dominant red signal (Ringo et al, 1977; Crocker et al, 1980). The ganglion cell responses of monkey are clearly distinguishable from those of cat in the degree of color opponency (Weinrich and Zrenner, 1984). Whatever subtle cone interactions may occur in the outer plexiform layer of the former species appear to be overridden by the stronger opponent interactions of the inner retina.

In the horizontal cell responses of monkey (Gouras and Zrenner, 1978) and rabbit (Dacheux and Raviola, 1982; Bloomfield and Miller, 1982) there is evidence of intermixing of rod and cone signals. Experiments to reveal more subtle cone interactions in these cells have not yet been performed. Similar to our findings in cat retina (Nelson et al, 1975; ibid, 1976; Nelson, 1977), in rabbit and mouse retinas horizontal cell axon terminals appear reserved for rod signals, whereas A- and B-type cell bodies reveal a mixed rod-cone physiology (Dacheux and Raviola, 1982; Bloomfield and

118

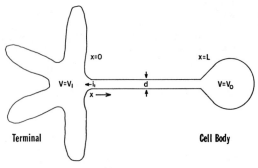

Fig. 8. Electrical model of the B-type horizontal cell. The attenuation of signals along the axon (of length $\underline{L}$) is described in the appendix. Definition of terms: $\underline{V}$, amplitude of an intracellular signal decrementing from the cell body, where it equals $\underline{V}_0$ to the terminal, where it equals $\underline{V}_1$; $\underline{x}$, distance along the axon increasing from left to right; $\underline{d}$, the diameter of the axon; $\underline{i}_i$, signal current exiting the axon to drive the signal voltage $\underline{V}_1$ by IR drop across the resistance of plasma membrane of the terminal.

Miller, 1982; Suzuki and Pinto, 1984). Evidence to date thus implies a great similarity among mammalian species in the outer retina. Although all other vertebrate divisions possess retinal horizontal cell types with azons, their connectivity with other neurons differs. In pigeon and turtle retinas, axon terminals of horizontal cells contact primarily cones and are not exclusive to rods (Mariani and Leure-duPree, 1977; Leeper, 1978). In telepstian retinas horizontal cell axon terminals have not been observed to contact photoreceptors at all. In turtle retina, as in mammalian species, the axon terminal and cell body regions of the axon bearing horizontal cell appear to be electrically isolated (Ohtsuka, 1983), and are distinguished by different receptive field sizes. A similar situation prevails in catfish retina (Davis and Naka, 1980). Thus although the general morphological and consequent electrical features of this cell type seems preserved among vertebrates, the specific connectivity is not. Connectivity and perhaps function thus appear more plastic than morphology in this class of vertebrate neurons.

Appendix: Signal attenuation along the B-type axon
The passive decay of voltage along an axon is described by the time independent cable equation:

$$\lambda^2 \partial^2 \underline{V}/\partial \underline{x}^2 = \underline{V} \qquad (1)$$

λ is the space constant, $[(\underline{d}/4)(\underline{R}_m/\underline{R}_i)]^{1/2}$, $\underline{V}$ is an intracellular signal voltage decrementing along the axon in the direction $\underline{x}$ (Fig. 8). In the following resting potential is not considered to be a part of $\underline{V}$. Although it is commonly taught that this second order differential equation has the solution $\underline{V}_0 e^{-\underline{x}/\lambda}$, like other differential equations, the cable equation is susceptible to a family of functional solutions, dependent on boundary conditions. What is not emphasized is that exponential voltage decay (above) is appropriate only to a semi-infinite axon, and need not apply to axons of finite length, with or without axon terminals. An ingenious and more general solution to the cable equation was proposed by Rall (1959):

$$\underline{V}/\underline{V}_1 = \cosh(\underline{x}/\lambda) + \underline{B}_1 \sinh(\underline{x}/\lambda) \qquad (2)$$

B_1 is a dimensionless conductance ratio, identified by Rall as the ratio of the conductance of the terminal (G_t) to the conductance of semi-infinite axon, $G_{inf} = (r_i \lambda)^{-1}$, where r_i is the resistance per unit length of the axon. The correctness of Rall's solution, as modified to suit the problem at hand, can be seen from the following argument: The signal current i_1 emerging from the axon at the juncture of axon and terminal $(x=0, Fig. 8)$ can be calculated from the longitudinal derivative of axonal voltage by $-1/r_i \, dV/dx$ or:

$$i_1 = (1/r_i)(V_1/\lambda)[\sinh(x/\lambda) + B_1 \cosh(x/\lambda)] \qquad (3)$$

Evaluated at $x=0$, this gives the simple result:

$$i_1 = V_1 (r_i \lambda)^{-1}(B_1) \qquad (4)$$

Since $B_1 = G_t/G_{inf}$:

$$i_1 = V_1 (r_i \lambda)^{-1}(r_i \lambda G_t) \qquad (5)$$

or:

$$i_1 = V_1 G_1 \qquad (6)$$

In other words the signal current flowing out of the axon exactly equals the current that the signal voltage V_1 will drive through the conductance of the axon terminal membrane. Thus at $x=0$ both current and voltage $(V/V_1=1)$ are continuous across the axon/terminal junction, showing the appropriateness of the Rall solution. Finally, since interest generally centers on the attenuation of signal between the cell body and the terminal, and not the voltage at various positions along the axon, expressing B_1 in fundamental units and assuming the same resistivity for axonal and terminal membrane (not a necessary constraint):

$$V_0/V_1 = \cosh(L/\lambda) + (2A_t/\pi)R_m^{-1/2}R_i^{1/2}d^{-3/2}\sinh(L/\lambda) \qquad (7)$$

G_t has been calculated from the surface area of the terminal (A_t) divided by R_m and L is the length of the axon. The attenuation (V_0/V_1) thus can be seen to depend linearly on the surface area of the terminal.

For a previously described B-type horizontal cell (Nelson et al, 1975) we have measured the surface area of the terminal (17,800 um^2), the cell body and dendrites (5100 um^2) and the length and diameter of the axon (330 um and 0.5 um^2 respectively). The cell is similar to that depicted in Fig. 1. Values of attenuation are calculated for different values of R_m (Table 1) using 70 ohm cm for R_i. The potent effect of the terminal in decreasing the signal transfer between the two ends of the cell can be seen by comparison to the 'sealed end' case where the terminal has been removed from the axon. The value of R_m given by Barrett and Crill (1974) for cat spinal motor neurons, 2000 ohm cm^2, yields a signal attenuation factor of 170 between cell body and terminal. Even values of R_m an order of magnitude higher than this yield the same conclusion. Very little signal voltage arising in the cell body will be seen in the terminal. For propagation of signals from axon terminal to cell body, the attenuation is about a factor of three less, owing to the lesser area of the cell body and dendrites. At 2000 ohm cm^2 the axonal space constant is 189 μm.

T A B L E 1

R_m ohm cm^2	V_0/V_1	'sealed end'
1,000	503	5.98
2,000	170	2.96
5,000	53	1.68
10,000	24	1.32
20,000	12	1.16
50,000	5	1.06

The values of attenuation (V_0/V_1) have been generated from equation 7 with the following parameters: R_i, 70 ohm cm; L, 330 um; A_t, 17,800 um^2 and d, 0.5 um. The 'sealed end' case is generated by using a 1 um^2 patch of membrane for A_t, removing the terminal and sealing the end of the axon with this patch. The attenuation of the axon is increased dramatically when connected to the axon terminal as compared to having a sealed end.

Weiler (1978) has suggested that the axon in fish horizontal cells may be active rather than passive and capable of regeneratively conducting graded slow potentials. The passive properties of the system have some bearing on his idea. It is reasonable to suppose that for a conducting axon to effectively drive the terminal, its active input resistance must match or be less than that of the terminal. For R_m = 2000 ohm cm^2 the resistance of the terminal being considered is 11 megohms. To achieve an 11 megohm input resistance for a semi-infinite axon of 0.5 um diameter requires an R_m for the active axon of 0.55 ohm cm^2. Cole (1972) found the resistivity of the active squid axon to be 5 ohm cm^2. An active horizontal cell axolemma would have to exceed the conductance of the active squid axolemma by an order of magnitude to drive the axon terminal by such a mechanism.

References:

Barrett, J.N. and W.E. Crill, J. Physiol (Lond) 239, 301-324 (1974).
Bloomfield, S.A. and R.F. Miller, J. Comp. Neur. 208, 288-303 (1982).
Boycott, B.B., L. Peichl and H. Wassle, Proc. R. Soc. Lond. B. 203, 229-245 (1978).
Cajal, S.R. y in The Structure of the Retina. S.A. Thorpe and M. Glickstein translators. (Charles C. Thomas, Springfield, Illinois) (1933).
Cole, K.S. Membranes Ions and Impulses, (University of California Press, Berkeley 1972), p. 521.
Crocker, R.A., J. Ringo, M.L. Wolbarsht and H.G. Wagner, J. Gen. Physiol. 76, 763-785 (1980).
Dacheux, R.F. and E. Raviola, J. Neurosci 2, 1486-1493 (1982).
Davis, G.W. and K.-I. Naka, J. Neurophysiol 43, 807-831 (1980).
Gallego, A., Vis. Res. (suppl 3) 11, 33-50 (1971).
Gallego, A., in Neural Principals in Vision S. Zettler and R. Weiler eds (Springer Verlag 1976) p. 26-62.
Gouras, P. and M. Hoff, Invest. Ophthal. 9, 388-399 (1970).
Gouras, P. and E. Zrenner International Congress Series No. 450, XXIII Concilium Ophthalmologicum K. Shimizu, J.A. Oosterhuis eds (Elsevier North-Holland, 1978) p. 379-384.
Kolb, H. J. Comp. Neur. 155, 1-14 (1974).
Kolb, H. J. Neurocytol. 6, 131-153 (1977).
Leeper, H.F. J. Comp. Neur. 182, 795-810 (1978).
Mariani, A.P. and A.E. Leure-du-Pree J. Comp. Neur. 75, 13-26 (1977).
Nelson, R. J. Comp. Neur. 172, 109-135 (1977).
Nelson, R., H. Kolb, E.V. Famiglietti and P. Gouras Invest. Ophthal. 15, 946-953 (1976).

Nelson, R. A.v. Lutzow, H. Kolb and P. Gouras Science 189, 137-139 (1975).
Niemeyer, G. J. Neurosci Meth. 3, 317-337 (1981).
Niemeyer, G. and P. Gouras Vis. Res. 13, 1603-1612 (1973).
Normann, R.A., I. Pearlman, H. Kolb, J. Jones and S. Daly Science 224, 625-627 (1984).
Ohtsuka, T. J. Comp. Neur. 220, 191-198 (1983).
Pearlman, A.L. and N.W. Daw Science 167, 84-86 (1969).
Rall, W. Exp. Neuro. 1, 491-527 (1959).
Ringo, J., M.L. Wolbarsht, H.G. Wagner, R. Crocker and F. Amthor, Science 198, 753-755 (1977).
Steinberg, R.H., Vis. Res. 9, 1345-1355 (1969).
Stell, W.K., D.O. Lightfoot J. Comp. Neur. 159, 473-502 (1975).
Suzuki, H. and L.H. Pinto Invest. Ophthal. Suppl. 25, 291 (1984).
Wassle, H., B.B. Boycott and L. Peichl, Proc. R. Soc. Lond. B. 203, 247-267 (1978).
Weiler, R., Cell Tissue Res. 195, 515-526 (1978).
Wienrich, M. and E. Zrenner, Ophthalmic Res. 16, 40-47 (1984).

Advances in Horizontal Cell Terminology Since Cajal
Antonio Gallego
Instituto de Investigaciones Oftalmologicas
"Ramon Castroviejo"
Universidad Complutense
Madrid, Spain

Cajal (1893) gave the name of "horizontal" to cells described initially by Muller (1851) with the name of "sternformigen zellen" (stellate cells). Muller cells were studied by several authors in the nineteenth century in the retina of vertebrates and described with different names. The predominant idea since Muller was that "sternformigen zellen" were supporting cells (neuroglia) of the retina organized into "membranes" (Krause, 1868), "perforata" and "fenestrata", and classified as "concentrische stutzzellen" by Schiefferdecker (1886). The years 1887 and 1888 must be recognized as a landmark in the knowledge of the structure of the nervous system and particularly of the retina. The structure of the retina was studied by Tartuferi (1887) with the Golgi method and by Dogiel (1888) with methylene blue vital staining but these authors, as well as other scientists who studied the retina previous to Cajal, were so deeply influenced by Gerlach's and Golgi's reticular theory about the organization of the nervous system, that in spite of the images they obtained, they "saw" anastomoses linking adjoining cells one to the other; therefore they described the plexiform layers as being "nets" or a continuous reticulum (The Golgi's "rete nervosa").

The studies which led Cajal to postulate his "neuron theory" were performed in 1887 and 1888. After he realized, using the Golgi method, that between the terminal arborization of the axon of one neuron and the soma or dendrites of neighboring cells there was not "continuity" but "contiguity" he decided to test such hypotheses in the bird retina (Cajal, 1988 a,b) and cerebellum (1888c). One year after, he published his classic paper "Connexion general de los Centros Nerviosos" (Cajal,1889) where he states the ideas known thereafter as the "Neuron Theory".

In 1893, Cajal published his masterpiece on the retina "La retine des Vertebres". Referring to the "Horizontal cells" (HCs) he concluded that "...these cells are neural in nature, and that they may be considered as neurons with very short axons, since the axon originates and finishes within the retina itself" (Cajal, 1893). Cajal subdivided his short axon Hcs into "external" and "internal" for the mammals and amphibian retina and in "brushshaped" and "stellate" for the avian and reptile retina. In the teleost retina he described three subtypes of HCs: "external", which corresponded to Krause's "membrane perforata", "medial" equivalent to Krause's "membrana fenestrata" and "internal" identified by Cajal as the "kernlose concentrische zellen" of Krause.

Cajal's contribution to the knowledge of the structure of the retina was of such great importance that his findings and concepts of the synaptic organization of the retina remain unquestioned over a period of 75 years, in spite of the several problems raised by himself in a paper written one year before his death (1933). In relation to retina's transverse neurons he discusses "the horizontal cell paradox" and the "enigma of the amacrine cells". Referring to horizontal cells he had concluded that they made contacts through their dendrites and axon terminal with the inferior endings of photoreceptors and because of his ideas of centripetal axonal conduction, he felt confused when obliged to admit that the "visual impulse" originated in some receptors was transmitted through these "tangential" neurons back to photoreceptors located at some distance forming a "vicious circle". In his own words, to

Neurocircuitry of the Retina, A Cajal Memorial
A. Gallego and P. Gouras, Editors

explain that "nonsense", Cajal stated that "the horizontal cells do not represent authentic visual pathways but energetic centers related to the articulation established by the rods and specific bipolars and reinforce signals transmitted by the pair of bipolar-ganglion cells".

A fundamental advance in the knowledge of the synaptic connections of HCs was achieved by Stell (1965, 1967) using a combination of Golgi stained HCs and electron microscopy; he demonstrated that triads in the photoreceptors of teleost retina were composed of a process of a bipolar cell as the central and processes of horizontal cells as the lateral elements. Stell's method has been highly effective in elucidating the synaptic connections between photoreceptors, bipolar and HCs in vertebrate retina.

The application of silver reduced impregnation (Gallego, 1953) and of the Golgi method to the entire retina, and its study in whole-flat mounted preparations gave a new perspective to retinal cells. In relation with synaptic organization of the outer plexiform layer (OPL), such techniques led to the discovery of axonless HCs and interplexiform cells, allowed a study with precision of Cajal's short axon HCs and gave valuable information about the diversity of retinal neurons, their dendritic and field sizes, lengths of their axons and the complexity of their branching patterns.

The correlation between electrophysiological and structural observations has been achieved by intracellular recording followed by various dye injections since the early demonstration by Kaneko (1970) that the source of S potentials were the HCs. The introduction of new dyes as Lucifer yellow, and particularly the use of horseradish peroxidase (HRP), to stain the intracellularly studied cells, followed by their analysis by light or electron microscopy, is improving our knowledge of the various cell types and of their synaptic relations.

Two categories of horizontal cells in tetrapod retina
The comparative study of the tetrapod retina (Gallego, 1976, 1982, 1983) leads to the conclusion that two different types of HCs have to be considered. Short axon horizontal cells (SAHC) and axonless horizontal cells (ALHC). These two types of HCs differ not only by their morphology but also by their connections with photoreceptors and probably by their function.

Since Polyak's (1941) description of the SAHC in the monkey retina, modern studies of Golgi stained whole-flat mounted retinas have shown that Cajal's varieties of the SAHC do not exist. Only one type of Cajal's SAHC has been found in mammals, birds, reptiles and amphibian retina. Cajal's "external" HC in mammals was actually the ALHC (Gallego, 1964, 1965) and in birds and reptiles Cajal's "stellate" HC was shown to be the axon ending of his "brush-shaped" HC (Gallego et al, 1975a; Gallego and Perez Arroyo, 1976). In the frog retina only one type of Cajal's SAHC has been recently described (Stephan and Weiler, 1981; Tarres and Baron, 1984). In all the tetrapod retinas studied the SAHC dendrites form the lateral component of the cone triads while the axon endings penetrate into the synaptic complex of rods in mammals (Kolb, 1970, 1974; Boycott and Kolb, 1973; Gallego and Sobrino, 1975) and in nocturnal birds (Gallego et al, 1975b; Tarres et al, 1984). In diurnal birds and reptiles (Gallego, 1976; Gallego and Perez Arroyo, 1976; Leeper, 1978) the dendrites of the SAHC contact also cone synaptic bodies while the axon endings contact not only rods but also some cone pedicles. In amphibians the connections of the SAHC have not been clearly established.

The dendrites and axon endings of this cell type overlap to a great extent but   gap-junctions between somas or dendrites of neighbor cells have only been described in the turtle retina (Witkowsky et al, 1983). The axon endings in birds (Gallego, 1975; Baron and Gallego, 1982) and reptiles (Gallego and P erez Arroyo, 1976; Leeper, 1978) form a well defined plexus located between the photoreceptor synaptic bodies and the somata of the HCs. Different animal classes and even species show morphological variations of this cell type which refer to the size of its dendritic arborization, to the number of cones connected to it, to the axon length and to the structure of the axon endings as well as the number and type of photoreceptors connected to it.

The ALHC was first described by Gallego (1964, 1965) in the cat retina and found afterwards in the retina of birds (Gallego, 1977, 1978; Mariani et al, 1977; Genis-Galvez et al, 1979) reptiles (Gallego and Perez Arroyo, 1976) and amphibians (Stephan and Weiler, 1981). Only one type of ALHC has been found in the mammal retina. The retina of birds and reptiles, and probably amphibians, has two or three subtypes of ALHC. In lower mammals this cell type builds a plexus which expands over the retina; neighbor cells establish large gap-junctions between one another. From the ALHC thin terminal fibers arise which penetrate into the cone synaptic bodies in all the tetrapod retinas studied (Lasansky, 1971; Kolb, 1974: Gallego, 1976; Leeper, 1978). The retina of primates is an exception among tetrapods. It has no ALHC but has instead a second type of SAHC which connects with cones both by its dendrites and by its axon endings (Kolb et al, 1980).

The two basic types of HCs are also found in fish retina. The SAHC studied by Stell (1972, 1975) shows two main differences compared with the same cell type in the tetrapod retina; its axon ends in a large, elongated structure, identified as Cajal's internal HC, located at the vitreal side of the inner granular layer with no apparent contact with photoreceptors and the somata form a plexus, as the ALHCs in tetrapod retina. Two or three layers of this cell type have been described in teleost retina in several species (Stell, 1967; Parthe, 1972; Weiler, 1977). In all cases the dendrites penetrate the cone pedicles; the connections of the axon terminal is unknown. The ALHCs in fish retina form one layer in teleost (Weiler, 1977) and two or three layers in the selachian retina (Stell and Witkovsky, 1973; Gallego, 1979). Wide gap-junctions are seen between the ALHCs which form a syncitium. The cell processes contact only rods.

A different functional role for each of the two categories of HCs can be suspected due to their different connections with photoreceptors: the SAHC contacts always cones by its dendrties and exclusively rods (in mammals) or mainly rods (in birds and reptiles) by its axon while the ALHC connects only cones in all tetrapod retinas studied.

Nomenclature of HCs

All HCs described by Cajal in the vertebrate retina were SAHCs and his classification by their location in the OPL as "external" and "internal" or by their shape as "brush-shaped" and "stellate" was generally accepted for seventy years. The ALHC was named initially "amacrine cell of the OPL" (Gallego, 1964); the name "amacrine" was used in its entymological meaning (without large fiber) as Cajal did when he discovered the amacrine cells of the inner plexiform layer. In subsequent studies using Golgi stainings of the entire retina each author named HCs without following a systematic nomenclature. The SAHC and the ALHC were studied by Dowling et al, (1966) in the rabbit and cat retinas and named "small" or "B" and "large or "A" respectively. Boycott and Dowling (1969) also named "A" and "B" two supposedly different types of axon bearing HCs of the monkey retina which were soon identified as a single cell type (Kolb, 1970). The classification into "A" and "B" HCs was again used by Fisher and Boycott (1974), in this case for the cat retina, the "A" cell being an ALHC and the "B" a SAHC. Other authors employ numbers to distinguish morphologically distinct types of HCs as Leeper (1978) in turtle, Stephan and Weiler (1981) in the frog. The nomenclature with numbers is regularly used since Stell (1967) used them for fish retina. HCs have also been named for their S potential responses as L1-HC and L2-HC (Simon, 1973) in the turtle; in this case the two differently responding HCs are in fact the soma and axon ending of the same SAHC.

The classification of HCs in SAHC and ALHC was introduced by Gallego (1976) in a comparative study of mammal and bird retinas. This classification of HCs could be enlarged to include their structural and functional properties. In those retinas where more than one subtype of each basic HC is found, they could be named: SAHC, type I, Type II... and ALHC, type I, II,. III... or they could be defined by their C or L responses to light. Following these rules the monkey HCs will be SAHC type I and type II, the cat and rabbit HCs will be classified as L-SAHC and ALHC and the turtle HCs will be subdivided in L-SAHC (H1 from Leeper) and C-ALHCs (H2, H3,H4) which could be further subdivided in R/G ALHC and G/B ALHC. In our opinion this approach to an HCs nomenclature facilitates general conclusions about the comparative anatomy of the OPL in different retinas and avoids the confusion produced when studying a particular retina.

Mammals HCs

Major differences have been found between the HCs in primate and subprimate retina. Cajal (1893), having not studied the primate retina, subdivided mammalion HCs into "external" and "internal". The first study of primate retina with the Golgi method was by Polyak (1941) who only found one type of HC in the monkey retina. Admitting Cajal's two types of HCs for the subprimate retina, the finding of a single type in the monkey reinforced his idea that "the structural pattern of the retina is much more complex than conceived by Ramon y Cajal" who had stated that "the only anatomical variations occur in the relative thickness of the layers and in the shape and size of the rods and cones". A single type of SAHC was also found in the subprimate retina by several authors (Dowling et al, 1966; Gallego, 1971a; Kolb, 1974; Fisher and Boycott, 1974). Thus Cajal's classification into "external and "internal" HCs is no longer tenable. The SAHC dendrites form the lateral components of the cone triads and its axon forms the synaptic complex of rods (Kolb, 1970; Fisher and Boycott, 1974).

The ALHC found in subprimate retinas (Gallego, 1964, 1965) shows some morphological differences among species. In all retinas studied their thin terminal fibers form the lateral component of cone triads (Kolb, 1970; Fisher and Boycott, 1974). Up to now the authors who studied the monkey retina have not been able to stain the ALHC with the methods used successfully in subprimate retina. The monkey retina has instead a second type of SAHC which differs in its morphology and synaptic connections from Cajal's HC (Gallego, 1977, 1978; Kolb et , 1980).

Subprimate retina (Fig. 1)

All the subprimate retinas studied have one type of SAHC and ALH. The SAHC was first described by Cajal (1893) in the retinas of cat, dog, rabbit, pig, sheep and ox. The SAHC morphology in subprimate retinas has been studied with the Golgi method and EM by several authors (Dowling et al, 1966; Gallego, 1971; Fisher and Boycott, 1974; Kolb, 1974) and more recently with injected Lucifer yellow or HRP after recording intra-

126

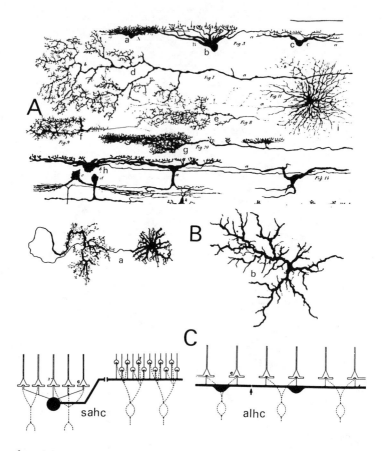

Fig. 1. Subprimate retina. A) Cajal drawings (1893): a, external HC, dog; b, c, internal HCs; axon endings: d, bull; e, dog; f, rabbit; g, bull seen in transverse section; h, HC bull. B) a, sahc of the newborn dog; b, alhc of the rabbit. C) connections with photoreceptors of sahc and alhc (arrow, gap-junction).

cellularly its responses to light stimuli (Dacheux and Raviola, 1982; Bloomfield and Miller, 1982).

To interpret the electrical responses of HCs the main morphological data needed are their synaptic connections, the anatomical field of their dendrites and axon terminal and the axon length. The anatomical field of the SAHC in the adult cat, dog and rabbit, is practically circular and 50 to 140 μm and does not show colaterals. The axon terminal covers a retinal area of 150 x 250 μm and contacts 3,000 to 4,000 rods (Gallego, 1971; Kolb, 1974; Fisher and Boycott, 1974).

Membrane contacts between the processes of SAHC and ALHC have been described (Gallego, 1971) but Lucifer yellow injected intracellularly fails to demonstrate intercellular dye transfer between the two cell types

(Dacheux and Raviola, 1982). The axon endings overlap frequently but do not show membrane contacts between one another. Lucifer yellow fails to transfer between axon endings of separate cells confirming the absence of coupling between these structures.

When comparing the anatomical and functional field sizes of the dendrites and of the axon endings some discrepancies appear. In the rabbit retina the field size of recorded electrical responses of the soma and dendrites is larger than the spread of the dendritic arborization but the axon ending receptive field is slightly larger than its anatomical spread (Dacheux and Raviola, 1982; Bloomfield and Miller, 1982). The difference in size of the anatomical and functional fields of the soma and dendrites could be explained by light scattering, electrical coupling between photoreceptors or contacts between processes of SAHC and ALHC. In our opinion there is the possibility that the axon ending signals may be transmitted antidromically to the cell body enlarging its functional receptive field but such a possibility can be discounted due to the different input of photoreceptor signals to the two structures and to computations in the cat retina of the electrotonic decay along the axon which indicate an electrical isolation between the soma and axon ending of the SAHC (Nelson et al, 1975).

The AlHC was first described by Gallego (1964, 1965) using a reduced silver impregnation of the entire cat retina. The ALHCs extend from the ora serrata to the pappila forming a well defined plexus, even in the area central is. The ALHCs in the dog (Honrubia, 1966) and in cat and rabbit retina (Honrubia and Elliot, 1969) were studied using Gallego's technique; two types "symmetric" and asymmetric" were found in the rabbit retina while in the cat a more regular and star-shaped appearance was observed (Leicester and Stone, 1967). The pleomorphism of ALHCs in the rabbit retina has been confirmed in cells injected with HRP (Dacheux and Raviola, 1982). By using the Golgi method in whole-flat mounted preparations the ALHC can be observed in isolation or by partial images of the plexus especially demonstratable by the neurofibrillar staining method (Dowling et al, 1966; Gallego, 1973, 1975, 1976; Kolb, 1974; Fisher and Boycott, 1974).

The cell processes cover, in the cat retina, a circular area which varies according to the location of the ALHC. In the peripheral retina the area has a diameter of 150-250 µm but in the area centralis the diameter is only 50 µm. In the rabbit retina the processes cover eliptic area of 70 x 300 µm in average size but circular areas are also found. This cell type contacts cone pedicles; its terminal knobs form the lateral component of cone triads (Kolb, 1974; Fisher and Boycott, 1974). Great overlapping of neighboring cells is always observed and wide gap-junctions between their processes have been described by EM and beautifully confirmed by the transfer of the intracellularly injected Lucifer yellow from one cell to many neighboring cells over a circular area 0.9 µm in diameter (Dacheux and Raviola, 1982).

Primate HCs (Fig. 2)

The monkey retina has two types of SAHC. The ALHC has not been found in primate retina. Type I of SAHC has been widely studied since its first description by Polyak (1941) and corresponds to the HC described by Cajal in other mammalian retina. The study of Golgi stained retinas shows a gradual transition of the morphology of the SAHC type I from the fovea to peripheral retina; the dendritic field increases with distance from the fovea. In the parafoveal area the dendritic field is circular with a diameter of 25 to 30 um; near the ora serrata the cell has thicker and longer dendrites which spread horizontally over 60-100 µm in oval shaped

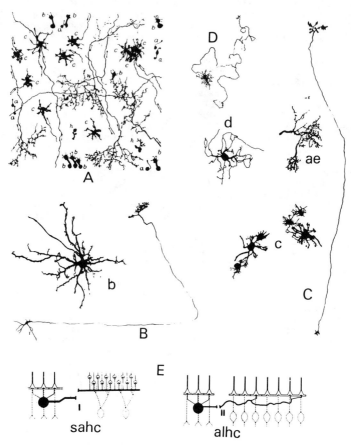

Fig. 2. Primate retina. A) Polyak drawing (1941) of HCs, monkey retina.
B) sahc type I of the peripheral retina, b, detail of the soma. C) sahc
type I of the parafoveal retina; c, detail of the soma, ie, axon ending;
D) sahc Type II, d, detail of the soma; E) connections with
photoreceptors of SAHCs type I and II.

areas. Each parafoveal SAHC type I contacts 6 to 9 cones and the most
peripheral ones up to 30-40 cones (Kolb, 1970; Boycott and Kolb, 1973).
The cell body has a 1 μm thick axon which runs straight without branching.
At its end the axon widens into a thicker process which branches out
several times. Thin fibers arising from these branches end in knobs which
penetrate rod spherules (Kolb, 1970; Gallego and Sobrino, 1975). The axon
length varies from 800 μm to 2,500 μm in different species of monkeys
(Ogden, 1974; Gallego, 1976a; Mariani, 1984)

The SAHC type II was found in the retina of several species of monkeys
and studied by light and EM (Gallego, 1977, 1978; Kolb et al, 1980). The
morphology of this cell type differs from the type I SACH. The dendrites
are very thin and in disorderly arrays. The very thin axon, 0.5 μm in
diameter, meanders over a distance of 400-500 μm giving off collaterals.

Due to the convoluted course, the axon terminal can be found at distances of 100 to 400 μm from the cell body. The dendritic field is circular near the fovea with diameters of 30 to 50 μm and with diameters of 50 to 60 at 7 mm from the fovea; near the periphery the dendritic field is more elliptical and 90 x 100 μm in diameter. The dendrite endings contact cones (10 to 22) forming the lateral component of triads (Kolb et al, 1980). The axon endings also form the lateral components of cone triads. Thus type II SAHC have different photoreceptor connections than type I cells contacting cones by both its dendrites and axon terminals. It therefore shows the same connections as the ALHC in the subprimate retina.

Birds HCs (Fig. 3)

In Cajal's first two papers (1888 a,b) on the structure of the avian retina he describes neural "stellate" or "subepithelial" cells and "brush-shaped" cells classified as neuroglia. In his 1893 paper he includes both cells among his short axon "horizontal cells". No studies were made of the avian HCs until the demonstration that Cajal's "stellate" cell is in fact the axon ending of the "brush-shaped" cell (Gallego et al, 1975). Thus birds as other tetrapods have only one type of SAHC. Two types of ALHCs have been described in the diurnal bird retina (Gallego, 1977, 1978; Mariani and Leure Dupre, 1977; Genis-Galvez, 1979; Baron and Gallego, 1982). There are differences between diurnal and nocturnal birds related not only to photoreceptors but to horizontal cells as well.

Diurnal birds

In gallinaceae and falconidae retinas one type of SAHC and two types of ALHCs have been described. The SAHC dendrites in gallinaceae have a circular field of 30 μm in diameter; in falconidae retina the dendritic field of the SAHC is elliptical. The 1 μm thick axon, is 100 μm long in the newborn chick, 600-800 μm in the falconidae and 700-900 in the owlet. The axon ends by a wide enlargement ramifying in thick branches which give off thin terminal fibers with isolated knobs. The dendrites contact double cones in the outer row of synaptic bodies of the OPL, the straight cones of the middle row and the oblique cones. The axon terminals penetrate the rod and some single cone synaptic complexes (Gallego, 2978; Tarres, 1982). The axon endings form a plexus by gap-junctions among themselves with the peculiarity that vesicles at either side of the junction are frequently seen (Baron and Gallego, 1982). Membrane contacts between the soma or dendrites of the SAHC have not been reported.

The ALHC type I is a characteristic cell of the gallinaceae and falconidae retina (Gallego, 1977, 1978; Genis-Galves et al, 1979; Baron and Gallego, 1982). In falconidae the cell has five to seven processes spreading at opposite ends in a horizontal plane. The area covered by the processes is a 120 x 25 μm rectangle. When several neighboring cells are stained in Golgi preparations, the intermingling of their cell processes as well as a parallel intertwining can be clearly seen. The processes give out very thin terminals which, without branching, reach the outer row of photoreceptor endings. The terminal fibers contact the synaptic bodies of double cones. Each cell contacts 16-24 cones in a 120 x 25 μm rectangular area.

The ALHC type II has also been described (Gallego, 1977, 1978; Mariani and Leure Deupre, 1977; Genis-Galvez et al, 1979; Baron and Gallego, 1982). It was already noted by Cajal (1888a), in cross-sections of several diurnal avian species, who made a brief description of it under the name of "stellate" or "subepithelial" cell (Fig. 3a). One of its long process was considered by Cajal to be an axon. Nevertheless, Cajal (1893) subsequently described the "brush-shaped" HC and its axon ending (Fig. 3d) thinking that its ending was an independent cell. He named it a "stellate"

130

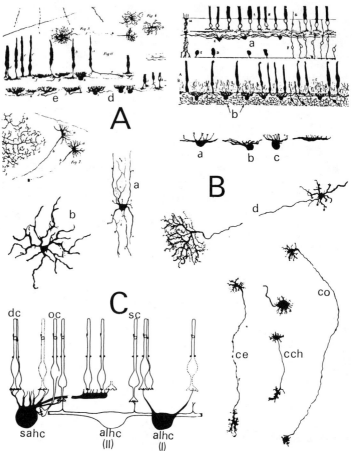

Fig. 3. Bird retina. A) Cajal drawings: a, stellate cell (1888a) of the chicken; b, "spongioblast of the 3rd variety", sparrow (1888b); c, brush-shaped HC of the hen; d, brush-shaped HC; e, HCs "aplaties" or stellate" (1893). B) HCs of bird retina: a, alhc type I; b, alhc type II; c, sahc, cch chicken, ce, eagle; co, owlet; d, sahc of the owl. C) connections of HCs with photoreceptors: dc, double cone; sc, straight cone; oc, oblique cone. sahc, short axon horizontal cell; alhc, axonless horizontal cell type I and II.

HC (Fig. 3e). It is clear from his drawings that the "stellate" cell of his 1888 paper is different from his "stellate" cell of the 1893 study.

The processes of the ALHC type II cover a circular area of 100 μm in diameter. The thin terminal fibers which arise from the processes end in a small cluster of two to four knobs at the level of the middle row of photoreceptors syhaptic bodies. Golgi EM studies have shown that the terminal knobs penetrate in the synaptic complex of the straight cones with a red oil droplet (Gallego, 1978).

Nocturnal birds   The retina of the owl (Tyto alba), a nocturnal bird, has more rods than diurnal birds. The cones have only colourless oil droplets and the synaptic bodies of photoreceptors are located at a single level of the OPL in contrast with the three levels found in diurnal birds. In the owl retina both SAHC and ALHC have been found (Tarres et al, 1984). The morphology of the owl SAHC is different from the same cell in the diurnal birds and similar to the SAHC of the mammal retina. The SAHC's six to eight dendrites cover an oval area of 50 x 70 μm. The 1 μm thick axon does not give off colateral branches and runs straight for a length more than 800 μm. The axon terminal is a profusely branched structure similar to the axon terminal shown by the SAHC in the primate (Fig. 3d). The contacts of this cell with photoreceptors have not been determined up to now but the similar numbers of rods in primate and owl retinas and the similar morphology of the SAHC suggests it will also contact rods.

The ALHC of the owl has been difficult to stain with the Golgi method. Only one type has been detected whose morphology corresponds to the type II ALHC found in diurnal bird retina. Its processes spread in a horizontal plane and divide once or twice to cover a circular area 125-150 μm in diameter. The thin terminal fibers found in the same cell type of diurnal birds have not been seen in the few stained owl cells. Only some isolated knobs were stained and found to contact cones. We do not yet know if these cells have so few terminal fibers or staining is incomplete.

Reptiles HCs.
    Cajal (1893) using Golgi and methylene blue methods studied the retinas of Lac erta viridis and muralis, Emys europea and Chameleon vulgaris. He described two types of SAHCs in the lizard retina: "brush-shaped and "stellate". He described the soma and dendrites of the "brush-shaped' cell stating that its short ascending dendrites reach the uppermost part of the OPL "where they contact   the 'feet' of 'straight' cones". The axon, arising form the lateral part of the body, as it progresses, gives rise to ascending spines terminating in a small swelling. Its destination "is still unknown to me", he wrote, but added the suggestion that "these axons terminate in free arborizations at a fairly great distance in the OPL". Cajal was also able to stain, with methylene blue, the "flattened stellate" HCs which showed a "crescent" shaped soma sending out divergent processes "that ascend obliquely to the OPL where they terminate after branching". The dendrite endings do not rise as high as those of the "brush-shaped" cell and seem to contact the "oblique" cones. One of the processes of the "stellate" HC was described by Cajal as an axon arising "from one end of these cells and which travels horizontally. Its termination is still unknown to me". He was not able to stain the axon endings and made only a reference to these structures suggesting that "they could correspond to certain processes arising from a fine horizontal fiber, as is sometimes found in the OPL of the lizard retina" (Fig. 4).

Few studies on the reptile retina HCs have been reported since Cajal's. According to Yamada and Ishikawa (1965) EM studies of the turtle retina revealed only one type of HC. Lasansky (1971) observed two types of HCs in the turtle retina, similar to those described by Cajal in the lizard. According to him all the processes of the HCs terminate as lateral components of cone triads; rods were not considered in his study. One axonless HC and only one type of short axon HC, "brush-shaped", were described by Gallego and Perez Arroyo (1976). The axon endings of the short axon HCs were described as a plexus located at the vitreal side of the OPL. Perez Arroyo (1978) described a second type of axonless HC and confirmed the existence of gap-junctions between them. EM study revealed that the endings established contacts with the synaptic bodies of rods and

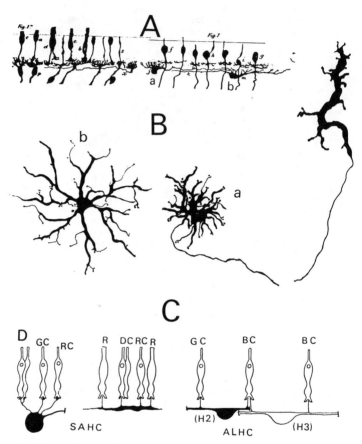

Fig. 4. Reptile retina. A) Cajal drawings (1893): a, brush-shaped HC; b, stellate HC of the Lacerta viridis. B) turtle Hcs: a, SAHC; b, ALHC. C) connections of HCs with photoreceptors in turtle; GC, green cone, RC, red cone: R, rod; DC, double cone; BC, blue cone; SAHC, short axon HC; ALHC, axonless HC.

single cones. Of the two types of axonless HCs, one shows a "bitufted" morphology (type I) and the other a "stellate" structure (type II) being similar to types I and II of the avian retina. In our opinion (Gallego, 1981), Cajal's "stellate" cell is the type II axonless HC of the turtle retina and has no axon, though one of the longer processes was erroneously identified by him as an axon.

A complete study of turtle's HCs, correlating their morphology and connections with photoreceptors with their electrical responses, has been made by Leeper (1978a). He described one type of SAHC (H1) and three types of ALHCs (H2, H3, H4). The dendrites of the SAHC establish contacts with red single cones and the red sensitive main member of the double cones as well as with the green single cones and the green sensitive accessory member of the double cones. The axon terminal contacts red cones, the main member of the double cones and rods.

The morphological features of Leeper's three ALHCs are similar to the ones of the ALHC initially described (Gallego and Perez Arroyo, 1976), and of type II ALHC from Perez Arroyo (1978). The cell described as type I ALHC by Perez Arroyo (1978) could be a morphologically different type of ALHC, similar to type I ALHC of the avian retina (Gallego, 1978) although it has possibly been confused with a SAHC of the peripheral retina as described by Leeper. There are no relevant morphological differences between the ALHCs described by Leeper as H2, H3 and H4. His study was made by intracellular recording followed by injection of Lucifer yellow. He compared these images with HCs stained with the Golgi method. The differences between H2 and H 3 refer to the photoreceptors they contact and as a consequence to their respective spectral responses; axonless H2 contacts green and blue sensitive cones and H3 blue sensitive cones only. In our opinion the existence of a third type of ALHC, Leeper's H4 is doubtful. The argument that H4 showed a dendritic field smaller than H2 and H3 in the same retinal area is not strong enough to classify such a cell as an independent type of axonless HC without knowing the response characteristics of the cell.

Both the dendrites and axon terminals of neighboring short axon HCs are interconnected by gap-junctions, studied in thin sections and freeze-fracture replicas by Witkovsky et al, 1983. The dendrites as well as the axon terminal possess gap-junctions but of different sizes, perikaryal gap-junctions were extremely restricted and found between the dendrites of neighboring cells whereas those of axon terminals were much larger. Actually, two different plexuses are formed at the OPL level by structures of the short axon HC, one by the soma and dendrites, the other by the axon endings. This morphological organization has a functional correlation of great interest as was found in the electrophysiological study of the turtle retina.

The turtle HCs give C and L responses to light stimuli (Saito et al, 1974). Two classes of L responses, supposedly produced by two different types of HCs, were recorded by Simon (1973) who distinguished them by their spatial properties: a large field HC (L2HC) and a small field HC (L2HC). The structures which give the L1 and L2 responses actually correspond to the soma (L2) and axon ending (L1) of a single SAHC as was unequivocally demonstrated by Leeper (1978). But the response characteristics of L1 and L2 differ sufficiently to consider them as separate functional units. The problem is whether or not these responses, which belong to the same neuron are functionally independent of each other. The spatial properties of L1 and L2 responses are not the only difference between them. The most reliable way to distinguish between L1 and L2 responses is the rod dominant response to dim stimuli showed by L1 (Leeper and Copenhagen, 1979) and the existence of antagonistic center-surround organization in the L2 response (Piccolino et al, 1981). The morphological and electrophysiological study (Norman and Kolb, 1981) of the SAHCs of the turtle visual streak reveals that receptive fields are smaller than they are in peripheral retina, elongated and oriented in the direction of the streak. Their orientation selectivity may have consequences on the receptive field properties of ganglion cells.

There is physiological evidence, supported by the EM studies of gap-junctions previously mentioned, of electrical coupling between L-HCs as suggested by Naka and Rushton (1967). In turtle retina the electrical coupling between L-HCs structures which give the L1 and L2 responses has been demonstrated by Simon (1973) with intracellular current injection showing that coupling was strong between the axon terminals and weak between the cell bodies. Piccolino et al, (1982) showed that when Lucifer yellow was injected through a microelectrode recording a small field L2

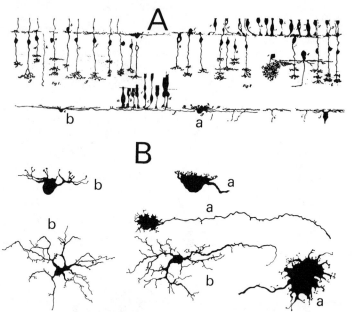

Fig. 5. Amphibian retina. A) Cajal drawings (1893). a, external HC; b, internal HC. B) HCs of the frog retina; a, SAHC; b, ALHCs.

response the dye slightly diffuses to other cell bodies and through the axon to the axon ending. According to them round spots, faintly stained, correspond to neighboring H1 cell bodies. They concluded that H1 soma is weakly coupled to other similar cell bodies. When the dye is injected through a microelectrode recording a large field L1 response an extensive network of axon terminals appeared stained suggesting that the coupling between them was strong. The difference in coupling efficiency accounts for the difference between the spatial receptive field properties of the L1 and L2 responses.

Amphibians (frog) horizontal cells

As in mammals, Cajal (1893) described in frog retina two types of HCs: "external" and "internal", different in the position and size of their soma and dendritic fields. These cells Cajal considered as neurons with very short axons. Previously Dogiel (1888) had described a single type of HC, "stellate", in the frog retina, but this cell does not look like an HC because it has a descending process directed toward the inner plexiform layer. Probably Dogiel's cell is a type of "interplexiform" cell studied recently in the rana ridibunda retina (Tarres and Baron, 1984) (Fig. 5). Recent studies of the HCs in frog retina have shown that it has the two basic types of HCs: a single type of SAHC, and probably two types of ALHCs as in the other tetrapods (Stephan and Weiler, 1981; Gallego, 1982; Tarres and Baron, 1984).

The SAHC has been identified with Cajal's "internal" HC. The dendritic field is circular and covers areas of 25-30 μm in rana ridibunda and 40-90 μm in rana temporaria. The size of the dendritic field is related to the distance of the ALHC from the optic disc. The axon, 0.6 μm in diameter has short collaterals, 4-30 μm long and a length of 200 to 800 μm. The axon terminal is an enlargement of the axon having a diameter of 3-4 um and a length of about 30 um. The ALHC can be identified with Cajal's "external" HC. It has been described in the rana temporaria (Stephan and Weiler, 1981) and rana ridibunda retinas (Tarres and Baron, 1984). The cell processes cover circular areas 70-160 um in diameter. From the processes emerge thin fibers which end in a cluster of small knobs at the level of the photoreceptor synapses. A second variety of ALHC has also been stained with the Golgi-Colonnier method. This cell has two or more longer processes, up to 100 um, spreading in opposite directions to give out small, thin fibers ending in tiny knobs (Tarres and Baron, 1984).

The connections of the two types of HCs have not been clearly established. According to Ogden et al (1982) the dendrites of the "internal" HC, that is the SAHC, contact both cones and rods but the receptors contacted by the axon endings have not been identified. Copenhagen and Reuter (personal communication) find that Lucifer yellow injected in the soma of a SAHC is transferred to neighboring cells. The SAHC body has a small rod driven and a larger cone driven receptive field. If these findings are confirmed the frog retina will be the only one, among tetrapods, where dendrites of the SAHC contacts rods. The connections with the photoreceptors of the ALHCs have not been established.

Horizontal cells and Cajal's neuron doctrine
As a consequence of the neuron doctrine the general organization of the central nervous system involved the transmission of impulses through chains of long axon neurons(Cajal, 1904), forming the main afferent and efferent pathways together with circuits of short axon neurons interneurons) of great complexity interacting with them (Lorente de No, 1933). The functional role of neurons without axons which form plexuses or "laminas" was not considered.

In the retina the description of "membranes" (perforata, fenestrata and stratum lacunosum) had been made before Cajal by several authors (Shiefferdecker, 1886) although they thought that these structures were formed by supporting cells (neuroglia). Cajal used the Golgi method which gives stains of isolated cells but fails to reveal with precision their relation to neighboring cells. Cajal emphasized the connections of individual neurons forming the visual pathways and neglected the "membranes": "I believe that the networks described by Krause (membrana fenestrata) and Schiefferdecker are only illusions that arise from the near impossibility of distinguishing the outlines of dendrites stained by current methods" (Cajal, 1893). It is understandable that Cajal's idea about the organization of the afferent pathways in the central nervous system and particularly in the retina made him consider connections formed by the HCs to be a "paradox" the "vicious circle" and the role played by neurons devoid of an axon, the amacrine cells to be an "enigma".

The discovery that HCs in some fish retina are electrically coupled (Mitarai et al, 1961; Naka and Rushton, 1967; Kaneko, 1971) and capable of wide spatial summation called attention to the plexus formed in fish by the HCs and to their possible functional role. Since the description of HCs plexus in the mammalian retina (Gallego, 1964) and of similar plexuses in other classes of tetrapods it was concluded that their existence is a general characteristic of the vertebrate retina with the probable exception of primates (Gallego, 1983) Fig. 6).

The existence of plexuses or "laminas" of HCs which form a functional syncitium located tangentially to the photoreceptor bipolar synapses

136

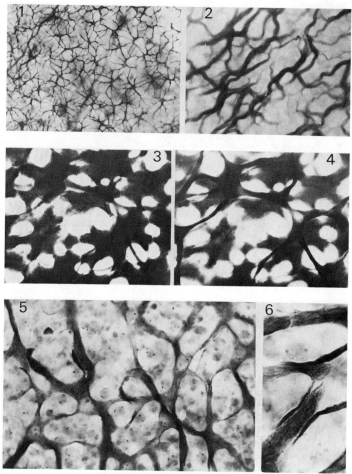

Fig. 6. Plexuses of HCS: 1) ALHC plexus of the cat retina. 2) Axon ending plexus of the SAHC in turtle. 3) plexus of the external HCs. 4) plexus of the medial HCs (Prionane glauca). 5) HCs plexus (Ginglymostoma cerratum). ç) details of the contacts of HCs in 5.

required us to reconsider the several schematic diagrams of the retina which have been used to interpret its organization in view of the great differences existing between the HCs and their organization in plexuses and connections with photoreceptors among classes, orders and even species.

The vertebrate retina has two basic types of HCs: SAHC and ALHC. In fish retina both types form plexuses. In birds and reptiles only the ALHC subtypes and the axon endings of the SAHCs form plexuses; the somata of the SAHCs do not, or only slightly. In lower mammals only the ALHCs form a plexus; neither the somata nor the axon endings of the SAHCs are coupled; in primate retina the two subtypes of SAHCs described do not form

plexuses. The functional study of the retina is mainly analyzed through
the behavior of individual cells but the function of the plexuses has not
been deeply studied. The carp retina has three SAHCs which connect with
cones and the ALHC which contact rods; these form plexuses at the OPL
level. The axon endings of SAHCs, which have no contact with
photoreceptors also form a plexus at the vitread side of the inner
granular layer.

In fish the S potentials originate in the soma of the SAHC and are
conducted along the plexus through gap-junctions. Those of the axon are
also conducted transversally by the plexus. In the carp the axon shows
the same three C-responses as the somata of SAHCs (H1, H2, H3) and as
these endings have no contact with photoreceptors, propagation of these
signals from the somata have to be admitted (Zettler and Weiler, 1981).
The functional role of the plexus formed by the axon remains unknown. If
functional contacts with amacrine or interplexiform cells (Naka, 1982) are
confirmed, the endings could be a link in a feedback from amacrines to HCs
through interplexiform cells. Another role of the axon plexus could be to
modify the excitability of the presynaptic fibers at the inner plexiform
layer by changes in the K^+ concentration of the intercellular space.
Changes in the membrane polarization of the axon endings, which form a
"lamina", imply fluxes of K^+ as the membrane currents of HCs which consist
of voltage dependent fast and slow K-currents, a K-current through the
anomalous rectifier and Ca-current as shown by Kaneko (1984) in the
isolated HCs of the carp retina. The K-currents may change the K^+
concentration at the "lamina" and modulate the liberation of
neurotransmitters at the IPL. The structure and location of the axon
endings may make them a useful model to study the function of plexuses,
independently of their connection with photoreceptors.

Signal spreading along HCs plexuses is supposed to be the mechanism
involved in the feedback to cones in turtle (Baylor et al, 1971),
pikeperch (Burkhardt, 1977) larval tiger salamander (Lasansky, 1981) and
carp (Murakami et al, 1978), the chromatic processing of cone signals
(Fuortes and Simon, 1974), and the adaptation of photoreceptors to changes
in retinal illumination (Byzov, 1969). Contrast discrimination (O'Bryan,
1973) are also functional properties of HCs supposed to be based on the
feedback on cones.

The transformation of the trichromatic process of cones into an
opponent color process in HCs (Svaetichin et al, 1965) has been explained
by several models based on the C responses of HCs being pre- and
postsynatpic to cones in the carp (Stell and Lightfoot, 1975) and turtle
(Leeper, 1978b). No color opponent responses have been recorded in
mammalian HCs. Both SAHC and ALHC give in mammals L-responses to light
stimuli (Nelson et al, 1975; Dacheux and Raviola, 1982; Bloomfield and
Miller, 1982). These findings make it difficult to understand the
functional role of the ALHC plexus in in the chromatic processing of the
cone signals in mammals. The few records obtained from HCs in primate
retina are also of the L-type. In primates no plexuses of HCs have been
seen. A very interesting suggestion has been made by Gouras and Zrenner
(1981) to explain the cone opponency seen in ganglion cells in the primate
retina, assuming that cone opponent interactions are developed in two
stages; a weak one which requires selective chromatic adaptation before it
is detectable and a strong one revealed under all conditions. The weak
stage of cone opponency is produced by horizontal cell interaction between
R and G cones, the strong one is mediated by amacrine interaction between
bipolar cells. Records from type II SAHC in primate retina have not been
obtained but we could expect R/G opponent responses as this cell is

connected with cones by its dendrites and axon terminal. Gouras and Zrenner's idea leads to the suggestion that in the course of evolution the chromatic process of cone signals has been shifted from the HCs plexuses, which play a main role in fish and reptiles, to the amacrine cells in mammals. The ALHC plexus in mammalian retina if not involved in the chromatic processing of cone signals could play a role in contrast detection, adaptation of photoreceptors to changes of illumination and movement detection.

Differences in the organization of the SAHCs among classes of vertebrates are relevant. In fish the somata and axon endings form plexuses but in primate retina the SAHCs appear as individual cells not coupled to each other or connected by their dendrites to cones and by its axon ending to rods. The problem of the axon conducting signals between the two structures has to be solved. If the axon conducts the signals originating at the dendrites or axon ending an antagonistic action between the cone and rod systems mediated by SAHC type I might be expected.

Great advances have been made in the knowledge of the horizontal cells since Cajal's fundamental study but the problem he raised when questioning the function of HCs, "related to the articulation established by the rods (visual cells) and the specific bipolars" has not been completely solved. We can expect that the wealth of information obtained at present with the help of structural, electrical and neurochemical techniques will bring us in the near future to the end of a road opened up by Cajal one hundred years ago.

References

Baron, M. and Gallego, A. in The Structure of the Eye. J.G. Hollyfield, ed, Elsevier North Holland, 1982) pp. 165-173.
Baylor, D.A., Fuortes, M.G.F. and O'Bryan, P.M., J. Physiol. Lond. 214, 265-294. (1971).
Bloomfield, S. A. and Miller, R.F. J. Comp. Neurol. 208, 288-303 (1982).
Boycott, B.B. and Dowling, J.E., Phil. Trans. R. Soc. Lond. B. 255, 109-194 (1969).
Boycott, B.B. and Kolb, H. J. Comp. Neurol. 148, 115-140 (1973).
Burkhardt, D.A. J. Neurophysiol. 40, 53-62 (1977).
Byzov, A.L. Neurosci. Transl. 14-62 (1969).
Cajal, S.R. Rev. Trim. Histol. Norm. Pat. 2, 317-322 (1888a).
Cajal, S.R. Rev. Trim. Histol. Norm. Pat. 2, 355-363 (1888b).
Cajal, S.R. Gaceta Med. Catal. August (1888c).
Cajal, S.R. La Medicina Practica Oct. 479-487 (1889).
Cajal, S.R. La Cellule 9-119 (1893).
Cajal, S.R. in Textura del Sistema Nervioso del Hombre y de los Vertebrados. Nicolas Moya. Madrid (1904).
Cajal, S.R. XIV Concilium Ophthalmologicum, Madrid pp. 1-19 (1933).
Dacheux, R.F. and Raviola, E. J. Neurosci. 2, 1486-1493 (1982).
Dogiel, A.S. Anat. Anz. 3, 133 (1888).
Dowling, J.E., Brown, J.E. and Major, D. Science 153, 1639-1641 (1966).
Fisher, S.K. and Boycott, B.B. Proc. R. Soc. Lond. B. 186, 317-331 (1974).
Fuortes, M.G.F. and Simon, E.J. J. Physiol. Lond. 240, 177-198 (1974).
Gallego, A. An. Inst. Farm. Esp. II, 171-176 (1953).
Gallego, A. Bull. Ass. Anat. XLIX, 624-631 (1964).
Gallego, A. Actualites Neurophysiol. Masson, Paris p. 5-27 (1965).
Gallego, A. Vis. Res. Suppl. 3, 11, 33-50 (1971).
Gallego, A. Trab. Inst. Cajal Invest. Biol. LXV, 227-257 (1973).
Gallego, A. Real Acad. Nac. Med. Inst. de Espana Madrid (1975).
Gallego, A. in Neural Principles in Vision F. Zettler and R. Weiler, eds (Springer Verlag, 1976) p 26-62.

Gallego, A.   Neurobiologia 25, 41-54 (1977).
Gallego, A.   Fundacion Juan March. Serie Universitaria, 52,   Madrid
(1978).
Gallego, A.   Norm. y Pat. A 3, 313-334 (1979).
Gallego, A.   in The S potential. B.D. Drujan and M. Laufer, eds Alan R.
Liss, New York 1982)pp. 9-29.
Gallego, A.   in Prog. in Sensory Physiol. 4, 83-114 (1983).
Gallego, A., Baron, M. and Gayoso, M. Vis. Res. 15, 1029-1030 (1975).
Gallego, A. and Perez Arroyo, M. in Structure of the Eye III E. Yamada and
S. Mishima eds, Jap. J. Ophthal 1976)pp 311-317.
Gallego, A. and Sobrino, J.A. Vis. Res. 15, 747-748 (1975).
Genis-Galves, J.M., Prada, F. and Armengol, J.A. Jap. J. Ophthal. 23,
378-387 (1979).
Gouras, P. and Zrenner, E. Vis. Res. 21, 1591-1598 (1981).
Honrubia, F.M. Arch. Soc. Oftal. Hisp-Amer. 26, 693-720 (1966).
Honrubia, F.M. and Elliot, J.H. Arch. Ophthal. 82, 98-104 (1969).
Kaneko, A. J. Physiol. Lond. 107, 623-633 (1970).
Kaneko, A. J. Physiol. Lond. 213, 95-105 (1971).
Kaneko, A. Proc. Int. Soc. Eye Res. III: 17 (1984).
Kolb, H. Phil. Trans. R. Soc. Lond. B. 258, 261-283 (1970).
Kolb, H. J. Comp. Neurol. 155, 1-14 (1974).
Kolb, H., Mariani,A. and Gallego, A. J. Comp. Neurol. 189, 31-39 (1980).
Krause, W. Wiss. Gottingen P. 163 (1968).
Lasansky, A. Phil. Trans. R. Soc. Lond. B. 262, 365-381 (1971).
Lasansky, A. J. Physiol. Lond. 310, 205-214 (1981).
Leeper, H.F. J. Comp. Neurol. 182, 777-794 (1978a).
Leeper, H.F. J. Comp. Neurol. 182, 795-809 (1978b).
Leeper, H.F. and Copenhagen, D.R. Vis. Res. 19, 407-412 (1979).
Leicester, J. and Stone, J. Vis. Res. 7, 695-705 (1967).
Lorente De No, R. Arch. Neurol. Psychiat. 30, 245-291 (1967).
Mariani, A.P. Int. Rev. of Cytol. 86, 285-320 (1984).
Mariani, A.P. and Leure-Deupre, A.E. J. Comp. Neurol. 175, 13-26 (1977).
Mitarai, G., Goto T. and Takagi, S. Sen. Proc. 2, 3750382 (1978).
Mitarai, G., Svaetichin, G., Vallecalle, E., Fatehchand, R., Villegas, J.
and Laufer, M. in The Visual System Neurophysiology and Psychophysics R.
Jung and H. Kornhuber eds, Springer Berlin 1961) p. 463-481.
Muller, H. Verhandl. d. Physik-Med. Gesells, Wurzburg 2, 216 (1851).
Murakami, M., Shimoda, Y., Nakatani, K., Miyachi, E. and Watanabe, S. Jap.
J. Physiol. 32, 911-926 (1982).
Naka, K.I. Vis. Res. 22, 653-660 (1982).
Naka, K.I. and Rushton, W.A.H. J. Physiol. Lond. 192, 437-461 (1967).
Nelson, R. Lutzow, Av., Kolb, H. and Gouras, P. Science 189, 137-139
(1975).
Normann, R.A. and Kolb, H. Vis. Res. 21, 1585-1588 (1981).
O'Bryan, M. J. Physiol. Lond. 235, 207-223 (1973).
Odgen, T.E. J. Comp. Neurol. 153, 399-428 (1974).
Odgen, T.E., Pierantoni, R. and Citron, M.C. in The Structure of the eye
J.G. Hollyfield ed, Elsevier North-Holland 1982) pp. 142-173.
Parthe, V. Vis. Res. 12, 395-406 (1972).
Perez Arroyo M. Doc. Thesis Univ. Comp. Madrid (1978).
Piccolino, M., Neyton, J. and Gerschenfield, H. (J. Neurophysiol. 45,
363-375 (1981).
Piccolino, M., Neyton, J., Witkovsky, P. and Gerschenfield, H. Neurosci.
Letters, suppl. 10, 387-388 (1982).
Polyak, S.L. The Retina Univ. Chicago Press. (1941).
Saito, T., Miller, W.H. and Tomita, T. Vis. Res. 14, 119-123 (1974).
Schiefferdecker, P. Arch. f. Mikrosk. Anat. 28, 305-396 (1886).
Simon, E.J. J. Physiol Lond 230, 199-211 (1973).
Stell, W.K. Anat. Rec. 153, 389-398 (1965).

140

Stell, W.K. Am. J. Anat. 120, 401-424 (1967).

Stell, W.K. J. Comp. Neurol 159, 503-520 (1975).

Stell, W.K. and Witkovsky, P. J.Comp. Neurol. 148, 33-45 (1973).

Stell, W.K. and Lightfoot, D.O. J. Comp. Neurol. 159, 473-502 (1975).

Stephan, P. and Weiler,R. Cell Tissue Res. 221, 443-449 (1981).

Svaetichin, G., Negishi, K. and Fatehchand, R. Symp on Physiol. and Exp. Psychol of Colour Vision, G.E.W. Wolstenholme and J. Knigh eds, Churchill Ltd. Lond 1965) pp. 178-207.

Tarres, M.A.G. Doc. Thesis. Univ. Complutense Madrid (1982).

Tarres, M.A.G. and Baron, M. Morfol. Norm. Pat. (1984) in press.

Tarres, M.A.G., Baron, M. and Gallego, A. Proc. Int. Soc. Eye Res. III, 23 (1984).

Tartuferi, F. Int. Monatsch. Anat. Physiol. 4, 421 (1887).

Weiler,R. Doc. Thesis. Universitat Munchen. (1977).

Werblin, F.S. and Dowling, J.E. J. Neurophysiol. 32, 339-355 (1969).

Witkovsky, P., Owen, W.G. and Woodworth, M. J. Comp. Neurol. 216, 359-368 (1983).

Yamada, E. and Ishikawa, T. Cold Spring Harbor Symp. Anat. Biol. 30, 383-392 (1965).

Functional Morphology of the Outer Plexifom Layer

Ken-Ichi Naka and Hiroko Sakai
National Institute for Basic Biology
Okazaki, Japan 444

The vertebrate retina is divided roughly into two layers, the outer and inner layers. In the outer layer the photons are caught and their energy is transformed into electrical signals in the receptor outer segments. The electrical signal is transmittted to the two second order neurons, bipolar and horizontal cells. The transaction of signals takes place in the receptor terminal into which the two second-order cells send their distal processes. Outside the receptor terminals horizontal cells are known to interact with bipolar cells to produce their receptive field surround. Horizontal cells may also interact with the receptors.

This paper summarizes our findings on the functional morphology of the distal layer of the catfish retina which we have been studying since 1968. We will show in this paper that the morphology of the catfish outer layer is similar to but much simpler than other teleost retinas. Signal processing in the outer plexiform layer is essentially linear for the input which is a (random) modulation of a mean illuminance but changes its characteristics to reflect the magnitude of the mean illuminance. This is Rushton's field adaptation in a generalized sense. We suggest that some of the subtle changes are produced through synapses we observe in the outer plexiform layer.

Materials and Methods
Materials used most were retinas from channel catfish, Ictalurus punctatus, but retinas from red-eared turtle, Pseudemys scripta elegans, were also used. Aldehyde fixation and standard procedures were taken for electron microscopy. Recordings were made conventionally and details of analytical procedure can be found elsewhere (Sakuranaga and Naka, 1985).

Morphology
The retina of catfish is shown in Fig. 1a in which the distal most layer, ONL (outer nuclear layer) is occupied by the receptors, and the INL (inner nuclear layer) is occupied by the bipolar, horizontal, and amacrine cells, one of which is marked A in the figure. The most prominent feature of the catfish INL, however, is the horizontal cells which constitute the large part of the layer. Catfish retina is a horizontal-cell preponderate retina. There are two types of horizontal cells, the cone and rod horizontal cells. They send their distal processes into the cone (marked C in Fig. 1b) and rod (marked R in Fig. 1b) receptor terminals. A recent study has indicated that the receptor terminals could be differentiated by the number of synaptic ribbons in the catfish retina; the cone terminals had multiple ribbons and the rod terminals had single ribbon (Hidaka and Christensen, personal communication). Otherwise the two terminals look very similar, although in other retinas their size and location are generally different. Because of the difference in their morphology the cone terminals are referred to as the cone pedicles and the rod terminals as the rod spherules (Sjostrand, 1961: Dowling and Werblin, 1969). The catfish cone terminals are very similar to those seen in other retinas but are much simpler in their organization. This is because the cone terminals are invaginated by one class of horizontal cells which are the luminosity type or red horizontal cells in other teleost retinas (Stell, 1976). This fact makes structural as well as functional analysis of catfish retinal circuit very attractive. Functionally this simple structure is the univariance response in the photopic range (Naka, 1969). There are ribbon synapses, usually less than 4 in a terminal, whose

Neurocircuitry of the Retina, A Cajal Memorial
A. Gallego and P. Gouras, Editors

142

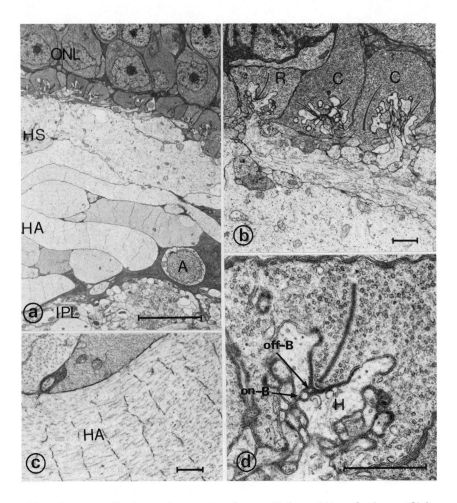

Fig. 1. a: Electron micrograph of a radial section of the catfish retina. ONL ; outer nuclear layer, HS: horizontal-cell soma layer, HA; horizontal-cell axon layer, A: amacrine cell, IPL: inner plexiform layer. Calibration is 10μm.
b: The outer plexiform layer of the catfish retina. Rod terminal (R) contains a single synaptic ribbon and cone terminals (C) multiple ribbons.
c: Cytoplasm of horizontal-cell axons (HA).
d: Synaptic ribbon complex in the rod terminal showing the spatial arrangement among horizontal cell, on-center and off-center bipolar cell processes. H: horizontal cell-B: off-center bipolar cell, on-B: on-center bipolar cell. Calibration is 1 μm for b-d.

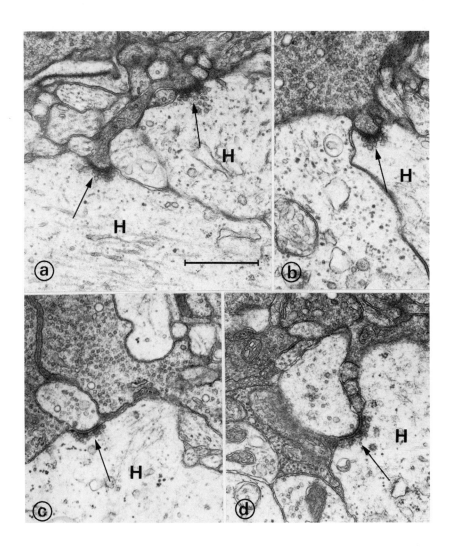

Fig. 2. Electron micrographs of the outer plexiform layer showing
conventional chemical synapses made by the horizontal cell.
Horizontal-cell processes (H) are presynaptic to vesicle-filled dark
processes similar to those found in receptor terminals in (a) and (b), and
presynaptic to bipolar-cell like dendrites in (c) and (d). Calibration is
the same through a-d, 1 μm.

lateral elements are from the cone horizontal cells and the central elements are from the bipolar cells. Generally the processes from the off-center bipolar cells come very close to the synaptic ridge whereas there is always an element, probably processes from off-center bipolar cells, between the synaptic ridge and the processes from the on-center bipolar cells (Sakai and Naka, 1983). In Fig. 1d an example is shown from a rod terminal. This receptor-bipolar cell arrangements have been seen in other teleost retinas (Saito et al, 1983). In catfish most bipolar cells invaginated both the cone and rod terminals. The distal processes from the horizontal cell are very prominent in the terminal and there are characteristic electron-dense particles in the interface between the receptor and horizontal cells.

The horizontal cells have two parts, their soma (HS in Fig. 1A) and axon (HA in Fig. 1A and c). The somas form a layer not unlike a layer of bricks and cement for bricks is gap junctions for the horizontal cells. In other retinas horizontal cells are interconnected through extensive gap junctions (Raviola and Gilula, 1975; Witkovsky et al, 1983). The horizontal cell somas often come into direct contact with the receptor terminals so that in catfish the outer plexiform layer is very poorly developed, a fact noted by Detweiler 40 years ago (Detweiler, 1943). The proximal part of the inner nuclear layer is occupied largely by the axons from the horizontal cell. The horizontal cell axons, which are connected with their somas by a thin fiber (Stell, 1975), have the typical fusiform structure with numerous neurofibriles which run parallel to the longitudinal axis. The axons often come into direct contact with the elements in the inner plexiform layer. It is very possible that the axons form conventional chemical synapses onto the elements in the inner plexiform layer.

In the outer plexiform layer there are two types of conventional chemical synapses characterized by aggregation of synaptic vesicles with specialized synaptic membranes (Sakai and Naka, 1983). One is made by the horizontal soma or dendrites back to the receptor telodendria (Fig. 2a, b) and the other is made by the horizontal cells onto some elements which are very like the bipolar cells (Fig. 2c, d). We believe that the horizontal synapses made onto the receptor terminals mediate the feedback pathway through which the dynamics of horizontal cell themselves were improved. For example a steady field of light, as we will show in the next section, enhances the dynamics of spot response. Most plausible mechanism for such an interaction is through the synapses we have shown here. Polarization of horizontal cells produces changes in the bipolar cells and the transmission is not electrical judging from the transmission's transfer function (Sakuranaga and Naka, 1985). The transmission is either sign inverting (for the off-center bipolar cells) or sign non-inverting (for the on-center bipolar cells). The synapses shown here are the most probable candidate for the transmission.

Physiology

In catfish both the receptor and horizontal cells produce sustained hyperpolarization to step inputs and form monophasic receptive fields which are approximated by a lamina. Naka and Rushton (1967) referred the lamina formed by the horizontal cells as the S-space in honor of Gunnar Svaetichin who discovered potentials from the horizontal cells in 1953 (Svaetichin, 1953). The idea of a space, very unique 20 years ago, has been accepted and many attempts have been made to define it mathematically (Marmarelis and Naka, 1971; Lamb and Simon, 1976). Within the space formed by the horizontal cells current injected into one point within a space evoked almost step-like potential changes, without any delay, from points more than 1 mm away from the site of current injection. Current

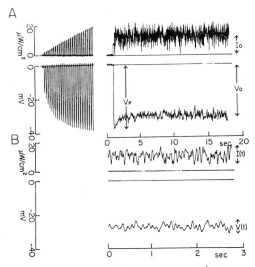

Fig. 3. The responses from a catfish horizontal-cell soma evoked by step and white-noise light (field) stimulus. In A are shown the responses evoked by step inputs whose magnitude was increased in a linear fashion and the initial part of the response evoked by a white-noise light stimulus. In B are shown a part of the steady state response to the white-noise stimulus. In the figure the upper traces were light signals and the lower traces were cellular responses. In B there are two response traces, one actual response and the other the prediction by the first order kernel. The DC and AC components in the stimulus and response are I_o, V_o, $(I(t)$, an $V(t)$. The initial peak is V_p.

injected into the horizontal cell soma produced potential changes in their axon. Thus in the catfish inner nuclear layer there are two spaces, one formed by the somas and the other by axons and two layers are connected electrically (Sakuranaga and Naka, 1985). In turtle there are two spaces but they receive independent inputs from the receptors (Fuortes and Simon, 1974).

In catfish both the cone and horizontal cells produce sustained hyperpolarizations to step inputs (Lasater, 1982; Naka, 1969) and the relationship between the input and the amplitude of the step-evoked responses is Michaelis-Menten, or Naka-Rushton (Naka and Rushton, 1966). This relationship is shown in Fig. 3A in which the responses from the horizontal-cell soma was evoked by a series of step inputs whose amplitude increased in a linear fashion. The contour line formed by the response peaks, Vp, was the Michaelis-Menten equation in a linear plot. The relationship between the amplitude of the step-evoked responses, Vp or Vo, and Io, is the absolute sensitivity (Naka et al, 1979; Sakuranaga and Ando, 1985). The equation or its modification has been used extensively since its conception in 1966 to describe static relationship between light input and responses from distal neurons (Baylor and Fuortes, 1970; Boynton and Whitten, 1970; Normann and Werblin, 1974).

In the natural environment visual stimulus is not a step or flash of light but is a (random) modulation of a mean illuminance which changes according to the time of a day and the season of a year. The depth of modulation is moderate and the changes in mean illuminance are so gradual that we do not notice the changes in our daily life. The absolute sensitivity, therefore, is an artificial measure. More important is a cell's response to modulation around a mean illuminance. One example of white-noise modulate light stimulus is shown in Fig. 3 together with the responses evoked by the stimulus. To a modulation around a mean illuminance horizontal cells, and receptors too, produce a response which is decomposed into two parts, the DC component, V_o, and the AC component, $V(t)$. The DC component is produced by the DC component in light stimulus, the mean illuminance I_o, and the AC component by the modulation, $I(t)$, around the mean. In white-noise analysis it is called the (first order or linear) kernel (Marmarelis and Naka, 1973). Light stimulus, unless it is given in dark, always has a mean on which an increment is imposed. The kernel is, therefore, a cell's incremental sensitivity which includes information on the response dynamics; the kernel is the generalized incremental sensitivity. Knowing the kernel or impulse response, it is possible to predict the cell's response to white-noise inputs. In Fig. 3B there are two response traces, one is the cell's actual response and the other the response predicted by the kernel obtained by crosscorrelation between the input, $I(t)$, and output, $(V(t)$. Except the occasional mismatches the two traces superposed on top of the other. In white-noise analysis the degree of mismatch is expressed by the mean square error (MSE) and the MSE for this particular record was 4.7%. The kernels could predict the response with rather high degree of precision. In other words the response was quite linear.

Changes in the mean illuminance brought forth changes in the kernels' amplitude as well as their waveforms: the (generalized) incremental sensitivity changed with changes in the mean illuminance. This is the field (light) adaptation. In the classical field adaptation only incremental sensitivity which corresponds to the kernel's amplitude was dealt with (Rushton, 1965). The field adaptation we observed through kernels included sensitivity as well as response dynamics. In catfish the amplitude of the kernels (or impulse responses) was the local slope of the Michaelis-Menten curve plotted on a linear scale (Naka et al, 1975). In Fig. 3A it is seen that the local slopes became less steep as the mean illuminance increased. (Note the stimulus had a uniform local slope.) In turtle horizontal cells their incremental sensitivity was Weber-Fechner like (Chappell et al, 1985). With changes in the mean illumiannce the waveforms of the kernels transformed from monophasic into biphasic and their peak response times became shorter. This is shown in Fig. 4 in which kernels were produced for four mean illuminance levels. In the figure the kernels were plotted either in the absolute scale (inA) or were normalized (in B). The numbers 0 through 4 indicate the log density of neutral density filters ehich attenuated the mean illuminance as well as the modulation. The 'depth of modulation' of white-noise stimulus remain unchanged. When the mean illuminance was increased we observed three changes: 1) The amplitude of kernels became smaller, 2) their peak response times became shorter, and 3) their waveform transformed from monphasic into biphasic. The first change was a decrease in the incremental sensitivity with an increase in the mean illuminance. The second and third changes were related to the response dynamics. As the mean was made brighter the cells responded to faster inputs (as indicated by the shorter peak response times) as well to changes in the inputs (as indicated by the biphasic waveform). Advantages in time resolution (frequency response) and sensitivity were balanced. The process of field adaptation is a very complex phenomena whose one facet is changes in the incremental sensitivity.

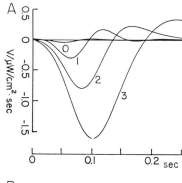

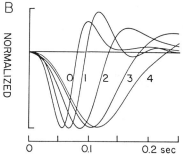

Fig. 4. The kernels from a turtle, Psudemys scripta elegans, horizontal cell obtained at four mean illuminance levels. In A, kernels are plotted on the absolute scale and in B they are normalized. Numbers 0 through 4 are the log neutral density filters interposed. MSEs were 5.5% for 0 log, 7.5% for 1 log, 2.2% for 2 log, 4.2% for 3 log, and 25.5% for 4 log kernels. The large MSEs for brighter inputs were due to the nonlinear component and the large MSE for the 4 log record was due to poor signal-to-noise ratio in the record.

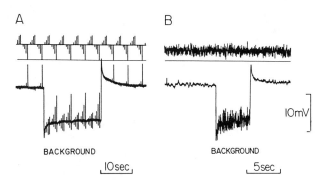

Fig. 5. Effects of a steady background illumination on the dynamics of the spot-evoked responses. The post of light has a diameter of 0.45 mm and the background covered the entire retinal surface. In A the spot was modulated by a series of incremental and decremental steps superposed on a steady illuminance and in B it was modulated by a white-noise signal. The presence of the background is indicated.

The fact that both the receptor and horizontal cells produced a sustained hyperpolarization to a step input posed a problem for neurophysiologists in whose mind hyperpolarization was always associated with some inhibitory process or IPSPs (inhibitory post-synaptic potentials (Slaughter and Miller, 1983). With the horizontal cells this problem can easily be overcome by assuming that potential changes were neutral: the idea of excitation or inhibition is relative to generation of spike discharges and in the other retinal layer where no spike discharge is produced there is no way to tell an excitatory process from an inhibitory process. Another problem associated with the horizontal cells is the problem of surround which has always been associated with the idea of lateral inhibition. Surround does not always act to suppress the center response and one example is shown in Fig. 5. In the experiments shown in the figure, the test stimulus was a spot of light, 0.45 mm in diameter, whose illuminance was modulated by incremental or decremental steps from a mean in 'A' and by a white-noise signal in 'B'. With a spot stimulus alone the horizontal cell responded poorly to these modulations. In the middle of traces in A and B a large steady field of light was added (indicated by BACKGROUND) while the spot stimuli were kept unchanged. The large background light produced a large steady hyperpolarization as we would expect from the idea of the S-space. What we did not expect was the great increase in the spot response to the in- or decrements or to white-noise modulation. A steady background greatly increased the incremental sensitivity of catfish horizontal cell. Under similar experimental conditions receptors did not show such dramatic increase in their incremental sensitivity (Kawasaki et al, 1984) and a similar increase in the incremental sensitivity was also seen in the turtle horizontal cells (Chappell et al, 1985). In the lower-vertebrate horizontal cells the central and surround regions act in a synergic fashion to increment the cell's incremental sensitivity. This increase in the incremental sensitivity could have been produced through the synapses made by the horizontal cells onto the receptor terminals (Sakai and Naka, 1983).

Bipolar cells on the other hand form biphasic or concentric receptive fields in which stimulation of the center and surround produced responses of opposing polarity. Receptive field profiles of both the on- and off-center bipolar cells are shown in Fig. 6 in which the cells' receptive field profiles were produced either by a sweeping bar or light or travelling random grating. The profiles plotted by the bar of light included the nonlinear interaction whereas those produced by crosscorrelation method (for the travelling random grating) were only for the linear part. The receptive field profiles produced by these two methods were very similar to show that no complex nonlinear interaction was involved in the generation of bipolar cells' biphasic (concentric) receptive fields (Davis and Naka, 1980). In some proximal neurons two methods produced very different receptive field profiles. Temporal inputs have also shown that the cells' response were quite linear (Naka et al, 1975). Current injected into the horizontal cell soma not axon produced potential changes in the bipolar cells. A depolarization of horizontal cell soma produced a depolarizing response from on-center bipolar cells and a hyperpolarizing response from off-center bipolar cells. The signal transmission from the horizontal to bipolar cell was also quite linear (Sakuranaga and Naka, 1985).

Bipolar cells, therefore, receive two independent inputs, one from a small number of receptors and the other from the horizontal cell soma. The former input produced the receptive field center and the latter receptive field surround. The signal transmission is either through sign inverting or sign no-inverting (sign conserving) synapses and that the

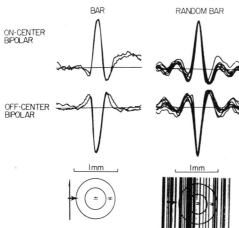

Fig. 6. Receptive field profiles of catfish bipolar cells plotted by a single moving bar and travelling random bars. In single bar data, individual traces were an average of seven repeated sweeps and the two traces for each cell were for the forward and reverse directions of the bar's sweep. In random bar data 10 correlograms from 10 cells were superposed. Receptive field profiles plotted by the two stimuli were similar and those from the on- and off-center cells were mirror images of each other.

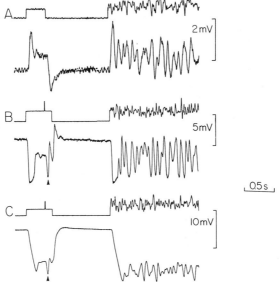

Fig. 7. Responses from catfish on- (A) and off-center (B) bipolar cells and a horizontal cell. Stimulus was a field of light with step or white noise modulation. In B and C the step of light had a superposed increment which produced incremental responses marked by arrows. The horizontal cell response had a large DC component, V_o, and a small AC component, $V(t)$. In bipolar cell the AC components, $V(t)$, were much larger compared with the DC components. The incremental response was biphasic in the bipolar cell.

signals in the horizontal cells are not excitatory or inhibitory; the signal is neutral as already suggested by Naka (1976). The idea of synaptic transmission without inhibitory or excitatory action has been generally accepted (Schaffer et al, 1982; Attwell et al, 1983). The direct inputs to the bipolar cells from the receptors are the local changes in illuminance and the horizontal cell inputs are the average of such changes over a large area produced by the S-space and are the global signal. In the bipolar cells difference between the two signals are produced to remove the large DC component, V_o, arising from the steady mean illuminance, I (Naka and Nye, 1971). In the other retinas horizontal cells are also thought to provide the receptive field surround of bipolar cells (Werblin and Dowling, 1969; Thibos and Werblin, 1978).

In catfish current injected into the horizontal cell soma, as in some other teleost and turtle retinas produced responses from the bipolar cells either through a sign-inverting or noninverting synapses (Marchiafava, 1978; Toyoda and Tonosaki, 1978; Toyoda and Kujiraoka, 1982). Through this arrangement the large DC potential in the horizontal and (receptors) is removed. This is shown in Fig. 7 in which responses from an on- and an off-center bipolar cells and a horizontal cell were evoked either by steps from dark or by a white-noise modulated light. It is seen that the large DC component, V_o, in the horizontal cell response is removed in the bipolar cell responses and that the cells were responding more vigorously to the modulation, I(t), and less to the mean, I_o, of the white-noise stimulus.

Conclusions

Catfish outer retinal layer shares the basic structural features with other retinas but is much simpler in structural as well as functional organization because there is only one class of cone horizontal cells and because the retina does not perform any complex chromatic information processing. The simple structure enabled us to identify two (chemical) synapses made by the horizontal-cell soma onto the receptor terminal and bipolar-cell dendrites. Signal processing in the outer layer is essentially linear but the response dynamics change with changes in the mean illuminance so that the cells responded optimally to modulation around a given mean. Experimental results show that the piecewise linearization was achieved by an active process (Chapell et al, 1985). What we have described in this paper is an extended version of the field adaptation originally conceived by Rushton (1965) and we propose to refer to the set of changes as the Rushtonian transformation to honor his imaginative contribution to our idea of adaptation. Another feature of the signal transmission in outer layer is that the transmissions are not in terms of excitation or inhibition. Transmission and synaptic interactions are through sign inverting or noninverting syanpses and results are subtraction of common mode signal (in bipolar cells) or an improvement in the frequency response (in horizontal cells). Signals in the horizontal cells are not excitatory or inhibitory but are neutral. Interpretation of morphology and physiology of the outer retinal layer must be made based on an entirely new concept.

Acknowledgements
Some of the data presented here were obtained in collaboration with Drs. M. Kawasaki and R.L. Chappell. We also thank Dr. M. Sakuranagan for the use of white-noise analysis routine.

References
Attwell, D., Werblin, S.F., Wilson, M. and Wu, S.M. J. Physiol. Lond. <u>336,</u> 313-333 (1983).
Baylor, D.A. and Fuortes, M.G.F. J. Physiol Lond. <u>207,</u> 77-92 (1970).

Boynton, R.M. and Whitten, D.N. Science 170, 1423-1626 (1970).
Chappell, R.L, Naka, K.-I and Sakuranaga, M. J. gen. Physiol (1985).
Davis, G.W. and Nkaa, K.-I. J. Neurophysiol. 43, 807-831 (1980).
Detweiler, S.R. Vertebrate photoreceptors, Macmillan, New York (1943).
Dowling, J.E. and Werblin, F.S. J. Neurophysiol. 32, 315-338 (1969).
Fuortes, M.G.F. and Simon, F.J. J. Physiol. Lond 240, 177-198 (1974).
Kawasaki, M., Aoki, K. and Naka, K.-I Vis. Res. in press (1984).
Lamb, T.D. and Simon, E.J. J. Physiol Lond 263, 257-286 (1976).
Lasater, E.M. J. Neurophysiol 47, 1057-1068 (1982).
Marchiafava, P.L. Nature 275, 141-142 (1978).
Marmarelis, P.Z. and Naka, K.-I. Biophys. J. 12, 1515-1532 (1973).
Naka, K.-I. Biophys. J. 9, 845-859 (1969).
Naka, K.-I. and Rushton, W.A.H. J. Physiol Lond. 185, 536-555 (1966).
Naka, K.-I. and Rushton, W.A.H. J. Physiol Lond. 192, 437-461 (1967).
Naka, K.-I., Nye, P.W. J. Neurophysiol 34, 785-801 (1971).
Naka, K.-I., Marmarelis, P.Z. and Chan, R.Y. J. Neurophysiol. 38, 92-131 (1975).
Normann, R.A. and Werblin, F.S. J. gen. Physiol. 63, 37-61 (1974).
Raviola, E. and Gilula, N.B. J. Cell Biol. 65, 191-222 (1975).
Rushton, W.A.H. Proc. Roy. Soc. B 162, 20-46 (1965).
Saito, T., Kujiraoka, T. and Yonaha, T. Vis. Res. 23, 353-362 (1983).
Sakai, H. and Naka, K.-I. Vis. Res. 23, 339-352 (1983).
Sakuranaga, M. and Naka, K.-I. J. Neurophysiol (in press) (1985).
Sakuranaga, M. and Ando, Y.-I. Vis. Res. in press (1985).
Schaffer, S.F., Raviola, E and Heuser, J.E. J. Comp. Neurol. 204, 253-267 (1982).
Sjostrand, F.S. in The Structure of the Eye (Academic Press, New York, 1961) pp. 1-28.
Slaughter, M.M. and Miller, R.F. Science 219, 1230-1232 (1983).
Stell, W.K. J. Comp. Neurol. 159, 503-520 (1975).
Stell, W.K. Invest. Ophthal. 15, 895-908 (1976).
Svaetichin, G. Acta Physiol. Scand. 29, Suppl 106, 565-600 (1978).
Thibos, L.N. and Werblin, F.S. J. Physiol Lond. 278, 79-99 (1978).
Toyoda, J. and Tonosaki, K. Nature 276, 399-400 (1978).
Toyoda, J. and Kjiraoka, T. J. gen. Physiol, 27, 131-145 (1982).
Werblin, F.S. and Dowling, J.E. J. Neurophysiol. 32, 339-355 (1969).
Witkovsky, P., Owen, W.G. and Woodworth, M. J. Comp. Neurol. 216, 359-368 (1983).

Neurotransmitters in the Retina of the Mudpuppy

Necturus Maculosus

A. Bruun, B. Ehinger and K. Tornqvist
Department of Ophthalmology
University of Lund
Lund, Sweden

Stable recordings can be relatively easy to obtain from cells in the mudpuppy retina because they are comparatively large and easily impaled with glass microelectrodes. The mudpuppy retina was therefore used already early on in studies on the electrophysiology of the retina, and it has subsequently been thoroughly studied by many investigators (Dowling and Werblin 1971; Wachtmeister and Dowling 1978; Wachtmeister 1980; Miller et al, 1981, 1982; Slaughter and Miller 1981, 1983a,b; Belgum et al, 1982).

Dopaminergic and indoleamine accumulating cells are known in the mudpuppy retina (Adolph et al, 1980). In addition, electrophysiological results have suggested that glycine and GABA are possible neurotransmitters in amacrine cells (Miller et al, 1977) as in most other animal species, and there are also reports suggesting that substance P and enkephalins may affect the neurotransmission in amacrines (Dick and Miller, Millet et al, 1981). This paper attempts to summarize the current knowledge of the localization of neurotransmitters in the mudpuppy retina and to compare it with what is known in other animals.

Methods

Studies on the neurotransmitter localization in the mudpuppy retina have involved formaldehyde induced fluorescence according to Falck and Hillarp, autoradiography and immunohistochemistry (Adolph et al, 1980 Bruun et al, 1985). Enzyme histochemistry has not been used to any significant extent, nor have microdissections or chemical assays of extracts. Exact identification of neurotransmitters is therefore not available at the present time.

The formaldehyde fluorescence method of Falck and Hillarp readily demonstrate endogenous catecholamines. Whenever chemical assays have been performed in other animal species the main catecholamine in the retina has been found to be dopamine (Ehinger 1982). There are therefore reasons to presume that dopamine is the main catecholamine also in mudpuppies.

Some simple amino acids like glycine, GABA, aspartic acid or glutamic acid are presumed to be neurotransmitters in the central nervous system and also in the retina of many species (Ehinger 1982). It is not yet possible to demonstrate the localization of the endogenous amino acid with direct methods. However, autoradiography can be used, because nerve cells often have a very active and specific uptake mechanism for their neurotransmitter which is then also effectively retained in unchanged form. Cells accumulating and storing (^{3}H)-GABA and (^{3}H)-glycine have been localized with this procedure in the mudpuppy. It should be noted that these amino acids can also be accumulated for reasons which may have little to do with neurotransmission.

Immunohistochemistry is the most recent procedure used for the localization of neurotransmitters. It is particularly useful for identifying substances of moderate to high molecular weight, such as the neuropeptides. The specificity of the reaction should always be examined carefully because the antibodies react with a given sequence of amino acid residues, whenever it occurs. In the worst case, a given antibody will

Neurocircuitry of the Retina, A Cajal Memorial
A. Gallego and P. Gouras, Editors

therefore demonstrate two widely different peptides equally well. On the other hand, minor variations in the structure of a peptide may not be of much consequence for its function, and if the antibody is also indifferent to this variation, meaningful results can be obtained also when the antibody "makes a mistake".

To test the specificity of the antisera the following controls were made: 1) 5-hydroxytryptamine antiserum diluted 1:500 was preincubated for 36 h at +4°C with a 30 mM solution of 5-hydroxytryptamine and related indoleamines; 2) The different peptide antisera in the appropriate dilutions were preincubated for 24 h with the respective antigen in excess (10-100 µg/ml). Only staining abolished by preincubation with the antigen was regarded as specific.

Mudpuppies of 20-30 cm total length were used in the studies summarized here. They were light adapted when killed.

Autoradiography
5 µCi (^{3}H)-glycine (1 µCi/ul) or 10 µCi (^{3}H)-GABA (1 µCi/ul) was injected intravitreally with precision syringes. After 2 h (^{3}H)-glycine) or 4 h ((^{3}H)-GABA), the animals were decapitated and the eyes were excised and processed for autoradiography.

It has been shown that accumulated glycine and GABA are metabolized only to a minor extent in the retina of both mammals and heterotherms (Goodchild and Neal 1970; Ehinger and Falck, 1971; Voaden et al 1974; Chin and Lam 1980). The distribution of radioactivity can therefore be regarded as representing mainly unchanged amino acid in stable cellular stores.

Results
In the following descriptions, the inner plexiform layer has for convenience been arbitrarily subdivided into five sublaminae of equal width. Such a sublamination is well accepted for many species, but has previously not been seen in the mudpuppy.

Dopamine
Fibers displaying the characteristic catecholamine fluorescence were seen in a close-meshed lattice in sublamina 1 of the inner plexiform layer, at the border to the inner nuclear layer (Fig. 1). As noted, dopamine is likely to be the main catecholamine, although this has not been directly established in the mudpuppy. Occasionally, individual fibers could be followed for several hundred microns. At times, fibers were also seen in other parts of the inner plexiform layer and very rarely as far out as the outer plexiform layer.

Cell bodies with catecholamine fluorescence were seen in the innermost part of the inner nuclear layer emitting the branches described above.

(^{3}H)-Glycine
Many amacrine cells accumulated (^{3}H)-glycine. There was also diffuse radioactivity throughout the inner plexiform layer, without any distinct sublayering (Fig. 1). Different amacrine cells were seen to have either high or low radioactivity, but there were also many cells with intermediate degrees of labelling. The most heavily labelled cells were usually seen in the middle of the inner nuclear layer but a few were also seen in the innermost part of the inner nuclear layer, next to the inner plexiform layer.

154

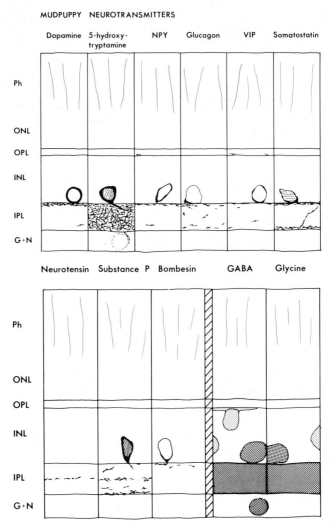

Fig. 1 Schematic representation of the distribution of neurons with different putative neurotransmitters. Dopamine was demonstrated with formaldehyde histofluorescence, GABA and glycine by uptake of the tritiated amino acid followed by autoradiography, and the others with immunohistochemistry. The resolution of autoradiography is less than with the other methods, and regions labelled by radioactive GABA or glycine are therefore stippled and do not show individual neuron processes. The two densities of stippling represent approximate differences in radioactivity. Ph, photoreceptor cells; ONL, outer nuclear layer; OPL, outer plexiform layer; INL, inner nuclear layer; IPL, inner plexiform layer; G+N, ganglion cell and nerve fiber layers.

A small proportion (about 5-10%) of the ganglion cells became radioactive; at times as much as the most radioactive amacrine cells, but usually less.

Glial Muller cells became only weakly radioactive, and with the exceptions already noted, there was no special accumulation of radioactivity in the outer plexiform layer or in the photoreceptors.

(^{3}H)-GABA

About 90% of the ganglion cells became strongly or moderately labeled by (^{3}H)-GABA. Radioactivity was also seen in cells in the middle and innermost parts of the inner nuclear layer (Fig. 1). The degree of labeling varied considerably. A subclass consisting of three to five strongly labeled cells per cross section of the eye could usually be distinguished in the innermost half of the inner nuclear layer. The inner plexiform layer also became homogeneously radioactive but at times with somewhat more radioactivity in its innermost part.

Horizontal cells (Fig. 1) were usually not well visible except after high doses of (^{3}H)-GABA and/or long exposure times, resulting in overexposure of structures in the inner half of the retina. The cell bodies were located in the outer row and their processes formed a sublayer in the outer plexiform layer. They may correspond to the H1 type in goldfish.

5-Hydroxytryptamine

Immunoreactive, fine varicose fibers were common throughout the inner plexiform layer without any distinct sublayering (Fig. 1). Occasionally fine varicose fibers could also be seen to reach into the ganglion cell layer encircling a ganglion cell. Only once in several hundred sections has a fiber been seen in the inner nuclear layer. No 5-hydroxytryptamine immunoreactivity was seen in any layer further outwards.

Immunoreactive cell bodies were seen (one or two per cross section of the whole eye) among the amacrine cells. They were comparatively large, but with only little cytoplasm like other amacrine cells in the mudpuppy. Rarely immunoreactive cells were also seen in the ganglion cell layer. They were of the same size as other ganglion cells and were seen to send their processes into the inner plexiform layer.

Neuropeptide Y (NPY)

Fine, varicose NPY-immunoreactive fibers appeared in a loose layer in sublamina 1 of the inner plexiform layer and in cell bodies with the position of amacrine cells (Fig. 1). Occasionally NPY-immunoreactive fibers were also found further inward in the inner plexiform layer. Rarely some fine varicose NPY-immunoreactive fibers were seen the outer plexiform layer (Fig. 1). No fibers were seen in the other layers of the retina.

Cell bodies with a narrow rim of NPY-immunoreactive cytoplasm appeared among the amacrine cells with a frequency of one, two or, rarely three per cross section of the eye (Fig. 1).

Glucagon

Glucagon-immunoreactive fibers appeared in sublaminae 1 and 5 of the inner plexiform layer and occasionally also in other sublayers (Fig. 1). Characteristically, the fibers were fine and tortuous and formed only rather indistinct sublayers.

One or two immunoreactive cell bodies were seen per cross section of the eye, among the amacrine cells. They showed immunoreactivity throughout their narrow rim of cytoplasm most intense in the parts facing the inner plexiform layer (Fig. 1).

A few immunoreactive cells were seen in the ganglion cell layer. Their general appearance was similar to that of the immunoreactive cells among the amacrine cells and they were seen to send their processes at least to sublayer 5. It was not possible to establish whether they also sent processes to other sublayers.

VIP (Vasoactive Intestinal Peptide)

Only weakly immunoreactive fibers were detected; the majority in sublamina 1 of the inner plexiform layer but also some in its other sublayers. In a few sites, immunoreactive fibers were also seen in the outer plexiform layer (Fig. 1). Only a few cell bodies were detected all along the amacrine cells and rather weakly fluorescing.

Somatostatin

Sublaminae 1 and 5 of the inner plexiform layer contained numerous fine, varicose somatostatin-immunoreactive fibers (Fig. 1). Fibers could also occasionally be seen in the other sublayers. No fibers were detected in the inner nuclear layer or any other layer further outward.

The somatostatin-immunoreactive fibers issued from immunoreactive cell bodies with the position of amacrine cells, up to three per cross section of the eye. A few immunoreactive cell bodies were also detected further outwards, roughly as far as to the middle of the inner nuclear layer.

Somatostatin-immunoreactive cell bodies were also detected among the ganglion cells and were seen to send fine varicose fibers to both sublaminae 1 and 5 in the inner plexiform layer. They were not seen to send any fiber to the nerve fiber layer.

Neurotensin

There was a sparse layer of fine, varicose neurotensin-immunoreactive fibers in sublamina 3 of the inner plexiform layer (Fig. 1). Fibers were rarely seen in sublaminae 1 and 5. Cell bodies were not seen.

Substance P

Sublamina 3 of the inner plexiform layer contained substance P-immunoreactive fibers in a rather dense lattice. Additional fibers were common in sublaminae 4 and 5, so that most of the immunoreactive fibers appeared in the inner half of the inner plexiform layer (Fig. 1). The fiber density of the different sublayers was somewhat variable.

Every cross section of the eye contained three to five substance P-immunoreactive cell bodies among the amacrine cells (Fig. 1). More rarely they were seen in the middle of the inner nuclear layer. The immunoreactive fibers of the inner plexiform layer were seen to emit from the perikarya without any hillock.

Substance P-immunoreactive cell bodies were also found among the ganglion cells. They were of the same general appearance as the immunoreactive amacrine cells and they sent their processes to the inner parts of the inner plexiform layer where they mingled indistinguishably with the processes from the immunoreactive amacrine cells. They were not seen to send any process to the nerve fiber layer.

Bombesin
       A few, thin bombesin-immunoreactive varicose fibers were observed in
sublamina 1 in the inner plexiform layer and cell bodies were seen in the
innermost part of the inner nuclear layer. The immunoreactivity was
concentrated to the dendrite hillock of the perikaryon.

Discussion
       The   histochemical   methods   for   demonstrating   the   various
neurotransmitters have all proven themselves useful in studies on many
species (Ehinger 1982). Nevertheless, it is worth re-emphasizing that
none of them by itself offers conclusive evidence that given substance is
a retinal neurotransmitter. Therefore, comparisons must always be made
with physiological, biochemical, pharmacological, or morphological results
obtained with independent methods.

       As already commented on, dopamine is the main catecholamine likely to
be present also in the mudpuppy retina. In most species, the dopaminergic
retinal neurons are a subclass of stratified amacrine cells (Ehinger
1982). Usually, the fibers are found in sublaminae 1, 3 and 5 in the
inner plexiform layer of heterotherm animals, and the the mudpuppy is
therefore somewhat unusual in this respect, having the dopaminergic
terminals almost exclusively in sublamina 1. Remarkably, this is the
organization seen in primates and some other mammals.

       There are good reasons to regard dopamine as a neurotransmitter in the
retina of all vertebrates (Ehinger 1982). However, its precise function
is not well known and the results with the mudpuppy suggest that this
animal should be useful for further investigations.

       Immunohistochemical methods have the advantage of demonstrating
directly the endogenous content of the substance under investigation. The
distribution of 5-hydroxytryptamine and various peptides has in the
mudpuppy been analyzed with this technique in our laboratory. However,
the selectivity of the antibody used in immunohistochemical work should
always be carefully examined. The 5-hydroxytryptamine antibody used for
the studies on the mudpuppy retina is the same as that used for many other
studies on tissues from the central nervous system in many species. It is
known to cross react to some extent with certain 5-hydroxytryptamine-like
substances   such   as   6-hydroxytryptamine,   5,6-dihydroxytryptamine,
5,7-dihydroxytryptamine, or bufotenine (Steinbush et al 1978; Steinbush
1981; Tornqvist et al 1983). However, these substances have not been
demonstrated as normal tissue constituents and are therefore usually
disregarded.

       Indoleamine accumulating neurons were previously demonstrated with
5,6-dihydroxytryptamine uptake and formaldehyde induced fluorescence
(Adolph et al 1980). The picture now obtained with immunohistochemistry
in normal animals is identical with the uptake studies. Biochemically,
5-hydroxytryptamine has also been detected in heterotherms (lizards,
frogs, and goldfish; Osborn 1982; Osborn et al 1982; Tornqvist et al
1983). There are thus good reasons to presume that the mudpuppy retina
also contains 5-hydroxytryptamine and that the distribution of the
5-hydroxytryptamine neurons is that described above.

       The function of the 5-hydroxytryptamine neurons in the retina is not
well known in any species. At present there can therefore be no
meaningful inferences concerning the mudpuppy.

       Glycine and GABA are now well accepted as neurotransmitters in the
brain and there is much evidence to suggest the same is the case for the

retina (Ehinger 1982). In the mudpuppy glycine and glycine antagonists were shown to affect the oscillatory potentials (Wachtmeister and Dowling 1978; Wachtmeister 1980) and other electrophysiological results suggests that glycinergic amacrine neurons are both of the OFF and the ON-OFF types (Cunningham and Miller 1980a,b; Frumkes et al 1981).

Autoradiography is the only practical method currently available for demonstrating cells that may use glycine or GABA as neurotransmitters. The uptake may well be an indicator also for other processes than neurotransmission because both amino acids participate extensively in the general metabolism of the cells. There are several examples that illustrate this (^{3}H)-GABA is not very useful as a marker in many mammals because all cells, glia included become radioactive. Only in a few species is the metabolism sufficiently faster in glial cells to make the radioactivity in them disappear first, so that $_3$(^{3}H)-GABA can be successfully used for labelling (Ehinger 1977). (^{3}H)-isoguvacine or, perhaps, (^{3}H)-muscimol may be better alternatives in certain species.

$_3$ Another example of the problems encountered with (^{3}H)-GABA and ^{3}H)glycine is the labelling of ganglion cells by the amino acids. This is seen also in the mudpuppy. Glycine and GABA are not likely to be neurotransmitters in these cells, and it would therefore seem that the ganglion cell labelling is not directly related to the as yet unknown neurotransmitter in these neurons. Similarly, many different classes of cells in the inner nuclear layer have been seen to be labelled with these amino acid if used in sufficiently high concentrations (Pourcho 1980, Freed et al 1983). Finally, it has recently been cliamed that (^{3}H)-GABA in reality labels the postsynaptic cell rather than the presynaptic one (Yazulla and Kleinschmidt 1983; Zucker et 1984), but there are also suggestions to the contrary (see paper by W.K. Stell in this book). Perhaps, technical problems such as different fixation protocols lie behind the contradictions. In any case, they clearly illustrate the difficulties with uptake studies.

$_3$ Despite the technical questions concerning the (^{3}H)-GABA or (^{3}H)-glycine uptake studies, the substances will label neurons from which they can again be released by light stimulation (Ehinger 1982). Most likely, therefore, GABAergic and glycinergic cells are to be found among the ones labelled by the respective amino acid.

(^{3}H)-glycine labels the whole of the inner plexiform layer, i.e. both the outer OFF and the inner ON layer. Electrophysiological studies suggest that there are glycinergic ON and ON-OFF neurons in mudpuppies (Cunningham and Miller 1980a,b; Frumkes et al 1981). If there are no glycinergic OFF neurons, the number of ON-OFF neurons must be comparatively high in order to explain why there is uniform labelling of the inner plexiform layer.

The labelling with (^{3}H)-GABA in the mudpuppy is similar to that seen in goldfish where large pyriform amacrine cells also become labelled. These cells have been identified as red-depolarizing (OFF), sustained cells (Marc et al, 1978). In the mudpuppy both amacrine and ganglion cells are affected by GABA, and GABA receptors must consequently be present (Miller et al 1981b). The electrophysiological results suggest GABA to involved mainly in the ON pathways, but also in ON-OFF neurons (Frumkes et al, 1981). The oscillatory potentials are also sensitive to GABA and GABA antagonists (Waxhtmeister and Dowling 1978; Wachtmeister 1980).

The situation is slightly different in the outer plexiform layer (Marc 1978). In goldfish, GABA is presumed to be neurotransmitter in horizontal cells associated with the red channel. However, in mudpuppy, electrophysiological work has failed to show any effect at the level of horizontal cells (Miller et al 1981a,b; Frumkes et al 1981). Instead an unidentified cell, called the G-cell, responded to GABA. The function of GABA in the mudpuppy outer plexiform layer clearly remains to be established.

The morphological and electrophysiological results thus all agree with what is known from other species and permit the suggestion that glycine and GABA are neurotransmitters also in the mudpuppy retina, most likely in subclasses of amacrine cells.

Somatostatin, cholecystokinin, enkephalins, substance P, VIP and glucagon have been identified chromatographically in extracts from the retina of different species (Humbert et al 1979; Rorstad et al 1979; Yamada et al 1980, 1981; Eskay et al 1981; Sagar et al 1982; Eskay and Beinfeld 1982; Ekman and Tornqvist 1985). Immunohistochemical analyses have suggested several more neuropeptides. The list of neuropeptides demonstrated in the mudpuppy retina is therefore not unusual. It currently comprises NPY, glucagon, VIP, somatostatin, neurotensin, substance P, enkephalins, cholecystokinin, and bombesin (Brecha et al 1984).

It is far from clear how the presence of the many neuropeptides in the retina should be interpreted. The following comments on the enkephalins may serve an example of the problem.

Enkephalinamide (a degradation resistant enkephalin agonist) was found to depress the ganglion cell firing in mudpuppy, but the effect could not be blocked by naloxone like a proper opioid response is expected to be (Dick and Miller 1981; Miller et al, 1982). On the other hand, the number of enkephalin neurons currently demonstrable is quite small. In goldfish, electrophysiological experiments demonstrated an enkephalin system (Djamgoz et al 1981) but only few neurons are presently demonstrable, like in the mudpuppy. Enkephalins have also been reported to modulate the release of (^{3}H)-dopamine from rabbit retinae (Dubocovich and Weiner 1983), but the only mammal in which significant numbers of enkephalin neurons have been seen is guinea-pig, and then only with a special antiserum, RA143 (Altschuler et al 1982, Ehinger and Tornqvist unpublished). There is thus a discrepancy between physiological or pharmacological and morphological results not only in the mudpuppy but in many other species, suggesting that retinal enkephalins may form quite a complex system.

Acknowledgements
      This work was supported by grants from the Thorsten and Elsa Segerfalk's Foundation, The Magn. Bergwall's Foundation, the A.O. Sward's Foundation, the Swedish Society for Medical Research, the Anna Lisa and Sven-Erik Lundgrens Stiftelse, the Helfrid and Lorenz Nilsson's Foundaion, the Faculty of Medicine, University of Lund and the Swedish Medical Research Council (Project 14X2321).

160

References
Adolph, A, Dolwing, J.E., Ehinger, B. Cell Tiss. Res. 210, 269-282 (1980).
Alm, P., Alumets, J., Hakanson, R., Owman, Ch., Sjoberg, N.O. Walles, B. Cell Tiss. Res. 205, 337-347 (1980).
Altschuler, R.A., Mosinger, J.L., Hoffman, D.V. Parakkal, M.H. Proc. Natl. Acad. Sci. USA 79, 2398-2400 (1982).
Belgum D.H, Dvorak, D.R., McReynolds, J.S. J. Physiol 326, 91-108 (1982).
Brecha, N. Eldred, W., Kuljis, R.O., Karten, H.J. Prog. Ret. Res. 3, 185-226.
Chin, C-A., Lam, DM-K J. Physiol. 308, 185-195 (1980).
Cunningham, R., Miller, R.F. Brain Res. 197, 123-138 (1980a).
Cunningham, R., Miller, R.F. Brain Res. 197, 139-151 (1980b).
Djamgoz, M.B.A., Stell, W.K., Chin, Ch-A, Lam, D.M.K. Nature 292, 620-623 (1981).
Dick, E., Miller, R.F. Neurosci. Letters 26, 131-135 (1981).
Dolwing, J.E., Werblin, F.S. Vis. Res. Supl. 3, 1-15 (1971).
Dubocovich, M.L. Weiner, N. J. Pharmacol. Exp. Ther. 114, 634-639 (1983).
Ehinger, B., Falch, B. Brain Res. 33, 157-172 (1971).
Ekman, R. Tornqvist, K. Invest. Ophthal. Vis. Sci. submitted (1984).
Eskay, R.L., Beinfeld, M.C. Brain Res. 246, 315-318 (1982).
Eskay, R.L., Furness, J.F., Long, R.T. Science 212, 1049-1050 (1981).
Freed, M.A., Nakamura, Y. Sterling, P. J. Comp. Neurol 219, 295-304 (1983).
Frumkes, T.E., Miller, R.F., Slaughter, M., Dacheux, R.F. J. Neurophysiol. 45, 783-804 (1981).
Goodchild, F., Neal, M.J. J. Physiol 210, 182-183 (1970).
Humbert, J., Pradelles, P., Gros, C., Dray, F. Neurosci. Letters 12, 259-263 (1979).
Marc, R.E., Stell, W.K., Bok, D. Lam, DM-K. J. Comp. Neurol. 182, 221-246 (1978).
Miller, R.F., Dacheux, R.F., Frumkes, T.E. Science 198, 748-750 (1977).
Miller, R.F., Frumkes, T.E., Slaughter, M., Frumkes, T.E. J. Neurophysiol. 45, 743-763 (1981a).
Miller, R.F., Frumkes, T.E., Slaughter, M., Frumkes, T.E. J. Neurophysiol. 45, 764-782 (1981b).
Miller, R.F., Slaughter, M.M., Dick, E. in Neurotransmitter interaction and compartmentation. (H.F. Bradford ed, Plenum Press, New York 1982) pp 735-752.
Osborne, N.N. in Biology of Serotonergic Transmission. N.N. Osborne ed, John Wiley & Sons, Chichester, New York, Brisbane, Toronto, Singagpore 1982) pp. 401-430.
Osborne, N.N., Nesselhut, T., Nicholas, D.A., Patel, S., Cuello, A-C. J. Neurochem. 39, 1519-1528 (1982).
Pourcho, R.G. Brain Res. 198, 333-346 (1980).
Rorstad, O.P., Brownstein, M.J., Proc. Natl. Acad. Sci. USA 76, 3019-3023 (1979).
Sagar, S.M., Rorstad, O.O., Landis, D.M.D., Arnold, M.A., Martin, J.B. Brain, Res. 244, 91-99 (1982).
Slaughter, M.M., Miller, R.F. Science 211, 182 (1981).
Slaughter, M.M., Miller, R.F. Science 219, 1230-1232 (1983a).
Slaughter, M.M., Miller, R.F. J. Neurosci. 3, 1701-1711 (1983b).
Steinbush, H.W.M., Verhofstad, A.A.J., Joosten, H.W.J. Neurosci. 3, 811-819 (1978).
Tornqvist, K., Hansson, Ch, Ehinger, B. Neurochem. Internatl. 5, 299-308 (1983).
Voaden, M.J., Marshall, J., Murani, N. Brain Res. 67, 115-132 (1974).
Wachtmeister, L. Acta Ophthalmol. (Copenhagen) 58, 712-725 (1980).
Wachtmeister, L., Dowling, J.E. Invest. Ophthal. Vis. Sci. 17, 1176-1188 (1978).

Pyriform Ab Amacrine Cells in the Goldfish Retina:
an EM Immunocytochemical/Autoradiographical Study

S. Yazulla, C.L. Zucker, J.L. Mosinger, K.M. Studholme
Department of Neurobiology and Behavior
State University of New York
Stony Brook, N. Y. 11794

An important problem in neurobiology is the identification of neurotransmitter interactions involving specific populations of neurons. One such population is the pyriform Ab amacrine cell in the goldfish retina. This cell type consists of a large cell body, a descending process and an extensive dendritic plexus restricted to the most proximal portion of the inner plexiform layer (IPL). Cajal (1933) described two subtypes of pyriform Ab amacrine cell which he referred to as amacrine cells of the fifth level. Though very similar, the two types appeared to differ in the thickness of the descending and distal dendrites (Fig. 1). Ab amacrine cells are labeled by markers associated with two putative neurotransmitters: gamma aminobutyric acid (GABA) and a peptide, somatostatin. Ab amacrine cells take up 3H-GABA with high affinity (Marc et al, 1978) and show somatostatin-like (SL) immunoreactivity (IR) (Yamada et al 1980). It is possible that 3H-GABA uptake and SLIR are restricted to each of the two subtypes of Ab amacrine cell described by Cajal (1933). Alternatively, Yamada et al (1980) advanced the suggestion that 3H-GABA uptake and SLIR may co-localize in the same Ab amacrine cells. This was an exciting idea considering the increasing examples of co-localization of markers for conventional neurotransmitters and neuropeptides (Lundberg and Hokfelt, 1983).

The observation that pyriform Ab amacrine cells take up 3H-GABA and that this uptake appears to be affected by lighting conditions has led to the suggestion that these Ab amacrine cells are GABAergic (Marc et al 1978). However, Zucker et al (1984) found that only 18% of the amacrine cell processes that show immunoreactivity to glutamic acid decarboxylase (GAD) also take up 3H-GABA. Since GAD is the biosynthetic enzyme for GABA, these data suggested that high affinity uptake of 3H-GABA per se was not a sufficient criterion to identify GABAergic neurons, at least not for goldfish amacrine cells. However, we did not identify the population of double labeled processes and thus, did not rule out the possibility that processes of pyriform Ab amacrine cells contributed to the population in which co-localization of these two markers occurred.

Possible involvement of pyriform Ab amacrine cells with dopaminergic neurons comes from the work of O'Brien and Dowling (1985) who demonstrated that dopamine stimulates a calcium-dependent release of preloaded 3H-GABA from the goldfish retina. These authors suggested that dopaminergic interplexiform cells (DA-IPC) made excitatory synaptic contact onto GABA-accumulating amacrine cells.

We have developed a double label radio/immuno technique (Eldred et al 1983) whereby we can simultaneously observe the distribution of radio-labeled transmitter indicators and immunoreactivity to particular antisera at both the light (LM) and electron microscopical (EM) levels. With this method we can study identifiable transmitter contacts between specific populations of neurons. Combined with electrophysiological and pharmacological data, one can begin to understand the circuitry by which neuronal processing occurs. In this communication, three experiments will be described in which we tested specific hypotheses regarding pyriform Ab amacrine cells that take up 3H-GABA: 1. are they immunoreactive for GAD (i.e. GABAergic), 2. are they immunoreactive for somatostatin, thus forming one or two subtypes, and 3. do they interact synaptically with

Neurocircuitry of the Retina, A Cajal Memorial
A. Gallego and P. Gouras, Editors

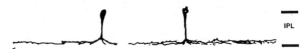

Fig. 1 shows schematic drawings, adapted from Cajal (1933, Plate I, Fig. 5, cells i and g), of two types of pyriform Ab amacrine cells which differ in the thickness of the descending and laterally extending dendrites which ramify in the most proximal portion of the inner plexiform layer.

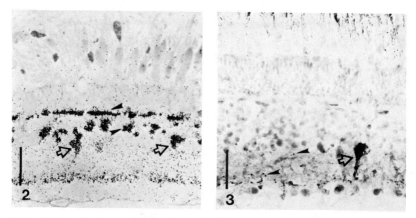

Figs. 2 and 3 show a comparison of 3H-GABA uptake and somatostatin-like immunoreactivity (SLIR). Bars indicate the thickness of the inner plexiform layer (IPL), approximately 35 μm. Fig. 2, A bright-field autoradiograph of a 1.5 μm Epon section of goldfish retina, exposed for 3 weeks. Note the heavy labeling in the most proximal IPL; uniform, light labeling is seen throughout the rest of the IPL. Two 3H-GABA accumulating cell bodies are seen (arrows), one of which has a thick process descending to the proximal IPL identifying it as a pyriform Ab amacrine cell. Horizontal cell bodies and axon terminals (arrowheads) also show heavy accumulation of 3H-GABA, Fig. 3, The immunohistochemical pattern of SLIR in a 10 μm cryostat section of a retina fixed in 4% paraformaldehyde. Fine punctate processes can be seen in the most proximal and distal IPL (arrowheads). A labeled pyriform Ab amacrine cell with its thick descending process is shown (arrow). This cell, although more fully visualized due to the thickness of the section, is similar to that seen in Fig. 2. Figures from Yazulla et al (1984).

dopaminergic IPCs, identified by immunoreactivity for tyrosine hydroxylase (TOH). This paper is based on several studies done in my laboratory (Yazulla et al 1984; Zucker, 1984; Zucker et al, 1984) as well as recent work in progress.

The methodologies that we use to process retinas for ultrastructural immunocytochemistry and electron microscopical autoradiography (EM-ARG) have been described in detail in previous work (Eldred et al, 1983; Yazulla et al, 1985; Yazulla 1981). However, a brief description is in order. Retinas were isolated from dark-adapted goldfish (Carassius auratus) 6 inch body length, incubated for 25 min in 0.4 uM 3H-GABA (Amersham, 35 Ci/mmol) in an oxygenated Ringer solution (pH 7.4), rinsed for 5 min in Hepes buffered Ringer solution, then fixed for 1 hour in 4% paraformaldehyde and 0.15% glutaraldehyde (pH 7.4), followed by overnight fixatation in 4% paraformaldehyde (pH 10.4). Treatment for 30 min in 1% sodium borohydride restored much of the masked immunoreactivity, and an ascending-descending buffered ethanolic series followed by freeze/thawing after careful cryoprotection was used to increase the penetration of immunological reagents (Eldred et al 1983). The tissue was then incubated in primary antiserum which was visualized by a PAP procedure. We used well characterized rabbit antisera directed against: human somatostatin-14 (DAKO) (1:500), catfish brain GAD (Su et al, 1979 1:750) and tryosine hydroxylase (Joh et al, 1979 1:750). After tertiary fixation in 1% osmium tetroxide and processing through Epon, retinas were processed for LM-ARG and EM-ARG as reference above.

The EM immunocytochemical procedure that we have developed results in complete infiltration of immunoreagents throughout retinal slices 50-500 um wide. Thus, our analysis is not restricted to an area only 5-10 um from a cut edge. This allows for a more rapid accumulation of data, avoidance of possible edge artefacts and a larger area within which to visualize the full extent of immunolabeled cells.

3H-GABA/Somatostatin

Figure 2 shows an LM-ARG of 3H-GABA uptake in goldfish retina processed for EM immunocytochemistry fixed with 0.15% glutaraldehyde. H1 horizontal cell bodies and axon terminals, pyriform Ab amacrine cells and the proximal IPL are labeled. This uptake pattern is qualitatively identical to that described previously utilizing higher concentrations of glutaraldehyde (Marc et al 1978; Yazulla 1981), indicating no selective loss of 3H-GABA from the retina due to fixation with low concentrations of glutaraldehyde. We have also seen labeled cell bodies in the ganglion cell layer (GCL, Fig. 7) which often can be as densely labeled as the pyriform Ab amacrine cells. It is possible that these represent displaced amacrine cells although ganglion cells cannot be excluded. Figure 3 shows a light micrograph of SLIR in the goldfish retina. Dendritic labeling can be seen at both the most proximal and distal borders of the IPL. A pyriform Ab amacrine cell with processes in the proximal IPL also is visible. Note the similarity between the Ab amacrine cells shown in Figures 2 and 3.

EM analysis of tissue double labeled for 3H-GABA uptake and SLIR showed that SL-immunoreactive processes in the goldfish IPL always contained large dense-cored vesicles (800-100 Å), within which most of the SL-immunoreaction product was concentrated (Fig. 4). SL-immunoreactive processes were not very common, appearing at a frequency of one process per 21 linear um. SL-immunoreactive synapses were even rarer, in agreement with Marshak et al (1984). EM-ARG analysis to determine possible co-localization of 3H-GABA uptake and SLIR was restricted to the most proximal 10 um of the IPL, the strata in which Ab amacrine cells arborize. Analysis comprised an area of 47,650 um2 which contained 31,000 silver grains and 222 SL-immunoreactive processes. Less than one percent (199) of the total grains in the area surveyed were within 3 half-distances (4,340 Å) of an SL-immunoreactive process. It was obvious that there were far more silver grains in the proximal IPL than could be

164

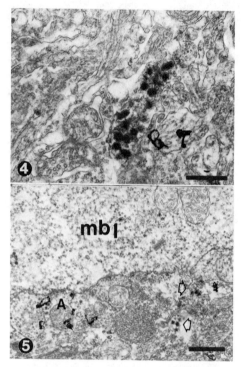

Figs. 4 and 5 show electron micrographs of tissue processed for both 3H-GABA autoradiography and somatostatin-like immunocytochemistry. Fig. 4, SLIR is seen in dense-cored vesicles throughout the labeled process. Two silver grains are seen over an amacrine cell process near an SLIR containing process. Note that the silver grains are within 2 to 4 half distances of the immunoreactive process but are likely to be associated with the underlying amacrine process. Calibration bar = 0.5 µm. Figure 5 shows an electron micrograph of 3H-GABA accumulating amacrine cell terminal (A) synapsing onto the proximal border of an Mbl bipolar cell terminal (mbl). Two SLIR processes are also shown (arrows); the upper one is making a synapse onto a possible 3H-GABA accumulating amacrine cell process that is juxtaposed with the bipolar terminal. Calibration bar = 1.0 µm. Figures from Yazulla et al (1984).

accounted for by SL-immunoreactive processes. Thus, in order to test for co-localization, only the 199 grains within 3 half-distances of SL-immunoreactive processes were considered in the analysis. Of these, only 9 grains were over an SL-immunoreactive process and only 52 were within one half-distance of a process. If SL-immunoreactive processes, with an average diameter of 1 um, were a uniform source of radioactivity, 50% of the grains within 3 half-distances would be expected to be over the confines of these processes (Salpeter and Bachmann 1972). However, only 4.5% were observed in this position, indicating that the two markers were not co-localized. Further evidence for non co-localization is provided by amacrine cells which take up 3H-GABA and make extensive synaptic contact along the proximal half of the axon terminal of mixed rod-cone (Mbl bipolar cells (Marc et al 1978). Such a synaptic arrangement is shown in Fig. 5. None of the grain-containing processes synapsing upon Mbl terminals were ever positive for SLIR. In addition, SL-immunoreactive process which did not contain 3H-GABA were often seen in the vicinity of the Mbl terminals. We thus concluded that 3H-GABA uptake and SLIR occur in spearate populations of pyriform Ab amacrine cells (Yazulla et al 1984).

3H-GABA/GAD
We found cell bodies in the ganglion cell layer which take up 3H-GABA almost as effectively as pyriform Ab amacrine cells (Fig. 7). Note that the ARG exposure for Fig. 7 is only one week, whereas for Figs. 6 and 8, the exposure is 3 weeks. The dendritic stratification of the labeled cells in the GCL, possibly displaced amacrine cells, is not known. There-

fore, it is possible that grain-containing synapses in the proximal IPL could belong to at least two types of amacrine cell, including pyriform Ab

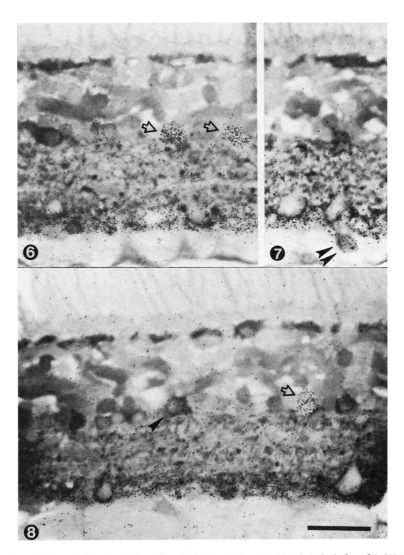

Figs. 6,7 and 8. LM-ARGs of goldfish retina double-labeled for 3H-GABA and GAD-IR, 5 μm sections. Incubation in 3H-GABA was done on eyecups rather than on isolated retinas in order to restrict uptake to the amacrine cells, thus eliminating confusion due to uptake by horizontal cell axon terminals (Yazulla, 1983). Thus, although Hl horizontal cells (H) show GAD-IR, they are not labeled with 3H-GABA. Arrows in Figs. 6 and 8 (3 week exposure) show pyriform Ab amacrine cells labeled with 3H-GABA but negative for GAD-IR. The double arrowheads in Fig. 7 (one week exposure) indicate a double-labeled cell in the ganglion cell layer, and the arrowhead in Fig. 8 indicates a lightly double-labeled amacrine cell. In addition, there are several GAD-IR positive amacrine cells which are not labeled with 3H-GABA. Calibration bar = 25 μm.

amacrine cells.   Since positive identification of the synaptic terminals
of pyriform Ab amacrine cells would be in doubt, the use of EM-ARG to
study co-localization of 3H-GABA/GAD-IR in these cells was ruled out.
This was not a problem in the previous section involving somatostatin
because co-localization of 3H-GABA uptake and SLIR was never seen.   We
therefore used LM-ARG by which cell body labeling with 3_H-GABA and GAD-IR
could be determined with relative ease.

Although at least two types of amacrine cell take up 3H-GABA in the
inner nuclear layer of goldfish retina, Ab amacrine cells are the largest
and most densely labeled cell type for a given autoradiographic exposure
(Marc et al 1978; Yazulla, 1981, Marc, 1982).   Thus, they are easily
identified at the LM level by their relative grain density and tear-drop
shape.   Figures 6 and 8 show LM-ARGs of tissue double-labeled for 3H-GABA
uptake and GAD-IR.   Figures 6 and 8 show clusters of grains in the
proximal INL in the postion and shape of pyriform Ab amacrine cells.   It
can be seen that the area under these grain clusters are not stained,
representing GAD-IR negative cell bodies.   In addition, there are GAD-IR
positive amacrine cell bodies located throughout the sections that do not
have overlying silver grains.   Pyriform Ab amacrine cells are not very
common, comprising only about 2.7% of the amacrine cell population in
goldfish retina (Marc 1982).   However, we found 60 pyriform Ab amacrine
cells that were positive for 3H-GABA uptake but negative for GAD-IR.
Occasionally we saw large cell bodies that were double labelled (Fig. 8,
arrowhead), but the relative grain density was less than that over
pyriform Ab amacrine cells in the same section (Fig. 8).   Some of these
large double labeled cells appeared pyriform in shape (not shown), but we
could not determine at what level in the IPL they ramified, i.e., levels
1,3, or 5.   After a one week exposure, double labeling was observed in
about 10% of the amacrine cells in the inner nuclear layer (Fig. 8, arrow),
including 75% of those taking up 3H-GABA but only 43% of those showing
GAD-IR.   Co-localization of 3H-GABA/GAD-IR also was observed in cell
bodies in the GCL (Fig. 7, double arrowheads).   There are no silver grains
over the GAD-IR positive horizontal cells because incubation in 3H-GABA
was done with an eyecup preparation which we have found restricts the
uptake of 3H-GABA to amarine cells (Yazulla, 1983).   This procedure thus
eliminates any confusion due to 3H-GABA uptake by the axon terminals of H1
horizontal cells which extend proximally to the level of amacrine cell
bodies (see Fig. 2).

3H-GABA/TOH
   In the final experiment we tried to determine the presence of synaptic
interactions between DA-IPCs and GABA-accumulating amacrine cells.   Figure
9 shows a DA-IPC labeled with anti-TOH in the goldfish retina.   This cell
type has an extensive plexus in the OPL and lighter plexes in the distal
and proximal borders of the IPL.   The stratification of DA-IPCs in the
proximal IPL overlaps that of pyriform Ab amacrine cells providing an
opportunity for synaptic interaction between the two cell types.   This
conjecture was investigated by EM analysis of tissue double labeled with
3H-GABA and TOH.   Amacrine cell processes labeled with 3H-GABA accounted
for 12% (n=12) of the input to and 10% (n=7) of the output from DA-IPCs.
Figure 10 shows a synaptic contact made by a DA-IPC onto a 3H-GABA labeled
amacrine cell process.   Unfortunately, based on the results just described
in the previous section, we are not certain as to whether the grain
containing processes contacting DA-IPCs belong to pyriform Ab amacrine
cells or 3H-GABA labeled cells in the GCL.

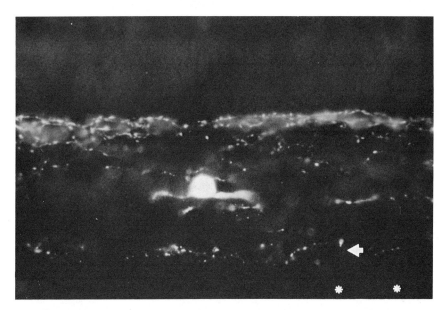

Fig. 9. Light micrograph of the immunocytochemical distribution of TOH in the goldfish retina. A large cell body belonging to a DA-IPC is seen along with its extensive plexus in the OPL and lighter plexes in the distal and proximal IPL (arrow). Calibration bar = 25 μm.

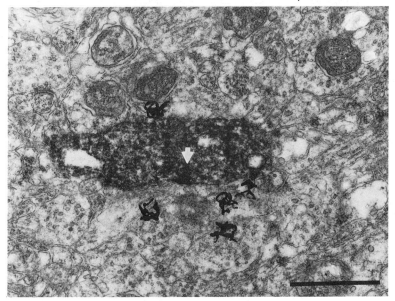

Fig. 10. Electron micrograph of a DA-IPC process in the IPL which is synapsing onto a 3H-GABA labeled amacrine cell process (arrow). Exposure time = 12 weeks, calibration bar = 1 um. Figure from Zucker (1984).

Discussion

We have used a double-labele radio/immunocytochemical technique to test three hypotheses regarding pyriform Ab amacrine cells, do they: 1. form single or multiple classes, 2. show co-localization of 3H-GABA uptake and GAD-IR, and 3. make synaptic contact with DA-IPCs. Conclusions are fairly straightforward for the first two problems but equivocal for the third.

Pyriform Ab amacrine cells that take up 3H-GABA are distinct from those that show somatostatin-like IR, although morphologically they are very similar. They may correspond to the two types described by Cajal (1933) (see Fig. 1), however, we have not been able to discern which type takes up 3H-GABA or shows SLIR. The role of two types of pyriform Ab amacrine cell in the fish retina is unknown. The dendrites of these cells are stratified in sublamina b, which has been related to "on" type neuronal activity (Famiglietti et al 1977; Stell et al 1977). The synaptic connectivity of the two cell types is different, suggesting separate functions. 3H-GABA Ab amacrine cells may affect the centripetal pathway in that they tend to contact the axon terminals of bipolar cells (Marc et al 1978). SLIR Ab amacrine cells, however, tend to contact other amacrine cells (Marshak et al 1984) and thus may be more involved in lateral interactions. The unique labeling of 3H-GABA and SLIR for different classes of Ab amacrine cells seems to provide a convenient method to further analyze their respective roles in retinal synaptic function. However, until the dendritic projection of 3H-GABA accumulating cells in the GCL is determined, caution must be exercised in using 3H-GABA uptake to identify synaptic terminals of Ab amacrine cells at the EM level.

The suggestion has been made that 3H-GABA Ab amacrine cells are GABAergic (Marc et al 1978; Marc 1982). However, we have shown that 3H-GABA Ab amacrine cells do not show GAD-like IR, suggesting that they may not synthesize GABA and therefore, may not be GABAergic. There is considerable evidence suggesting that goldfish Hl horizontal cells are GABAergic (see Discussions in Yazulla 1983 and Lam and Ayoub 1984). Hl cells take up 3H-GABA avidly but do not stain for GAD as intensely as some GAD positive amacrine cells. Thus, reduced staining for GAD-IR does not necessarily eliminate a neuron as being GABAergic. It is curious that of the three cell types in the goldfish retina that show the greatest uptake for 3H-GABA, only cell bodies in the GCL and Hl horizontal cells show GAD-IR, whereas Ab amacrine cells do not show GAD-IR at all. It is possible that these cell types contain different isozymes of GAD that are differentially recognized by the antisera we have used. However, double labeled amacrine cells are indeed observed, although they are less labeled with 3H-GABA than Ab amacrine cells. Some double labeled amacrine cells appear to be pyriform in shape. It is possible that they represent a rare third subtype of pyriform AB amacrine cell. Alternatively, they may correspond to any of the other types of pyriform amacrine cells which ramify throughout the IPL (Cajal 1933). Our observation that the vast majority of pyriform amacrine cells that take up 3H-GABA do not show GAD-IR, raises serious questions regarding the relevant criteria to identify GABAergic neurons in goldfish retina. Currently we favor the hypothesis that GAD-IR is a better indicator of GABAergic neurons and suggest that Ab amacrine cells are not GABAergic. The puzzling issue as to the possible role and reason why these cells possess a high affinity uptake mechanism for GABA remains to be determined.

In our third series of experiments were able to provide clear anatomical support for the biochemical study of O'Brien and Dowling (1985) which predicted synaptic input from DA-IPCs onto GABA accumulating amacrine cells. They demonstrated that the application of dopamine evoked calcium-dependent release of preloaded 3H-GABA from the goldfish retina. We found that approximately 10% of the synaptic output of DA-IPCs in the proximal IPL is onto amacrine cell processes that take up 3H-GABA. However, it is uncertain as to whether the 3H-GABA release reported by O'Brien and Dowling (1985) originated from pyriform Ab amacrine cells or cells in the GCL, both of which show a similar degree of 3H-GABA uptake. If the presence of GAD-IR rather than 3H-GABA uptake is taken as the indicator of GABAergic neurons, then processes of the double labeled (3H-GABA/GAD) cells in the GCL would appear to be the likely synaptic target of the DA-IPCs and consequently, the source of dopamine stimulated 3H-GABA release. We cannot rule out the possibility that pyriform Ab amacrine cells also are contacted by DA-IPCs. However, until the meaning of 3H-GABA uptake in the absence of GAD-IR is determined, the functional significance of such an interaction would be unclear.

The understanding of retinal circuitry is a complex undertaking requiring the combined efforts of anatomical, biochemical and electrophysiological studies, interpreted within the constraints of the psychophysical ability of the system under investigation. Such a large multidisciplinary information base exists for the goldfish visual system, thus making it an excellent preparation for study. Over the past several years we have utilized a combined immunocytochemical/autoradiographical procedure to study the synaptic circuitry of specific neuronal populations. In this communication we have illustrated the power and usefulness of this approach utilizing pyriform Ab amacrine cells which offer a number of advantages. They are large, relatively rare, unistratified (which restricts the area to be analyzed) readily labeled with transmitter markers, and lend themselves to several straightforward hypotheses. We tested these hypotheses and found that pyriform Ab amacrine cells form at least two, possibly three, sub types, and may not be GABAergic. Their involvement with DA-IPCs was less clear. The approach described here appears to work best when one is dealing with a population of neurons which consist of a single type, such as dopaminergic IPCs, or those, which although consisting of at least two types, have spatially segregated dendrites, such as cholinergic amacrine cells of bird (Baughman and Bader, 1977) and rabbit (Masland and Mills 1979). This eliminates the confusion in interpretation such as we encountered with the multiple types of GABA accumulating "amacrine" cells in the goldfish retina. Despite this limitation, much information regarding synaptic interaction between identified populations of neurons can be obtained using combined immunocytochemistry and autoradiography at the EM level.

Acknowledgements

We express our appreciation to Dr. Tong Joh who supplied us with anti-TOH and Dr. Jang-Yen Wu who supplied us with anti-GAD. This work was supported by NIH Grant EY 01682.

References

Baughman, R.W., C.R. Bader Brain Res. 138, 469-485 (1977).
Eldred, W.D., C. Zucker, H.J. Karten and S. Yazulla J. Histochem. Cytochem. 31, 285-292 (1983).
Famiglietti, E.V., A. Kaneko and M. Tachibana Science 198, 1267-1269 (1977).
Joh, T.H., C. Geghman and D. Reis Proc. Natl. Acad. Sci. USA 70, 2767 (1973).
Lam, D.M.K. and G.S. Ayoub Vis. Res. 230, 433-444 (1984).

Lundberg, J.M. and T. Hokfelt Trends Neurosci. 6, 325-329 (1983).

Marc, R.E. Vis. Res. 22, 589-608 (1982).

Marc, R.E., W.K. Stell, D. Bok and D.M.K. Lam J. Comp. Neurol 182, 221-246 (1978).

Marshak, D.W., T. Yamada and W.K. Stell J. Comp. Neurol 225, 44-52 (1984).

Masland, R.H. and J.W. Mills J. Cell Biol. 83, 159-178 (1979).

O'Brien, D.E and J.E. Dowling Brain Res (in press) (1985).

Ramon y Cajal, S. The structure of the retina. (translated S.A. Thorpe and M. Glickstein) Charles C. Thomas Springfield (1972).

Salpeter, M.M. and L. Bachmann in Principles and Techniques of Electron Microscopy V. 2 (M.A. Hayat ed, Van Nostrand Reinhold, N. Y. 1972) pp. 221-279.

Stell, W.K., A.T. Ishida and D.O. Lightfoot Science 198, 1269-1271 (1977).

Su, Y.Y.T., J.-Y. Wu and D.M.K. Lam J. Neurochem. 33, 169-179 (1979).

Wu, J.-Y. in Immunohistochemistry (A.C. Cuello ed, John Wiley and Sons, N. Y., 1983) pp. 159-192.

Yamada, T., D. Marshak, S. Basinger, J. Walsh, J. Morley and W. Stell Proc. Natl. Acad. Sci. USA 77, 1691-1695 (1980).

Yazulla, S. J. Comp. Neurol 200, 83-93 (1981).

Yazulla, S. Brain Res. 275, 61-74 (1983).

Yazulla, S., J. Mosinger and C. Zucker Brain Res. 321, 352-356 (1984).

Yazulla, S., K. Studholme and C. Zucker J. Comp. Neurol 231, 232-238 (1985).

Zucker, C.L. Ph.D. Thesis, State University of N. Y. Stony Brook (1984).

Zucker, C.L., S. Yazulla, and J.-Y Wu Brain Res. 298, 154-158 (1984).

Putative Peptide Transmitters, Amacrine Cell Diversity
and Function in the Inner Plexiform Layer

William K. Stell
University of Calgary
Department of Anatomy
Calgary, Alberta, Canada

As Cajal in particular was early to recognize, the vertebrate retina
is a part of the central nervous system well suited to studies of local
circuit functions, in which we may identify synaptic pathways and probable
sites of neuronal interactions. It converts spatio temporally variant
patterns of light stimulation into spatially and temporally coded patterns
of nerve impulses carried to the brain by optic nerve fibres. The
functional vocabulary of optic fibres, which are axons of retinal ganglion
cells, is somewhat limited (i.e. ON, OFF, ON-OFF) and highly invariant
from species to species. Thus it is possible, in theory as well as in
practice, to learn much about the principles of visual information
processing by focusing experimental attention on those few retinas that
are most convenient for study, including those of fish and mudpuppies
(Dowling, 1979).

Ganglion cell activity is governed directly by synaptic inputs from
bipolar and amacrine cells. Ganglion cells appear to be driven primarily
by excitatory responses to bipolar cell inputs, ON cells being excited by
ON bipolars in the light and OFF cells being excited by OFF bipolars in
the dark (Naka, 1976; Miller and Dacheux, 1976; Werblin, 1979). Changing
impinging illumination also modulates ganglion cell sensitivity through
activation of inhibitory amacrine cell influences (Werblin, 1979), and by
way of centres in the brain through activation of retinopetal (efferent)
fibres.

It has been known for some time that such "conventional"
neurotransmitters as acetylcholine, amino acids and biogenic amines are
well represented in the inner retina. Recent discoveries that a number of
different amacrine cell types, as well as efferent fibres, contain
neuroactive peptides(Stell et al, 1980, 1984) have profoundly affected our
appreciation of the pathways impinging upon ganglion cells. The
objective of this paper will be to review what is known about
neurotransmitter systems in the inner plexiform layer of the goldfish
retina. From such obscure and fleeting glimpses of reality we may begin
to comprehend the roles of conventional and peptide neurotransmitters in
processing of visual information in the retina.

Amacrine Cells
    Amacrine cells were discovered by Cajal (1892). In Golgi preparations
he observed cells with somata mainly in the more proximal (inner) portion
of the inner nuclear layer (INL) and neurites in various levels of the
inner plexiform layer (IPL). He coined the term "amacrine" from the Greek
(a + makros = no axon) to recognize their single most remarkable feature.
Because amacrine cells seemed to be structurally well placed to interact
with both bipolars and amacrine cells, Cajal reasoned that they must
modify bipolar-to-ganglion-cell transmission. His observation of many and
varied amacrine cell types in fish, frog, lizard, bird and domesticated
mammals has been confirmed many times over in the intervening century.
Kolb, for example, deduces from her Golgi preparations that there may be
at least 20 types of amacrines in the cat's retina (Kolb et al, 1981).
Physiologists, however, have become skeptical of this as their electrical

recordings have revealed only a few classes of amacrine cell response (see below).

Electron microscopical studies confirmed Cajal's impression of the uniqueness of amacrine cells by substantiating that their neurites are both presynaptic and postsynaptic to other neurons throughout their length. Indeed, early studies gave the impression of a great profusion of contacts: bipolar-amacrine, amacrine-bipolar, amacrine-ganglion, amacrine-amacrine, often in reciprocal and serial clusters - as if amacrine cells were interconnected indiscriminately all over the place (Dowling and Werblin, 1969; Dubin, 1970). More recent studies, however, have demonstrated the obvious: that amacrine cells are highly selective and individual in their contact patterns, just like other neurons, (Famiglietti and Kolb, 1975; Marc et al, 1978; Marshak et al, 1984).

Amacrine cells electrical activities were first described reliably by Werblin and Dowling (1969). By intracellular recording and dye-marking in the mudpuppy they found a single functional cell type with a cell body in the innermost INL. This cell responded with transient depolarizations (EPSPs) at ON and OFF and generated also smaller, briefer depolarizations shown subsequently to be either large, global somatic spikes or small, local dendritic spikes (Miller, 1979; Werblin, 1979). The transiency of the ON and OFF EPSPs has been ascribed variously to: (a) recurrent amacrine cell inhibition of excitatory bipoalr cell input (Dowling, 1979) (b) nonlinearity (inherent transiency) of postsynaptic response of amacrine cell membrane to sustained bipolar cell excitation (Werblin, 1979); or (c) interaction of simultaneous ON and OFF bipolar cel inputs, the OFF being delayed slightly with respect to the ON (Miller, 1979). Injection of current into bipolar cells while recording from ON-OFF amacrines, which ought to resolve this question, seems not to have been done (Naka, 1977). In the catfish, there is some doubt whether this transient, little or non-spiking, neuron is an amacrine at all, since polarizing it with extrinsic current causes no response in known ganglion cells (Chan and Naka, 1976; Naka, 1977). Inhibitory transmission from ON-OFF "amacrines" to ganglion cells has, however, been invoked as a central feature in most models of IPL circuitry (Dowling, 1979; Miller, 1979; Werbliu, 1979).

Electrophysiological investigations in fish, however, have revealed amacrine cells of another type. In goldfish, Kaneko and Hashimoto (1969) and Kaneko (1970, 1973) recorded from sustained hyperpolarizing (OFF) and depolarizing (ON) units whose responses to small spots resembled those of bipolars but which lacked an opponent surround; dye injection confirmed that some of these were amacrines. The transient ON-OFF amacrines were found to be influenced only by pathways from red-sensitive cones, whereas the sustained hyperpolarizing amacrines were found to be colour-opponent (red-OFF, green-ON). In catfish, Chan and Naka (1976) described a class of sustained-responding INL/IPL neurone believed to be genuine amacrine cells (type "N" of Naka, 1977). The ganglion cell response to amacrine cell polarizations suggested that sustained amacrines of either type are inhibitory to ON ganglion cells and excitatory to OFF ganglion cells; whether the pathways are mono- or poly-synaptic was not determined (Chan and Naka, 1976). Miller (1979) and Werblin (1979) assume the existence of sustained amacrines in amphibian and mammalian retinas and incorporate them into their circuit models, even though they have been unable to obtain recordings from them.

Candidate Neurotransmitter Systems in Goldfish Inner Plexiform Layer
    No retinal neurotransmitter system, with the possible exception of GABA in teleostean cone horizontal cells, meets fully the criteria for a

bona fide transmitter. Given the difficulty of recording from amacrine cells, which are the presumed targets of many putative inner plexiform layer (IPL) transmitters, convincing evidence of transmitter function may be long in coming. This is particularly true for the neuropeptides, which are widely assumed to mediate hormone-like as well as transmitter-like functions.

The main purpose of this section, therefore, will be to draw inferences about synaptic pathways and functional circuitry of neurochemically defined IPL units. In a sense, neurotransmitter-like functions will be assumed. The reader is referred to recent reviews of retinal transmitter systems (Brecha, 1983) for further documentation and analysis. Although this section will concentrate on goldfish, I shall have the audacity to include data on a closely related animal, the carp, which represents a separate genus, and occasionally others.

"Conventional" Transmitters

Gamma-aminobutyric acid (GABA)

Quite unexpectedly GABA, long accepted as a neurotransmitter in the retina and elsewhere, has become a focus of intense controversy. On the one hand, localization of (^{3}H)-GABA uptake by autoradiography (Lam and Steinman, 1971; Marc et al, 1978) revealed a single class of heavily labeled amacrine cells ramifying in the proximal one-fifth (layer 5) of the IPL. These cells, called type Ab, were shown to be both pre- and post-synaptic to the axon terminals of type b1 mixed rod-cone bipolar cells, and modulation of net GABA uptake by coloured light suggested that they might be the red-depolarizing, green-hyperpolarizing units assumed to generate the surround of double-colour-opponent ganglion cells (Marc et al 1978; Marc 1980). Excitatory (chemical or electrical) synaptic contacts from Ab to Ab amacrines, required for such wide area summation, have not been observed but may comprise such a small fraction of Ab synapses that they would be easily overlooked. Recently Yazulla and his associates (Zucker et al 1984) have claimed that the GABA-accumulating Ab amacrines do not contain the GABA-synthesizing enzyme, GAD; but this claim, based upon negative evidence, is contradicted by the finding that GABA-uptake and GAD-immunoreactivity can be co-localized to AB amacrines (Ball and Brandon 1984). Ab amacrines therefore may constitute a GABA-ergic network that interconnects the output terminals of type b mixed bipolars, and thereby generates receptive field surrounds of ON-centre double-colour-opponent cells. Some physiological data (Negishi et al 1978; Djamgoz et al 1981; Glickman et al 1984) support this view, although the recent report of Schellart et al (1984) might suggest that the surround/opponent pathways are inhibited by, but do not utilize, GABA. The Ab amacrines are closely analogous to the type 1 cone horizontal cells, as each constitutes a GABA-ergic network interconnecting the afferent axon terminals (bipolar or photoreceptor) within its synaptic layer.

Marc et al (1978) reported that they sometimes found many lightly GABA-labelled cells in addition to the few heavily labeled Ab amacrines. Yazulla and his co-workers have been helpful in calling attention to this population of cells and questioning its significance. Three relevant facts have emerged: first, that dry-mount autoradiographical receptor localisation results in diffuse labeling of most of the IPL, largely attributable to nonsynaptic receptor sites (Yazulla 1981); second, that (apart from the GABA-accumulating Aa amacrines) the level of GABA uptake is a poor indicator of the presence of GABAergic synapses (Yazulla 1981); and third, that within the low-uptake part of the IPL, the localization in depth of synaptic GAG immunoreactivity and GABA agonist binding are indistinguishable. These findings are consistent with physiological observations that exogenous GABA influences responses of all ganglion cells, irrespective of response type (Negishi et al 1978; Glickman et al 1981; Schellart et al 1984), as well as pathways impinging upon dopminergic interplexiform cells (Negishi et al 1983), and therefore that GABA-sensitive receptors are operative at all depths of the IPL (Famiglietti et al 1977). Given the apparent peculiarities of the putative GABA system in the distal IPL (Yazulla and Brecha 1980), it is open to question whether GABA is the proper substrate for either the uptake of the syanptic binding system, and in any event why there is so much nonsynaptic GABA binding. These concerns will resurface shortly in regard to other putative transmitter systems (glycine, acetylcholine). A recently published study demonstrates that the GABA-accumulating AB amacrines are not identical to the somatostatin-immunoreactive Ab amacrines, to which they are very similar morphologically (Yazulla et al 1984).

Glycine

Although it shares with GABA a widespread reputation as a ubiquitous inhibitory neurotransmitter, the role of glycine in the goldfish retina remains rather obscure. Marc et al (1978) reported that (3H)-glycine uptake labels many small cell bodies in the amacrine cell layer and diffusely labels processes in the distal two-thirds (at least) of the IPL. In size and distribution the glycine-transporting structures resemble the population of GAD-immunoreactive cells that are labeled poorly by GABA uptake, but the possibility of identity has yet to be explored experimentally. The glycine-accumulating somata comprise about 20% of all somata in the amacrine cell layer; their neurites in the IPL are mainly pre- or post-syanptic to unlabeled (non-glycine) amacrines (Marc and Lam 1981a; Marc 1982). Marc and Lam (1981a) also rediscovered Cajal's (1892) "small stellate cell", identifying it as a new glycine-accumulating interplexiform cell type with both pre- and post-synaptic relationships in the OPL and unknown relationships in the IPL. Physiological studies (Negishi et al 1981) reveal glycine-responsive inhibitory mechanisms in both the OPL and IPL, and presumably at all levels of the IPL since ganglion cells of all response types are affected. Because local application reveals actions in the OPL and IPL to be opposite (Negishi et al 1978) application by superfusion bath results in effects that change over time (Negishi et al 1978) and may therefore appear weak, unclear or inconsistent (Glickman et al 1981). In sum, glycine appears to be a good condidate for the transmitter of the most prevalent interneurons in the amacrine cell layer, as well as for a class of interplexiform cell. In both plexiform layers it acts primarily upon other horizontally conducting interneurons rather than upon cells of the vertical through-pathway (photoreceptor-bipolar-ganglion cell). Since the effects of exogenous glycine in the two plexiform layers differ, one may guess that the output of the target horizontal cell in the OPL is sign-inverting or inhibitor, whereas that of the target amacrine(s) in the IPL is sign-conserving or exictatory.

Marc (1980) has proposed that the glycine-accumulating Aa amacrines mediate the opponent surround of red-OFF-centre double-colour-opponent ganglion cells just as GABA-accumulating Ab amacrines may do for red-ON-centre cells. It is worthy of note, however that the two cell systems differ remarkably in cell size, cell density and synaptic contact patterns (glycine-Aa: small cells, closely packed, mostly amacrine-amacrine synapses; GAGA-Ab: larger cells, widely spaced, mostly amacrine-bipolar syanpses). Therefore significant asymmetries may be expected in circuit functions of these two cell groups, and perhaps of the surrounds of ON- and OFF-centre ganglion cells.

Dopamine

Catecholamines, visualized by the formaldehyde-condensation method of Falck and Hillarp, were the first putative neurotransmitters to be localized in the retina. The discovery of the dopaminergic interplexiform cell of teleosts (Ehinger et al 1969) was a particularly noteworthy accomplishment. The structure of the cells, which appears to be very similar in all teleostean species studied to date, is well illustrated for goldfish by Ehinger and Floren (1976, 1978); scattered processes appear in the distal and mid-IPL (roughly, layers 1 and 3), and a thicker and richer arborization is found in the proximal IPL (layer 5). The dopamine cells, which also accumulate labeled exogenous dopamine (Sarthy and Lam 1979; Marc 1980, 1982), are larger than but approximately equal in number or density to the indoleamine-accumulating cells (Negishi et al 1981; Marc 1982). The dopamine cells are interplexiorm, with axonal synaptic endings on horizontal cell somata (Dowling and Ehinger 1978), whereas the indoleamine cells are conventional amacrines (see below). The dopamine cells are pre- and post-synaptic exclusively to non-dopamine, non-indoleamine amacrine cells (Dowling and Ehinger, 1978) and clearly avoid contact with the large axon terminals of type b bipolars even though both are most numerous in IPL layer 5 (Marc 1980).

The physiological action of dopamine on type 1 (L-type) cone horizontal cells is well documented: small, erratic changes in membrane potentials and conductance (Hedden and Dowling 1978) accompanied by a substantial increase in cytoplasmic cAMP (Lasater et al 1983) and uncoupling of intercellular gap junctions (Laufer et al 1981; Teranishi et al 1984). In a percid teleost, Eugerres, dopamine-mediated horizontal cell responses are evoked as well by application of carbachol or substance P (Laufer et al 1981), and the same agents reduce visibility of dopamine-induced histofluorescence (Negishi et al 1980), indicating that pathways from cholinergic and substance P-immunoreactive amacrine (see below) impinge upon the dopaminergic interplexiform cells. Indoleamine pathways also appear to exert an excitatory influrnce on these cells, as does dopamine itself (Kato et al 1982, 1983) whereas GABa probaly inhibits them (Negishi et al, 1983). Electrophysiological studies of the action of dopamine on amacrine cells (Hedden and Dowling 1978) further promote the notion that the dopamine cells interact in the IPL primarily with transient amacrines, as cholinergic, small GABA-ergic, and substance P-immunoreactive cells may be presumed to be. Hedden and Dowling suggest that the dopaminergic interplexiforms, whose net action in the OPL is to reduce the influence of the surround, do so by responding to activity of transient amacrines in the IPL. Since transient neurons are responsive mainly to spatial and temporal change, it may not be surprising that Glickman et al (1982) observed little effect of exogenous dopamine on ganglion cell responses to stationary, long-lasting spots and annuli.

It has been assumed for many years that dopamine is the only catecholamine present in intrinsic retinal neurons. But recent evidence for adrenergic amacrine cells in the rat (Hadjiconstantinou et al 1984) suggests that they should be sought in teleosts. Preliminary analyses of extracts from goldfish retina by HPLC, in my laboratory (Muske, personal communication), suggest indeed that epinephrine is present in this animal as well.

Indoleamines

Although synthesis of 5-hydroxytryptamine (5HT, serotonin), a common indoleamine transmitter, has not been detected (Lam 1975), the presence of indoleamine (including 5HT) accumulating neurones in the goldfish retina is well documented. Histofluorescence, uptake-plus-autoradiography, and immunocytochemistry of 5HT have shown the indoleamine neurones to be smaller than but equal in number or spatial density to the dopamine interplexiforms; to arborize thickly in layer 1 of the IPL (in the outermost stratum which is unlabeled by glycine uptake), and more thinly layers 3 and 5; and to lack axonal projections to the outer plexiform layer (Ehinger and Floren 1976, 1978; Marc 1980, 1981; Negishi et al 1981; Osborne et al 1982; Holmgren-Taylor 1983). It has been suggested that dopamine and indoleamine cells may be paired (Negishe et al 1981). Indeed, there is evidence that dopamine cells have indoleamine receptors (Kato et al 1982, 1983) through layers 1, 3 and 5, the IPL arborization patterns of dopamine and indoleamine cells being rather complementary. Electron-microscopical analysis (Holmgren-Taylor 1983) shows an overwhelmingly prevalent pattern of conventional pre- and post-synaptic contacts with non-indoleamine amacrines, plus a minor bipolar cell component, independent of level in the IPL. It has been stated, however, that synaptic contacts between dopamine and indoleamine neurones are not observed in the goldfish IPL (Dowling and Ehinger 1978).

Acetylcholine

The presence of acetylcholinesterase in the IPL of teleostean retinas was observed long ago (Francis 1953). More recently, biochemical (Ross and McDougal 1976) and immunocytochemical studies of the acetylcholine-synthesizing enzyme, choline acetyltransferase (ChAT) (Tumosa et al 1984; Tumosa et al 1983, 1984a,b) have firmly established that ChAT-containing neurones with somata in the amacrine and ganglion cell layers contribute a dense plexus of fibres to layers 2 and 4 of the IPL. The neurones that have been identified as ChAT-containing are clearly amacrines; ganglion cells have not yet been shown to contain ChAT (Ross and McDougal 1976; Tumosa et al 1984a,b).

Putative nicotinic acetylcholine receptors have been localized throughout the goldfish IPL, in fact predominantly in layers 1, 3 and 5, by means of α-bungarotoxin labeled with ^{125}I (Schwartz and Bok 1979) or HRP (Zucker and Yazulla 1982). Electron microscopy of the HRP conjugate, however, showed that this trilaminar localization indicates non-synaptic binding (Zucker and Yuzulla 1982), probably to bipolar cells (Schwartz and Bok 1979). The distribution of synaptic binding sites, which comprise only 16% of all binding sites, more nearly approximates the laminar pattern of ChAT-positive neurites; this is particularly true of the syanapses upon bipolar cells, the density of which peaks at the 30% (ca. layer 2) and 70% (ca. layer 4) levels of the IPL. The broader distribution of synapses involving amacrine or ganglion cells as post-syanptic elements shows instead a single peak at the 60% level (ca. layer 3-4) of the IPL. Overall the distributions of synaptic ACh and GABA receptors (Yazulla, 1981) are very similar.

Physiological studies have confirmed the role of cholinergic transmission. As expected from their arborization in mid-IPL (Famiglietti et al 1977), cholinergic cells appear to be involved primarily in responses of transient ON and especially ON-OFF cells (Glickman et al 1981). The majority of ganglion cells activated by ACh have ACh receptors themselves (Glickman et al 1982). The pathways are usually excitatory and the receptors muscarinic for OFF ganglion cells (Negishi et al 1980) and physiological experiments (Laufer et al 1981).

Acidic Amino Acids

Given the evidence that photoreceptors may release glutamate or a closely related compound, that photoreceptors and bipolar cells are closely related in structure and function, and that some bipolars in non-teleostean species have been reported to contain large amounts of the appropriate sysnthesizing enzymes, an important role for pathways utilizing acidic amino acids in the teleostean IPL could be anticipated. Marc and Lam (1981b) demonstrated autoradiographically that uptake of radiolabeled aspartate produces labeling of many bipolar and amacrine cell bodies, and diffusely throughout the IPL. There seems otherwise to be no useful information on this point at present. Studies using a putative marker for glutamate/aspartate suggest that in the guinea pig retina, amacrine rather than bipolar cells may utilize such substances (Altschuler et al 1982), but comparable studies remain to be done in goldfish.

Neuropeptides - Substance P

Immunoreactive substance P (SP) was identified by chromatography and radioimmunoassay in carp by Eskay et al (1981). These authors found three separate substances P-like peptides, none of which was identical to substance P or any other tachykinin tested. It should not be surprising, then, that different antisera have yielded different results. Brecha et al (1981), using a monoclonal antibody, demonstrated a single class of substance P-immunoreactive amacrine cell with a monostratified arborization in the mid-IPL (layer 3) and, rarely, a poorly stained plexus in layer 5; whereas Li et (1983), as well as Stell et al (1985) using polyclonal antisera, observed substance P-immunoreactive processes in IPL layers 1 and 3. Our observations (Stell et al 1985 and unpublished) revealed only a single type of SP-IR processes in layer 1 were shown to be identical to the LHRH- and FMRFamide-IR efferent fibres of the terminal nerve (Stell et al 1984). Differential recognition by different antisera indicates that the Sp-like peptide in the terminal nerve differs from the SP-like peptide(s) in the amacrine cells (Stell et al, in progress). Preliminary results of double staining suggest that the SP-immunoreactive amacrines are also neurotensin-immunoreactive (Stell and Chohan, in progress).

Physiological studies indicate a tranmitter-like role for substance P-like peptides, not unlike the role proposed for acetylcholine (in spite of the non-overlapping IPL distributions of the cells that contain them). Exogenous substance P was found to excite most ON and ON-OFF ganglion cells, often even in the presence of Co^{+2}, whereas it often inhibited OFF cells (Glickman et al 1980, 1982; Djamgoz et al 1983). Some ganglion cells were found to be excited directly by both substance P and ACh, but blocking experiments showed that they did so through separate receptor systems (Glickman 1980). Substance P pathways also converge on dopamine cells (Negishi et al 1980, Laufer et al 1981). The possibility remains to be explored that the differences we have found recently between SP-like peptides in amacrine cells and efferent fibres (see above) may be coupled to different receptor systems as in other tissues (Hunter and Maggio 1984) and thereby account for some of the complex actions of exogenous substance P observed in the phyisological studies.

Glickman et al (1982) observed that "the long latency of the substance P effect (30-40s) and the long duration of its action (up to 15 min) make it unlikely that substance P mediates the light response of ganglion cells. It is more likely that substance P is involved in changing the excitativity of the retina, perhaps during the process of adaptation, when retinal sensitivity must be reset."

Neurotensin

Li et al (1983) indicate that some antisera to neurotensin stain cells ramifying in IPL layers 1 and 3. Using four different antisera to neurotensin we have been unable to replicate the staining of fibres in IPL layer 1 (Stell and Chohan, unpublished). The cells that ramify in layer 3 are identical in appearance to the SP-immunorective amacrine cells. As indicated above, preliminary results suggest that the substance P-like and neurotensin-like peptides are co-localized to the same amacrine cells.

Somatostatin

Immunoreactive somatostatin, possibly corresponding to mammalian somatostatin-14 and -28, was demonstrated by RIA and localized by immunofluorescence to as many as four types of neurone in goldfish retina by Yamada et al (1980). According to these authors, the neurites ramified in IPL layers 1 and 5. Tornqvist et al (1982) reported a "less well defined layer" in IPL layer 3 as well, which may well be processes of ASb amacrines in transit to layer 5, but observed none of the immunoreactive neurones seen in the ganglion cell layer by Yamada and co-workers. We (Stell and Chohan, unpublished) nevertheless have reproduced this observation of Yamada et al (1980) repeatedly, using different antisera.

The EM-immunocytochemical study of Marshak et al (1984) proved by ultrastructural criteria that the somatostatin-immunoreactive cells are amacrines, and showed that they are both pre- and post-syanptic primarily to other (non-somatostatin) amacrines; they also make a significant contribution to the synaptic inputs of ganglion cells in both layers 1 and 5. It appears then that putatively somatostatinergic amacrine cells in the goldfish retina play similar roles in sustained-ON and OFF pathways, acting upon both amacrine and ganglion cells. Preliminary electrophysiological studies in my laboratory by Djamgoz in 1983 indicated that somatostatin may indeed act specifically in pathways to sustained ON- and OFF- rather than transient ON-OFF ganglion cells, but further details of the mechanism of action of somatostatin and its consequences for visual information processing are lacking.

A study recently published by Yazulla et al (1984), and reported at this Symposium, has shown that the somatostatin-immunoreactive AB amacrines are not identical to the GABA-accumulating Ab amacrines. We have confirmed the segregation of somatostatin- and GAD-immunoreactivity by immunofluroescent double-labeling techniques (Stell and Chohan, unpublished).

Enkephalin

The pentapeptides, Met[5]- and Leu[5]-enkephalin, are so ubiquitous and well known that it was logical to expect them to be at work in the goldfish retina especially after enkephalin-immunoreactive amacrine cells were observed in pigeon retina by Brecha et al (1979). Djamgoz and Stell (1980) found that exogenous opiate agonists influenced most of the ganglion cells in goldfish retina, exciting ON cells and inhibiting OFF cells; the effects were rapid and reversible, and were blocked presynaptically by Co^{++} as well as postsynaptically by naloxone. Djamgoz et al (1981) observed also that the effect of naloxone alone implies the existence of an endogenous opioid transmitter, and showed that this transmitter disinhibits ON ganglion cells by inhibiting intermediary GABA amacrines. These data are consistent with a widely held view that enkephalin is (mainly) inhibitory (e.g. Mudge et al 1979; Pepper and Henderson 1980) and that its apparently excitatory effects for example upon hippocampal neurones, are mediated through inhibition of an intermediary, inhibitory neurone (Nicol et al 1980).

While enkephalin-like immunoreactivity has been localized to amacrine cells in a great many species (Brecha and Karten 1983), the nature of the opioid element in goldfish retina remains obscure. To date only scattered enkephalin-immunoreactive neurites have been seen, mainly in IPL layers 1 and 5, and it is not known whether they represent intrinsic (retinal) or extrinsic (centrifugal) neurones (Stell et al 1981). Although synthesis and release of Met^5-enkephalin have been reported for goldfish retina (Su and Lam 1982), since the quantities were small it remains possible that the major opioid peptide in goldfish retina has not yet been identified.

Vasoactive Intestinal Peptide
Vasoactive intestinal peptide (VIP) is a potent vasodilator substance, 28 amino acids long, first isolated from porcine gut. It is reported to occur widely in both peripheral and central nervous systems of many species, including the retina in some cases (Brecha and Karten 1983). The evidence for its existence in goldfish retina is indirect: exogenous porcine VIP in micromolar concentrations causes a depolarizing increase in membrane conductance and a marked increase in cyclic AMP in isolated carp cone horizontal cells (Lasater et al 1984; Watling and Dowling 1983). VIP and dopamine act upon horizontal cells via different receptors, since VIP effects are not blocked by dopamine antagonists; and VIP, unlike dopamine, does not reduce the electrical coupling among the horizontal cells.

Tornqvist et al (1982) and Stell and Chohan (unpublished) have been unable to demonstrate immunoreactivity for VIP, or the related peptide PHI, in cells or fibres in the goldfish retina.

Watling and Dowling (1983) report that attempts at immunocytochemical localization "in collaboration with other groups... have revealed a few specific VIP-immunoreactive cells and processes which are confined, however, almost exclusively to the inner nuclear and (inner) plexiform layers (Marshak, personal communication; Terenghi, et al personal communication)". They discuss several interesting possibilities. "Piscine VIP" may differ in amino acid sequence from porcine VIP at sites critical for antibody recognition; if so, such "piscine VIP" may either co-exist with dopamine in the I1 interplexiform cells and be co-released in the OPL, or it may be released from an ordinary amacrine cell in the IPL but act at a distance (Jan et al 1984). Alternatively exogenous VIP may be acting at a receptor whose natural (endogenous) ligand is not even "piscine VIP" but some other peptide, yet to be identified. These interesting speculations await proper empirical testing.

Glucagon
A substance related to the gut and pancreatic forms of mammalian glucagon has been localized to cells in goldfish retina, with somata in the amacrine cell layer and processes in IPL layer 1 and rarely 3 (Marshak et al 1983; Stell and Chohan, unpublished). These cells were said to differ in morphology from amacrine cells described using any other transmitter-specific markers, and testing by means of double-labeling has in general born this out (Stell and Chohan, unpublished, but see next section). Em-immunocytochemical analysis (Marshak, personal communication) indicates that the glucagon-immunoreactive neurites in IPL layer 1 are presynaptic to processes of amacrine and ganglion cells in approximately the ratio 2:1; synaptic inputs to the glucagon cells are completely unknown. No information is yet available on the function of glucagon pathways.

Corticotropin Releasing Factor
Preliminary studies (Sakanaka et al in progress) have revealed a single class of cells with somata in the amacrine cell layer and neurites in IPL layer 1. Double-labeling studies, to determine whether these are a separate class from the glucagon-immunoreactive cells, remain to be done.

Thyrotropin Releasing Hormone
Thyrotropin releasing hormone (TRH), a tripeptide, was the second neuropeptide (after substance P) to be detected in retina. While its

presence in mammalian retina remains in dispute, substantial amounts of TRH-like immunoreactivity have been detected in frog and eel retinas by radioimmunoassay (Eskay et al 1980). We have also detected significant amounts of TRH-like material by RIA in goldfish retina (Marshak et al unpublished). Binding and release experiments in bovine retina have demonstrated interactions of exogenous TRH with type D3 dopamine receptors (presumed autoreceptors; Reading 1983), and TRH receptors have been identified in sheep retina (Burt 1979). One may suppose that mammalian retinas, at least, contain an analogue of TRH that is recognized well by membrane receptors but not antisera. In frogs and fish, however, genuine TRH may be present, but in amounts insufficient (given the peculiar chemical structure of the peptide) to be stainable immunocytochemically. No results of physiological studies on TRH in the retina have yet been reported.

Pancreatic Polypeptides/Neuropeptide Y

Neuropeptides of this family, distinguished by a sequence of 36 amino acids ending in -Arg-Phe-Nh$_2$ are of great interest currently as they occur widely in central and peripheral nervous systems. The goldfish retina has a single class of amacrine cell containing peptide(s) in this family (Muske and Stell 1984; Muske et al 1984). By immunocytochemical criteria the peptide resembles most closely neuropeptide Y (NPY), and avian pancreatic polypeptide (APP). The cells appear to be true amacrines, having cell bodies in the amacrine cell layer, neurites ramifying in IPL layers 1, 3 and 5, and no fibres in the optic nerve. The NPY-immunoreactive neurones closely resemble dopamine interplexiform cells in their disposition in the IPL (except that their neurites are somewhat finer and more branching), but their spatial density is lower and somata are smaller than those of dopamine dopamine cells, and no NPY-like immunoreactivity is detected around the horizontal cells. Double staining for NPTY and tyrosine hydroxylase proves that NPY-immunoreactive cells comprise a different population from dopamine interplexiform cells (Muske et al in preparation). Physiological studies of NPY action have not yet begun, although similarities in structure of some members of the PP/NPY family to the molluscan cardioexcitatory peptide, FMRFamide and its relatives (see below), leave open the possibility that some actions of exogenous FMRFamide (Stell et al 1984; Walker and Stell in preparation) may be explained by binding of FMRFamide to PP/NPY postsynaptic sites.

EFFERENT FIBRES

The only retinopetal (efferent retinal) pathway identified conclusively so far is the one originating in the terminal nerve (Stell et al 1984). Fibres in this pathway are immunoreactive for the molluscan cardioexcitatory peptide, FMRFamide (but not pancreatic polypeptides or NPY; see previous section) and the decapeptide, luteinizing hormone-releasing hormone (LHRH). EM-immunocytochemistry shows that these efferent fibres end primarily upon amacrine cell somata and dendrites (Ball and Stell, 1983). Exogenous salmon brain LHRH, which may be identical to the endogenous LHRH-like peptide, and FMRFamide, which quite clearly is not identical to any of several FMRFamide-immunoreactive compounds separated chromatographically from extracts (Parkinson et al in progress) act to modify ganglion cell sensitivity and evoked activity polysynaptically, through amacrine cell intermediaries. The action of LHRH is slow, prolonged, and powerfully desensitizing, whereas the action of FMRFamide is rapid, brief, and little desensitizing. Sensitivity of the goldfish retina to both LHRH and FMRFamide is seasonal, being higher in the actively reproductive season (winter-spring). The disappearance of FMRFamide and LHRH immunoreactivity in the retina two weeks after optic nerve crush (Muske et al 1984) suggests a useful approach to test the possibility that other neuropeptide systems - such as opioids and TRH -

may be associated with efferent fibres. In fact, we have used this approach recently to confirm the localization also of a substance P-like peptide to efferent fibres (Stell et al 1985).

Ganglion Cells

Not a single ganglion cell tranmitter has been positively identified in the goldfish retina. Acetylcholine has been suspected for some time Freeman et al 1980; Schmidt and Freeman, 1980), but attempts to identify cholinergic ganglion cells by a combination of backfiling and ChAT immunocytochemistry (Tumosa et al 1984b) or by changes in biochemical activity of ChAT in deafferented tectum (Ross and Godfrey, 1984) so far have yielded only negative results. The elegant studies of Kuljis et al (1984) on the frog retina indicate that some frog ganglion cells may be peptidergic and suggest a fruitful approach to this question in fish.

Discussion

It has been known for many years that a wide variety of structurally distinctive amacrine cells is to be found in the cyprinid fish retina. Cajal (1892), for example, illustrated about a dozen and a half amacrine cell types in the carp. Cajal's classification was based largely upon the appearance of cell in vetical (transverse) section, in which the branching patterns of neurites within a particular IPL sublayer are difficult to appreciate. Ammermuller and Weiler (1982), therefore, studied amacrine cells in whole, flat-mounted carp retinas, arriving at a classification scheme having only three main classes and six sub-classes. Even this is more than the variety of cells observed by intracellular recording and marking with micropipettes, according to which only three response types (ON, OFF, ON-OFF) and 3-6 morphological types of amacrines have been observed (Famiglietti et al 1977; Murakami and Shimoda 1977; Downing 1983; Djamgoz et al 1984). These data have led to "skepticism that the large number of apparent morphological subclasses is attributable to the proclivity of anatomists to classify neurons by trivial differences in structural detail" (Stell et al 1980).

Such skepticism is clearly refuted by the ability of neurochemically selective methods to label a wide variety of amacrine cells. In goldfish, for exaple, the number of cell types identified so far by histofluorescence, uptake-autoradiography, or immunocytochemistry - about a dozen and a half - nearly equals the number discerned by Cajal in his Golgi preparations. In many instances, furthermore, it is easy to assign a recently-discovered neurochemical signature to one of Cajal's cell types (compare Figs. 1 and 2 and Table I).

A major reason for focusing upon retinal transmitter systems is the unqiue suitability of the retina for parallel anatomical, physiological, biochemical and pharmacological investigations. The wealth of evidence for neuropeptides in the retina, therefore, is encouraging for further study. With rare exceptions, however, neuropeptide experiments in the retina - as elsewhere in the CNS - have succeeded only in showing that the tissue contains a substance recognized by antiserum raised to another (presumably similar) synthetic substance of known structure, or that it responds functionally to such a synthetic substance. Rarely has the synthetic, exogenous transmitter candidate been shown to be identical (or non-identical) to the true, endogenous transmitter. Almost as rarely have the neural connections of the presumed peptidergic (or even non-peptidergic) retinal neurones been analyzed in sufficient detail and specificity to allow a functional interpretation of "peptidergic" circuitry to be made.

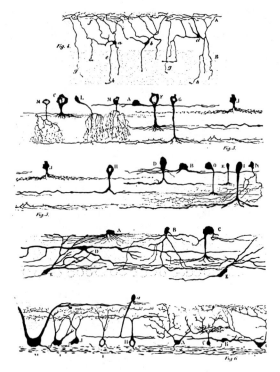

Fig. 1. Drawings of neurones in carp retina, impregnated with silver chromate (rapid Golgi method) and sectioned vertically. Compare Table I and Figure 2 (After Cajal, 1892).

Daw et al (1982) have outlined with particular clarity an appealing classification of transmitter roles in retinal function. First, the neurotransmitters of photoreceptors, bipolar cells and ganglion cells "simply carry the message from a neuron at one level of processing to a neuron at the next level". Second, the neurotransmitters of some horizontal and amacrine cells (for example, GABA and glycine) create "trigger features" of ganglion cells – that is, they restrict the range of stimulus properties that will be sufficient to evoke a postsynaptic response. Third, neurotransmitters in some pathways may effect much more subtle alterations ("modulations") in stimulus effectiveness, without radically changing the response type or trigger features. Acetylcholine and biogenic amine-releasing amacrine cells are mentioned as candidates for such roles. "So what is left for peptides?" ask Daw et al; answering, "Nobody knows".

Before undertaking this review, I subscribed to a view closely akin to the view of Daw et al that "maybe the peptides modulate the action of the dopamine cells, and the dopamine cells modulate the action of the acetycholine cells, and the acetylcholine cells modulate the action of...", and so forth. But this survey of the body of data available, while admittedly revealing far less than we would like to know about such fundamental issues, has produced a surprising conclusion.

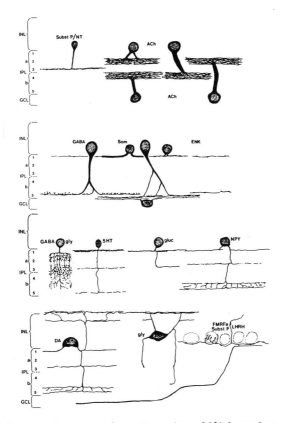

Fig. 2. Schematic drawings of neurones in goldfish retina, as inferred from neurochemical labeling studies. Subst P = substance P; NT = neurotensin; ACh = acetylcholine; GABA = gamma-aminobutyric acid; Som = somatostatin; ENK = enkephalin; glyc = glycine; 5HT = 5hydroxytryptamine (serotonin); gluc = glucagon; NPY = neuropeptide Y; DA = dopamine; FMRFa = Phe-Met-Arg-Phe-NH$_2$; LHRH = teleostean luteinizing hormone-releasing hormone. Compare Table I and Figure 1.

The surprise is that the circuitry of retinal neurones which contain conventional (non-peptide) neurotransmitter candidates differs so little overall from the circuitry of putatively peptidergic neurones. GABA and acetylcholine to be sure, may act directly upon ganglion cells in many instances; but so may the peptides substance P, somatostatin, and glucagon. Opioids, LHRH and FMRFamide-like peptides may well be employed more or less exclusively in amacrine cell interactions; but so, apparently, are serotonin, dopamine and glycine (excepting their action upon horizontal cells). One might conclude, therefore, that neuropeptides are every bit as likely to be neurotransmitters in the retina as any of the more conventionally accepted candidates. One may also speculate, following the line of reasoning suggested by Marshak, Ariel and Dowling (1984), that amacrine cells containing peptides or biogenic amines are concerned largely with "simple" ON or OFF pathways employing a low density of uncomplicated synaptic contacts, whereas amacrine cells containing acetylcholine or amino acids (or stubstance P!) are concerned largely with

184

T A B L E I

Amacrine Cells and Putative Neurotransmitters in Goldfish Retina

Cell Type Designation	Presumed Transmitter	IPL Layer	Cajal Figure	Inputs from BC	AC	Outputs to BC	GC	AC
GabAb	GABA	5	5(I)	+		+		
AChA(a/c)	ACh	2	5(C)			27%	few	few
AChA(b/d)	ACh	4	5(F)			27%	11%	36%
SPA(3)/NTA(3)	SP/NT	3	5(H,O)	56%	44%	0%	52%	48%
SAa(1,1)	SS)-13,128)	1	5(A)	12%	88%	5%	42%	53%
SAb, SGb	SS(-14,-28)	5	5(G)	11%	89%	8%	34%	58%
GlAa	Glucagon	1,3	5(B)	0	0	0	34%	66%
GabAa	GABA/Gly?	1-4	5(LMN)			19%	3%	57%
GlyAa	GABA/Gly	1-4	5(LMN)		+	rare	rare	+
IAA	5-HT	1,3,5	6(A)	6%	94%	12%	0	88%
I1-IPC	DA/VIP?	1,3,5	2(C)	0	+	occ.	0	+
12-IPC	Gly	?	4(abd)					
PPA	NPY	1,3,5	2(B)					
CRFA	CRF	1	5(B)					
TRHA?	TRH	?						
ENKA	ENK	1,5						+
EF(NT)	"FMRFamide"	1		0	0	0	0	+
	LHRH							
	"Subst. P"							
Trans +/-	?	1,3						

Summary of neurochemically identified cell types in goldfish retina (see Fig. 2) listing putative neurotransmitters, layers of stratification in the inner plexiform layer (IPL), similar cells described by Cajal (1892; see Fig. 1), known or inferred inputs and outputs.

functionally "complex" pathways employing a high density of complex synaptic contacts.

What we know least about, of course, is precisely what the peptides do at their presumed sites of action. The data available reveal tantalizing glimpses of possibly unique functional attributes: unusually delayed or prolonged actions (substance P, LHRH); action at a distance, without immediate contact (VIP); presynaptic modulation of release (TRH); and regulation of transmitter and receptor processing. For the most part it appears that a realistic appreciation of the visual role of neuropeptides - and indeed of amacrine cells themselves - awaits the results of a multitude of detailed studies on the synaptic interconnections, visual processing functions, and synaptic chemistry of the inner plexiform layer, as well as of subcellular regulatory mechanisms common to retinal and nonretinal neurones. We may expect substantial progress on all these fronts within the next few years.

References

Altschuler,R.A., J.L. Mosinger, G.G. Harmison, M.H., Parakkal and R.J. Wenthold. Nature 198, 657-659 (1982).
Ammermuller, J. and R. Weiler Cell Tiss. Res. 220, 699-723 (1981).
Ball, A.K. and C. Brandon Invest. Ophthal. Vis. Sci. Suppl 26, 1985.
Ball, A.K. and W.K. Stell Invest. Ophthal. Vis. Sci. Suppl. 24, 66 (1983).
Brecha, N. in Chemical Neuroanatomy P.C. Emson ed, (Raven Press, N. Y. 1983) pp. 85-129.

1983) pp. 85-129.
Brecha, N. S.C. Sharma and H.J. Kare=ten Neurosci. 6, 2737-2746 (1982).
Birt. D/R/ Exp. Eye Res. 29, 353-365 (1979).
Cajal, S.R. y. Cellule 9, 121-225 (1892).
Chan, R.Y. and K.I. Naka Ves. Res. 16, 1119-1129 (1976).
Daw, N.W., M. Ariel and J.H. Caldwell. Retina 2, 322-331 (1982).
Djamgoz, M.B.A., J.E.G. Downing and D.J. Prince Biochem. Soc. Trans. 11, 686-689 (1983).
Djamgoz, M.B.A., W.K. Stell, C.-A. Chin and D.M.K. Lam Nature 292, 620-623 (1981).
Dowling, J.E. in The Neurosciences. F.O. Schmitt and F.G. Worden eds. (MIT Press, Cambridge MA 1979) pp. 163-181.
Dowling, J.R. and B. Ehinger. Science 188, 270-273 (1975).
Dowling, J.R. and B. Ehinger. Proc. Roy. Soc. Lond. B. 201, 7-26 (1978).
Dowling, J.E. and F.Ş. Werblin J. Neurophysiol. 32, 315-338 (1969).
Downing, J.E.G. Ph.D. Thesis, Univ. London. Imperial College of Science and Technology (1983).
Dubin, M.W. J. Comp. Neurol. 140, 479-506 (1970).
Ehinger, B., B. Falck and A.M. Laties. Z. Zellforsch. 97, 2950297 (1969).
Ehinger, B. and I. Floren. Cell Tiss. Res. 175, 37-48 (1976).
Ehinger, B. and I. Floren. Exp. Eye Re. 26, 321-328 (1978).
Eskay, R.L., J.F. Furness and R.T. Long. Science 212, 1049-1051 (1981).
Eskay, R.L., R.T. Long and P.M. Iuvone. Brain Res. 196, 554-559 (1980).
Famiglietti, E.V., Jr., A. Kaneko and M. Tachibana Science 198, 1267-1269 (1977).
Famiglietti, E.V., Jr., H. Kolb Science 194, 193-195 (1976).
Francis, C.M. J. Physiol. Lond. 120, 435-439 (1953).
Freeman, J.A., J.T. Schmidt and R.E. Oswald Neuroscience 5, 929-942 (1980).
Glickman, R.D. and A.R. Adolph. Invest. Ophthal. Vis. Sci. Suppl 18, 33-34 (1979).
Glickman, R.D. and A.R. Adolph. Joint Fall Mtng. APS/CZS, Abstracts (1980).
Glickman, R.D., A.R. Adolph and J.E. Dowling. Invest. Ophthal. Vis. Sci. Suppl 19, 281 (1980).
Glickman, R.D., A.R. Adolph and J.E. Dowling. Brain Res. 234, 81-99 (1982).
Hadjiconstantinou, M., A.P. Mariani, P. Panula, T.H. Joh and N.H. Neff Neurosci. 13, 547-551 (1984).
Hankins, M.W. and K.H. Ruddock Neurosci. Lett 44, 1-6 (1984).
Hedden, W.L. and J.E. Dowling Proc. Roy. Sco. Lond. B. 201, 27-55 (1978).
Holmgren-Taylor, I. Cell Tiss. Res. 229, 317-335 (1983).
Hunter, J.E. and J.E. Maggio. Eur. J. Pharmacol. 105, 149-153 (1984).
Jan, Y.N., C.W. Bowers, D. Branton, L. Evans and L.Y. Jan. in Molecular Neurobiology. Cold Spring Harbor Symp Quant. Biol 48, 363-374 (1983).
Kaneko, A. J. Physiol Lond. 207, 623-633 (1970).
Kaneko, A. J. Physiol Lond. 235, 133-153 (1973).
Kato, S., T. Teranishi, C.H. Kuo and K. Negishi J. Neurochem. 39, 493-498 (1982).
Kato, S., K. Negishi, T. Teranishi and K. Sugawara. Vis. Res. 23, 445-449 (1983).
Kolb, H., R. Nelson and A. Mariani. Vis. Res. 21, 1081-1114 (1981).
Kuljis, R.O., J.E. Krause and H.J. Karten. J. Comp. Neurol. 226, 222-237 (1984).
Lam, D.M.K. Nature 254, 345-347 (1975).
Lam, D.M.K. and L. Steinman Proc. Nat. Acad. Sci. USA 68, 2777-2781 (1971).
Lasater, E.M., K.J. Watling and J.E. Dowling Science 221, 1070-1072 (1983).
Laufer, M., K. Negishi and B.D. Drujan Vis. Res. 21, 1657-1660 (1981).

Li, H.B., D.W. Marshak and J.E. Dowling. Invest. Ophthal. Vis. Sci. Supp. 24, 222 (1983)

Marc, R.E. in Colour Vision Deficiences V. G. Verriest, ed. (Adam Hilger Ltd., Bristol 1980) pp. 15-29.

Marc, R.E. Vis. Res. 22, 589-608 (1982).

Marc, R.E. and D.M.K. Lam J. Neurosci. 1, 152-165 (1981a).

Marc, R.E. and D.M.K. Lam Proc. Nat. Acad. Sci. USA 78, 7185-7189 (1981b).

Marc, R.E., W.K. Stell D. Bok and D.M.K. Lam. J. Comp. Neurol. 182, 221-246 (1978).

Marshak, D., M. Ariel and J.E. Dolwing Invest. Ophthal Vis. Sci. Suppl 25, 284 (1984).

Marshak, D.W., J.E. Dowling and T. Yamada Invest. Ophthal. Vis. Sci. Suppl 24, 223 (1983).

Marshak, D.W., T. Yamada and W.K. Stell. J. Comp. Neurol. 225, 44-52 (1984).

Miller, R.F. in The Neurosciences. F.O. Schmitt and F.G. Worden, Eds (MIT Press, Cambridge, MA 1979) pp. 227-245.

Miller, R.F. and R.F. Dacheux J. Gen. Physiol. 67, 679-690 (1976).

Murakami, M. and Y. Shimoda J. Physiol Lond. 264, 801-818 (1977).

Muske, L.E. and W.K. Stell Invest. Ophthal Vis. Sci. Suppl 25, 284 (1984).

Muske, L.E., W.K. Stell and K.S. Chohan Soc. Neurosci. Abstracts 10, 839 (1984).

Naka, L.-I. Invest. Ophthal. 15, 926-935 (1976).

Naka, K.-I. J. Neurophysiol. 40, 26-43 (1977).

Negishi, K., S. Kata and T. Teranishi Neurosci. Lett. 25, 1-5 (1981).

Negishi, K., S. Kato, T. Teranishi and M. Laufer. Brain Res. 148, 67-84 (1978a).

Negishi, K., S. Kato, T. Teranishi and M. Laufer. Brain Res. 148, 85-93 (1978b).

Negishi, K., M. Laufer and B.D. Drujan. J. Neurosci. Res. 5, 599-609 (1980).

Negishi, K., T. Teranishi and S. Kato. Neurosci. Lett. 37, 261-266 (1983).

Osborne, N.N., T. Nesselhut, D.A. Nicholas, S. Patel and A.C. Cuello J. Neurochem. 39, 1519-1528 (1982).

Reading, H.W. J. Neurochem. 42, 1587-1595 (1983).

Ross, C.D. and D.A. Godfrey. Soc. Neurosci. Abstracts 10, 575 (1984).

Ross, C.D. and D.B. McDougal, Jr. J. Neurochem. 265, 521-526 (1976).

Sarthy, P.V. and D.M.K. Lam. J. Neurochem. 32, 1269-1277 (1979).

Schellart, N.A.M., H.F. VanAcker and H. Spekreijse Neurosci. Lett. 48, 31-36 (1984).

Schmidt, J.T. and J.A. Freeman. Brain Res. 187, 129-142 (1980).

Schwartz, I.R. and D. Bok. J. Neurocytol. 8, 53-66 (1979).

Stell, W.K., K. S. Chohan and N. Brecha. Soc. Neurosci. Abstracts 7, 94 (1981).

Stell, W.K., K.S. Chohan and A.L. Kyle Invest. Ophthal Vis. Sci. Suppl 26, (1985).

Stell, W.K. D., Marshak, T. Yamada, N. Bre=cha and H. Karten. Trends in Neurosci. 292-295 (1980).

Stell, W.K., S.E. Walker, K.S. Chohan and A.K. Ball. Proc. Nat. Acad. Sci. USA 82, 940-944 (1984).

Su, Y.-Y. T. and D.M.K. Lam. Invest. Ophthal. Vis. Sci. 22, 179 (1982).

Tornqvist, K., R. Uddman, F. Sundler and B. Ehinger. Histochem. 76, 137-152 (1982).

Tumosa, N., F. Eckenstein and W.K. Stell Neurosci. Lett 48, 255-259 (1984).

Tumosa, N., W.K. Stell and F. Eckenstein Invest. Ophthal. Vis. Sci. Suppl 24, 223 (1983).

Tumosa, N., W.K. Stell and F. Eckenstein Invest. Ophthal. Vis. Sci. Suppl 25, 284 (1984a).

Tumosa, N., W.K. Stell and F. Eckenstein Soc. Neurosci. Abstracts 10, 575 (1984b).

Walker, S.E. and W.K. Stell Soc. Neurosci Abstracts 10, 837 (1984).

Watling, K.J. and J.E. Dowling. J. Neurochem. 41, 1205-1213 (1983).

Werblin, F.S. in The Neurosciences F.O. Schmitt and F.G. Worden, eds (MIT Press, Cambridge, MA 1979) pp. 193-211.

Werblin, F.S. and J.E. Dowling J. Neurophysiol 32, 339-355 (1969).

Yamada, T., D. Marshak, J. Morley, J. Hershman, J. Walsh, S. Basinger and W. Stell. Proc. Nat. Acad. Sci. USA 77, 1691-1695 (1980).

Yazulla, S. J. Comp. Neurol. 200, 83-93 (1981).

Yazulla, S. and N. Brecha. Invest. Ophthal. Vis. Sci. 19, 1415-1426 (1980).

Yazulla, S., K.M. Studholme and C.L. Zucker. J. Comp. Neurol. 213, 232-238 (19).

Zucker, C. and S. Yazulla. J. Comp. Neurol 204, 188-195 (1982).

Zucker, C., S. Yazulla and J.-Y Wu. Brain Res. 298, 154-158 (1984).

Functional Organization of Amacrine Cells in the
Teleost Fish Retina

M.B.A. Djamgoz, J.E.G. Downing, E.Wagner*
H.-J. Wagner* and I. Zeutzius*

Cellular Neurobiology Laboratory
Imperial College
London, England

Institute of Anatomy & Cell Biology*
University of Marburg
Marburg, West Germany

Amacrine cells are 'axonless' units found in all vertebrate retinas (Cajal 1893). They form the second laterally organized system of interneurones in the retina, having their cell bodies at the proximal margin of the inner nuclear layer, and their synaptic connections within the inner plexiform layer (Stell 1972). One of their main functions is to participate in the processing and the integration of the sensory information present in the visual image being focused on the retina. They also influence directly both bipolar and ganglion cells, and are thought to critically control bipolar to gangion cell transmission, the final link in the 'through' pathway of signal propagation in the retina (Dowling 1979).

The synaptic pathways directly associated with amacrine cells are illustrated in Fig. 2. One of the main set of inputs to amacrine cells is derived from the bipolars, with which reciprocal connections are made (Witkovsky and Dowling 1969). Amacrine cells are also extensively coupled to each other via chemical and electrotonic junctions thereby forming a network that seems to encompass the entire retina (Kaneko 1973; Werblin 1972; Witkovsky and Dowling 1969; Djamgoz and Ruddock 1978b; Naka and Christensen 1981). Other synaptic pathways associated with amacrine cells include two-way connections with the interplexiform cells (Dowling and Ehinger 1975), and inputs from the horizontal cell axon terminals (Naka 1976, 1982; Marshak and Dowling 1984). Finally, amacrine cells provide some one-half of the synaptic inputs to ganglion cells (Witkovsky and Dowling 1969). These inputs are mediated through chemical synapses, and are largely inhibitory (Miller 1979). Amacrine cells are thus thought to generate the antagonistic peripheral zone of the ganglion cell receptive fields (Dowling 1979).

In this article, we shall review our work on the amacrine cells of a common European cyprinid fish, the roach (Rutilus rutilus), and the work done on other teleosts including closely related species such as goldfish and carp. Where significant results have been obtained in other vertebrates, and no counterpart exists in teleost fish, these will also be cited. In order to maximize our understanding of the functional organization of amacrine cells, we have adopted a multi-faceted approach. Relevant technical details are given in the publications listed amongst the references.

Electrophysiological Aspects

Light-evoked Responses
In the roach retina, we could initially classify the light-evoked electrical responses of the amacrine cells into three categories; 'sustained depolarizing', 'sustained hyperpolarizing', and 'transient'. Sample records of these responses illustrating a variety of features that we have observed are shown in Fig. 2. The waveforms of some sustained responses appear to be relatively smooth (Fig. 2 al, a3), whilst others

Neurocircuitry of the Retina, A Cajal Memorial
A. Gallego and P. Gouras, Editors

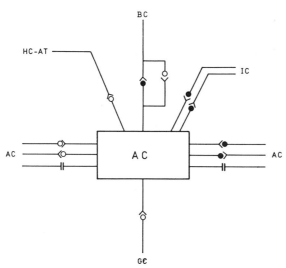

Fig. 1. The synaptic pathways associated with amacrine cells in teleost
fish retinas. Chemical synaptic connections are denoted by the
arrowhead/circle symbol; electro (gap) junctions are indicated by the
capacitor-like symbol. Inverted arrowheads denote presynaptic terminals
at excitatory and inhibitory synapses, respectively; crossed circles
denote interplexiform (IP) cell contacts where the functional identities
of the chemical synapses are not yet known. AC, amacrine cell; GC,
ganglion cell; HC-AT, horizontal cell axon terminal; BC, bipolar cell.

exhibit 'on' or 'off' transients, light-dependent membrane noise or
oscillations (Fig. 2 d1, a2,d3, c4). The transient amacrine cell
response clearly has three components: brief membrane depolarizations at
the onset and the offset of the light flash, and a sustained (D.C.)
component in between (Fig. 2 a6,b6). The durations of the transient
depolarizations appear to be variable (range 50-300 ms) giving the cells
either a brisk or sluggish time course of response (Fig 2 a5,b5,c5). The
D.C. component, if present, can be depolarizing or hyperpolarizing (Fig. 2
a6,b6). Some transient amacrine cell responses also incorporate
oscillations of membrane potential or spike-like activity, and
light-dependent membrane noise (Fig. 2 a7,b7). Another
interesting response component is the after-potential. Most commonly,
sustained depolarizing and transient responses are accompanied by a large
negativity at the offset of the light stimulus (Fig. 2 c1,c7). In some
sustained hyperpolarizing units, the after-potential can be 100 ms or
longer in duration, and several mV's in amplitude.

The question of amacrine cells generating 'action potentials' is
important, and if so, this would be a significant clue to their mode(s) of
functioning. Toyoda et al, (1973) have included some clear
spike-generators amongst their sustained units. None of our
morphologically identified sustained amacrine cells was associated with
spike trains. Murakami and Shimoda (1977) and Mitarai et al (1978), who
have also carried out electrophysiological studies of morphologically
identified amacrine cells, do not refer to spike activity in sustained
units. We have frequently impaled sustained units generating spike
activity, but these were later found to be ganglion cells. The large

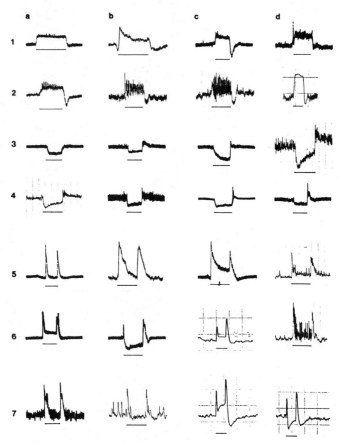

Fig. 2. A catalogue of light-evoked amacrine cell responses recorded in roach retinas. In each case, a 1mm diameter, 620 nm, 300 ms long test light stimulus (approximately 1 μW/mm^2) was used; its presentation is indicated by a horizontal bar beneath each response trace. Rows 1 and 2, sustained depolarizing responses; rows 3 and 4 sustained hyperpolarizing responses; rows 5-7, transient on-off responses. The response amplitudes illustrated are in the range of 10-20 mV, calibration bars have been omitted for clarity.

membrane depolarizations in the transient units, however, appear sometimes to be accompanied by a few spikes (Fig. 2 a7; see also Kaneko 1970); Murakami and Shimoda 1977). Kaneko and Hashimoto (1969) have shown that these spikes have a considerably longer duration (10 ms) compared with ganglion cell spikes (1-2 ms). Importantly, Murakami and Shimoda (1977) have found that non-spiking transient amacrine cells can be made to generate a spike by hyperpolarizing the membrane potential. This implies that the relatively course microelectrodes used for intracellular staining (see later) cause sufficient membrane damage and depolarization to inactivate the spike-generating mechanism. We do not know whether this is also true for the sustained units. Murakami and Shimoda (1977) have also

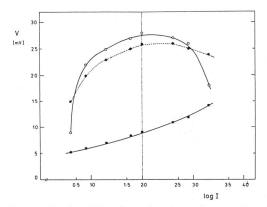

Fig. 3. V-log I relationships for the three components of the transient amacrine cell response. V, response amplitude (mV); log I, log relative illumination level, fixed arbitrarily as 0.0 for the dimmest stimulus used. Full and empty circles denote the values for the on and the off transients, respectively; squares refer to the D.C. component.

shown that the transient amacrine cell spikes are classical 'Hodgkin-Huxley' type sodium-dependent action potentials, since they were abolished by treating the retina with tetrodotoxin, similarly to the situation in the mudpuppy (Miller and Dacheux 1976).

Our three tier classification of the light evoked amacrine cell responses is in general agreement with schemes of Kaneko (1970, 1973), Toyoda et al (1973) Murakami and Shimoda (1977), Mitarai et al (1978) and Naka et (1978). It would be worth nothing, however, that the three types of response, in fact, possess some common features. Thus, sustained units can also have transient components, and vice versa, and all three can incorporate light-dependent membrane noise, oscillations and after potentials. Further, we have shown earlier that following brief, localized irradiation of the retina with a laser beam, purely sustained units can be made to generate transient responses (Djamgoz and Ruccock 1979a). Taken together, the existing evidence would suggest that the three electrophysiological types of amacrine cells may, in fact, be a homogenous group of neurones, and that their different response components represent differences in their synaptic connectivity, receptive field organization, and functional specialization, analogously to the different classes of horizontal cell (Stell and Lightfoot 1975). In order to understand better the functional significance of these light evoked electrophysiological response characteristics, we have concentrated on the transient amacrine cells, which incorporate most, if not all, of these characteristics.

<u>Operating Ranges</u>
A typical set of 'input-output' (responses voltage, V, vs. relative stimulus intensity, log I) relationships for the three response components of a transient amacrine cell is shown in Fig. 3. A number of conclusions can be reached from an examination of this data. The transients are associated with sharply rising V-log I curves, their operating ranges being less than 2 log units. The sustained component, on the other hand, has a much more gradually rising relationship, and a wider operating range, around 3 log untis, similarly to S potentials. Thus, both the on

192

being less than 2 log units. The sustained component, on the other hand, has a much more gradually rising relationship, and a wider operating range, around 3 log units, similarly to S potentials. Thus, both the on and the off transient depolarizations appear to be driven by a high gain mechanism enabling them (i) to have an absolute threshold level of illumination, at least 1log unit lower than the threshold for sustained component, and (ii) to be self-facilitatory for regenerative such that for a given stimulus intensity, a relatively large signal amplitude can be produced. Another interesting property of the transient components in that light stimuli brighter than that necessary to elicit a saturation response result in sub-maximal response amplitudes being generated. This indicates that the transient responses are also capable of rapid adaptation.

Spatial Organization
Both sustained and transient amacrine cells in goldfish have been shown to summate their signals over a retinal area of at least 2.5 mm in diameter (Kaneko 1973). We have shown that the lateral spread of signals in the amacrine cell layer of the roach retina is much more sensitive to local CoCl$_2$ application than the spread of S potentials in the horizontal cell layer (Djamgoz and Ruddock 1978b). This has been attributed to chemical coupling of the amacrine cells. Consistently with this suggestion, Witkovsky and Dowling (1969) have shown that serial, chemical synapses are found amongst amacrine cell processes in carp retina. Naka and Christensen (1981), on the other hand, have provided electrophysiological and ultrastructural evidence that amacrine cells of catfish may also couple through electrotonic (gap) junctions. It is not yet certain whether the chemically-coupled amacrine cells all use the same transmitter or different transmitters. Biochemical release experiments have shown that there are excitatory and inhibitory synaptic interactions between chemically unlike amacrine cells. Thus, putative enkephalinergic amacrine cells inhibit the GABAergic cells in goldfish retina (Djamgoz et al 1981). In turn, the latter and the glycinergic cells are inhibitory to cholinergic amacrine cells in rabbit retinas (Neal 1984). In the same retina x-MSH have been shown to excite the GABAergic cells (Bauer and Ehinger 1980). Although several neurotransmitter agonists cause the release of dopamine in a variety of retinas, it is not certain to what extent amacrine cells are involved (Kata et al 1983).

The other aspect of spatial organization is concerned with centre-surround antagonism. Although bipolar cells receptive fields are clearly centre-surround antagonistic (Kaneko 1970; Kaneko and Tachibana 1983), there are conflicting reports about the amacrine cells. Kaneko (1973; goldfish) and Murakami and Shimoda (1977; carp) have not observed centre-surround antagonisms in amacrine cells. Toyoda et al (1973) have reported, however, that some one-half of the sustained units encountered in the carp retina have such an organization. Mitarai et al (1978; carp) have also found some biphasic receptive field organization OTable 1). In catfish retina, Naka and Ohtsuka (1975) and Naka et al (1975) initially maintained that amacrine cells had monophasic receptive fields. Subsequently, Davis and Naka (1980) have shown that a large, antagonistic surround field does in fact exist. This seems to be true also in the roach retina, where using simple spot and annulus shaped test stimuli, we have observed that some centre-surround antagonisms also exists in the D.C. component of both sustained and transient units.

Taken together, the available electrophysiological, and morphological (see later) data suggest that amacrine cells may have more complex receptive fields than previously thought. The precise shapes and dimensions of these receptive fields are yet to be determined, however.

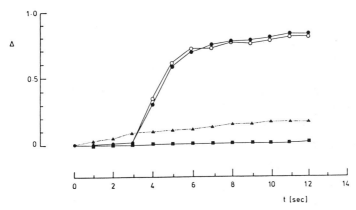

Fig. 4. Time course of recovery of maximal light-evoked response amplitudes of retinal interneurones following brief (0.1s), localized irradiation of the retina with a laser flash (647.1 nm; 0.13 W/mm^2); normalized maximal response amplitudes, expressed as a fraction of the corresponding pre-irradiation value. The laser flash was presented at t = 0. Full and empty circles, on and off components of a transient amacrine cell; squares, D.C. components; triangles, L_1/H_1 type S potentials (horizontal cell responses).

Sensitivity and Adaptation

As already noted, the light-evoked response characteristics of the transient amacrine cells would make them ideal for the control of sensitivity and adaptation in the retina. This high gain sensitivity control mechanism also manifests itself in the light-evoked amacrine cells responses during recovery of the retina from a brief intense bleaching light or when a steady background field of light is presented to the retina. The latter experiment was first carried out in the retina of the carp by Kaneko and Hashimoto (1969). They showed that during continuous application of background illumination, the transient amacrine cell response amplitudes, elicited by test light flashes, initially decrease but within about a minute or so, gradually recover to their original levels. A comparable phenomenon has been demonstrated in the retina of the roach by Djamgoz and Ruddock (1978a). This is illustrated in Fig. 4. When the retinal area covered by the test light flashes is irradiated briefly with a laser beam, the membrane potential of the transient amacrine cell is clamped for some seconds in a state of light adaptation, from which it gradually recovers. Within 10-20 seconds of the irradiation, the transient responses elicited by the test light flashes return to their full pre-irradiation levels. The sustained component, on the other hand, remains suppressed. Under these conditions, the L_1/H_1 type horizontal cell (and presumably cone photoreceptor) responses also lose much of their sensitivity, recovering no more than some 20% of their pre-irradiation response levels. This result again indicates that the transient components of amacrine cells are driven by relatively high gain (presumably synaptic) mechanism(s), compared with the slow (sustained) components and S potentials. This property enables the transients to retain their normal response levels under conditions when neurones of the distal retina have lost much of their sensitivities.

It might be relevant to note here that a similar sensitivity control phenomenon is apparent in ON-OFF ganglion cell responses (Werblin and Copenhagen 1974), and that substance P might be involved in this proves (Glickman 1982; Djamgoz et al 1983). Thus, we have found that application of 1 μM substance P to roach retina, following pre-treatment with an anti-peptidase cocktail, induces the following effects in ON-OFF ganglion cells (i) the dark- and light-dependent activities of the cells are enhanced; (ii) the absolute thresholds of light-evoked responses are increased by more than a log unit of illumination level; and (iii) the maximum response levels of the cells are more than trebled (Djamgoz et al 1983). It is not yet certain whether this mechanism originates in the corresponding amacrine cells or results from peptidergic transmission from amacrine to ganglion cell. Retinal amacrine cells contain most, if not all, of the neuroactive peptides in the central nervous system. On the whole, the physiology of retinal peptides is very poorly understood at present, but the quantitative results with substance P are an encouraging start in this direction.

Colour Coding

The chromatic organization of amacrine cells in the cyprinid fish retina was first described by Kaneko (1973). The sustained units of the goldfish were found to be colour coded similarly to the biphasic S potentials, but they were hyperpolarizing to long, and depolarizing to short wavelength lights. The transient type amacrine cells were found to be driven mainly by the red-sensitive cones (Kaneko and Hashimoto 1969).

Amacrine cells of the roach retina appear to have some novel features, as regards their chromatic organization. Most of the morphologically identified sustained amacrine cells of the roach do not appear to generate clearly colour coded, opposite polarity responses (Djamgoz 1978). The on and the off components of the transient amacrine cells are driven mainly by the red-sensitive cones in control retinas. Following laser irradiation, however, spectrally selective shifts in the quantum spectral sensitivity functions of these components have been observed thereby indicating that inputs from green- and or blue-sensitive cones may also be present (Djamgoz, 1978; Djamgoz and Ruddock 1983).

An interesting result concerns colour coding by the sustained component of the transient amacrine cells. We have found that in some 15% of these cells impaled randomly in the roach retina, the D.C. component is depolarizing to long, and hyperpolarizing to short wavelength lights (Djamgoz 1978; Djamgoz Ruddock 1983) (Fig. 5). In the rest of the units we have studied, the sustained component was monophasic (depolarizing), and its quantum spectral sensitivity was driven either by the red-sensitive cones alone or together with additional cone input(s). We have observed transient amacrine cells with colour-coded D.C. components also in the goldfish retina (unpublished work carried out in the laboratory of W.K. Stell). One of the figures in Kaneko (1973) also demonstrate the same effect. Mitarai et al (1978) have found that the D.C. components of sustained and transient amacrine cells encode colour extensively. Thus, 3 out of 7 sustained, and 6 out of 20 transient amacrine cells with a D.C. component were found to have a variety of combinations of spectral response (Table 1).

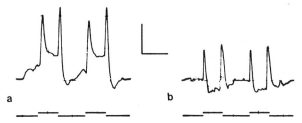

Fig. 5. Light evoked responses of a transient amacrine cell elicited by flashes (0.5s duration; approximately 1 μW/mm^2) of 446 nm (a) and 656 nm (b) light spots (0.6 mm diameter). Theresponses clearly demonstrate the colour-opponent D.C. component. Calibration bars 5 mV and 0.5s. (modified from Djamgoz and Ruddock 1983).

TABLE 1

Chromatic organization of sustained amacrine cell responses (+, depolarizing; - , hyperpolarizing) in the retina of the carp. Stimuli were red, R (640 nm), green, G (540 nm) and blue, B (460 nm) spots (0.7 mm diameter) and annuli (1.3 mm i.d., 2.0 mm o.d.) Modified from Mitarai et al (1978).

CENTRE			SURROUND		
R	G	B	R	G	B
+	+	+	−	+	+
+	−	−	−	−	−
+	−	−	−	−	+
+	−	+	−	−	−
−	−	+	−	−	−
−	+	+	−	−	−

Motion Detection

Motion sensitivity of certain ganglion cells in vertebrate retinas has been well documented (Barlow et al 1964). Amacrine cells are generally believed to have a crucial role in generating this function, although motion sensitivity of amacrine cells themselves has not been studied in detail (Miller 1979). Possible movement sensitivity of amacrine cells has been inferred from their anatomical features. Witkovsky and Dowling (1969); Dowling (1968, 1979); Dowling and Werblin (1969) have demonstrated that serial, chemical (i.e. one-way transmitting) synaptic connections frequently occur amongst amacrine cell dendrites in fish and amphibian retinas, thereby suggesting a role in motion detection. Miller (1979) has put forward a general model for the synaptic basis of motion sensitivity and directional selectivity of ganglion cells based on (i) amacrine to amacrine, and amacrine to ganglion cell inhibition, and (ii) bipolar to ganglion, and bipolar to amacrine cell excitation. Mariani (1982) has suggested, on the basis of their circularly asymmetrical dendritic fields, that the axon-bearing, association amacrine cells of the bird retina might mediate directional selectivity.

Direct electrophysiological evidence for motion sensitivity of the amacrine cells has been provided by Naka (1980) and Werblin (1970). In the retina of the catfish, Naka (1980) has found that a class of amacrine cell (Type BN) responds much more efficiently to a bar of light moving vertically in the fish's visual field than horizontally. The directional response of the cell comprises a sequence of depolarizing, hyperpolarizing and depolarizing membrane potentials. These cells' dendritic fields also demonstrate circular asymmetry, being selectively elongated along the fish's horizontal view. Werblin (1970) has shown that certain amacrine cells of the mudpuppy retina are transiently sensitive to the movement of a small spot of light across their receptive field boundaries. Thus, on-centre cells respond only as the scanning spot enters the field; off-centre units respond only as the spot leaves the field. Both types of unit are unresponsive to the spot as it traverses the middle of the field.

Morphological Aspects

There seems to be no doubt that retinal amacrine cells are a functionally very diverse group of interneurones. In order to attempt to correlate their electrophysiological response characteristics with their cellular morphologies and synaptic organizations, we have been carrying out a series of intracellular staining experiments using horseradish peroxidase (HRP) - filled microelectrodes. Up to this stage of our experiments, we have used relatively coarse micropipettes (tip resistances in the range 200-500 $M\Omega$, HRP-filled/40-60 $M\Omega$, KCl-filled) to obtain good staining. This has limited the time that could be spent on the electrophysiological characterization of the cells, and has probably resulted in selective impalement of those amacrine cells with relatively large somata and/or thick neurites (see later). We have, however, noted the following properties for most of the stained cells. (i) Light-evoked response type. This was decided using a small, red light spot (Fig. 2 legend for further details). Amacrine clels were thus classified, as described at the beginning of this article, into sustained depolarizing (SA^+), sustained hyperpolarizing (SA^-) and transient (TA); (ii) Colour coding. This was determined using 4 spectrally different test stimuli peaking at 454 nm, 534 nm, and 674 nm. (iii) Spatial organization. This was tested by recording and comparing a cell's response to small (0.5 mm diameter) and large (3 mm diameter) spot stimuli. Some of the sustained (SA) units appeared to have antagonistic surround receptive fields, and there was some indication of antagonistic centre- surround organization in the D.C. component of some TA's. Spatial summation was more commonly observed, however, in the amacrine cells studies.

We have so far successfully stained 45 amacrine cells (19 SA^+, 8 SA^- and 18 TA). We have studied their morphological details by light microscopy, and supplemented these observations by some Golgi-stained material. Our results on the morphological characteristics of functionally identified amacrine cells are summarized in the following sections.

Morphological Features of Amacrine Cells in the Plane of the Retina

Prior to radial sectioning of the stained cells and/or post-fixation with osmium for electron microscopy, the cells were examined in retinal whole mounts. From a qualitative assessment, the tangential views of all the cells appeared to fall into two groups irrespectively of their light-evoked response characteristics (Fig. 6; Table 2 Djamgoz et al 1984).

TABLE 2

Classification of amacrine cells. SA^+, SA^- , sustained depolarizing, and hyperpolarizing cells, respectively; TA, transient on-off cells.

Functional Class		Morphological Class	
		Type I n (%)	Type II n (%)
SA^+	19 (100%)	7 (37%)	12 (63%)
SA^-	8 (100%)	6 (75%)	2 (25%)
TA	18 (100%)	14 (78%)	4 (22%)
Total	45 (100%)	27 (60%)	18 (40%)

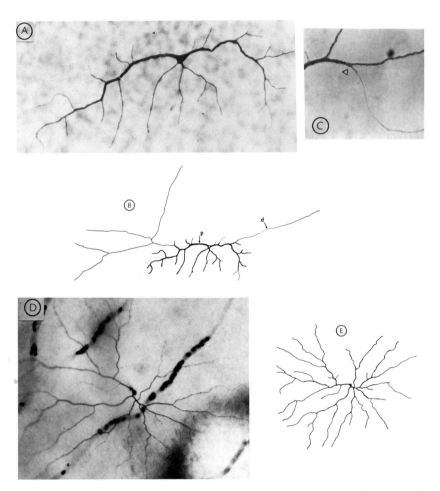

Fig. 6. Morphological classification of amacrine cells into Types I and
II. A.B, Wholemount photograph and camera lucida drawing, respectively,
of a Type I cell showing clearly p- and d-type dendrites. C, higher
magnification photograph of the junction between p- and d-type dendrites,
indicated by an arrowhead. D,E, wholemount photograph and camera lucida
drawing, respectively, of a Type II amacrine cell. Calibration bars 100
μm.

Type I amacrine cells have relatively large cell bodies (> 10 μm
diameter), and two types of dendrite. The main (p-type) dendritic field
comprises a number of neurites emerging from the cell body, and organized
proximally with respect to the cell body. The p-type dendrites and their
branches are at least 1 μm in thickness and terminate abruptly giving the
cells a chunky appearance. In most Type I cells that we have examined, a
distinctly different type of dendrite is also present. The latter arise
from branches of p-type dendrites, and project distally from the cell
body. We have termed them d-type dendrites. These are considerably
thinner than p-type dendrites, being usually less than 0.5 μm in diameter,
and gently tapering towards their terminations. In order to ensure that

d-type dendrites represent true cell processes, and not artefacts of staining, we have carefully examined their points of emergence from the corresponding cells under high magnification. Fig. 6c shows a typical junction between p and d-type dendrites, confirming the structural continuity of these processes. Although only 83% of the Type I amacrine cells stained had d-type dendrites, it is likely that these are, in fact, a common morphological feature of all Type I cells, and that the minority proportion represent incompletely or faintly stained cells.

Type II amacrine cells have similar size cell bodies to type I cells, which probably explain why they also have been successfully inpaled with the microelectrodes used for the present study. Their dendrites, however, are all gently tapering from the cell body towards their points of termination, where they are usually much thinner than 0.5 μm, giving the cells a fine spidery appearance. The dendrites of Type II amacrine cells appear to form a homogenous population with circularly symmetrical dendritic fields extending up to 1.3 mm in diameter.

Possible functional Significance of p- and d-type Dendrites

We have observed a maximum of 3, and most frequently 2 primary d-type dendrites per Type I amacrine cell. Each primary d-type dendrite we have seen is 1.6 mm, and between their extreme points, the overall dendritic field of a Type I amacrine cell could span up to 2.96 mm. Since, as already noted, it is not yet certain that all amacrine cells generate action potentials, the mechanism(s) by which slow signals are propagated over such long distances is unclear. One possibility is that relatively distant dendritic branches of these amacrine cells are, in fact, electrically isolated from each other (Ellias and Stevens 1980).

The p-type dendritic field of Type I amacrine cells are circularly asymmetrical and more or less eliptical, with the long and the short axes measuring 430 = 22 μm and 263 + 19 μm, respectively (means = SEM: n=19) (ranges 267-598 μm and 83-392 μm, respectively). The long axes of the cells have a preferred orientation in the retina, subtending an angle of $91 + 3^{\circ}$ (mean + SEM; n=21) at the optic disc. d-type dendrites also appear to have a similar orientation. The average angle which primary d-type dendrites subtend at the optic disc is $95 = 4^{\circ}$ (mean + SEM; n=37). Thus, both the p-type dendritic fields, and d-type dendrites are more or less tangentially oriented with respect to the optic disc.

The functional significance of the preferred orientation of Type I amacrine cells in the roach retina is also not yet clear. It is plausible that such dendritic field asymmetry and preferred orientation may be related to the motion sensitivity and directional selectivity of the cells's receptive fields (Naka 1980; Bloomfield and Miller 1982). Alternatively, these features may be the result of constraints in the growth of the eye and the retina. Johns (1981) has shown that during eye growth, the density of the cells in the inner nuclear and ganglion cell layers decreases. It would follow from this that during growth amacrine cell dendritic fields might become elongated with an orientation bias, as observed.

Golgi-stained Amacrine Cells

The Types I and II amacrine cells characterized in the present study by HRP filling correspond to the giant and the stellate amacrine cells, respectively which Cajal (1983) described in the retinas of several lower vertebrates. His drawings of Type I cells in the carp retina, however, do not show any d-type dendrites, whilst similar cells in the reptilian retinas appear to stain completely (Kolb 1982). In view of the known wider morphological diversity of amacrine cells observed in previous Golgi

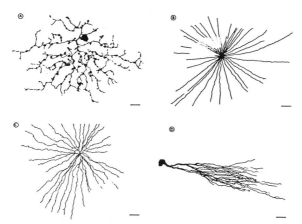

Fig. 7. A sample of amacrine cells of the roach retina stained with Golgi method. Calibration bars 10 μm (A, C, D) and 50 μm (B).

studies, we were surprised to find that we could impale and stain only the two types of amacrine cell. We have, therefore, processed a few roach retinas for Golgi staining of the neurones to see if and what other types of amacrine cell might be found. Not surprisingly, we have observed several different types of amacrine cell, and some of these are shown in Fig. 7. Some of the cells (Fig. 7a,d) have relatively large cell bodies (10 um diameter) similar to Type I amacrine cells. The fact that we have not impaled them with out HRP-filled microelectrodes suggests that there are relatively few of these cells in the roach retina. The asymmetrical cell shown in Fig. 7d is very similar to the glucagon-containing amacrine cells of the rabbit retina (Brecha and Karten 1984). The cell shown in Fig. 7b is clearly a starburst amacrine cell, which has been observed in the retinas of several vertebrates, and shown to be cholinergic (Famiglietti 1983; Stell, this volume). The dendritic field of this cell is much bigger than those of the others (note the different scale bar). The cell shown in Fig. 7c appears to correspond to a Type II amacrine cell. Thus, staining amacrine cells by intracellular injection of HRP and the Golgi technique gives complimentary results, and a more complete catalogue of the cell types than provided by either method. We are now in the process of further complimenting this catalogue by staining the cells immunohistochemically, as well.

Organization of Amacrine Cells Within the Layering of the Retina
On the basis of the layering of their dendrites within the inner plexiform layer (i.p.l.), Cajal (1893) divided the amacrine cells of all vertebrate retinas into two main types:

(i) Diffuse amacrine cells with dendrites that ramify and terminate throughout the full vertical extent of the i.p.l. and
(ii) Stratified amacrine cells whose arborizations are confined to one (monostratified) or more (bi-stratified or multi-stratified) distinct levels. By examining the cells in retinal wholemounts and noting the focal depth of the different dendritic layer(s), we have classified our population of functionally identified amacrine cells according to Cajal's scheme, and found the following generalizations:

1. Transient amacrine cells are mostly bi-stratified, multi-stratified or diffuse; only a few are monostratified (see later);
2. Sustained amacrine cells are never bi-stratified or

multi-stratified; they are mostly mono-stratified.

3. Type I cells are never diffusely stratified;

4. Type II cells are never bi-stratified or multi-stratified i.e. they are either diffuse or manostratified.

In the carp retina, Cajal (1893) distinguished 13 different types of amacrine cell based on the layering of their dendrites at the different levels of the i.p.l. He suggested that the i.p.l. was made up of a number of (perhaps 5) sub-strata to enable functionally related bipolar, amacrine and ganglion cell dendrites to be anatomically matched by being confined to one or more of these stratum and thus to form specific synaptic inter-connections. Famiglietti and Kolb (1976) have put forward a simplified version of this scheme in which the i.p.l. is considered to be made up of two sub-laminae only, with the distal half (sub-lamina A) subserving hyperpolarizing responses, and the other (sub-lamina B) depolarizing ones. This hypothesis has been tested in the retina of the carp and found to be true (Famiglietti et al 1977). We have repeated the test for the amacrine cells of the roach retina using our population of 45 units. The results are shown in Fig. 8, the procedure used being outlined in the lengend. Thus, the dendrites of the SA^- maacrine cells are confined to sub-lamina A, whilst those of SA^+ units are found within sub-lamina B. The transient amacrine cell dendrites, on the other hand, are clearly stratified in both sub-laminae.

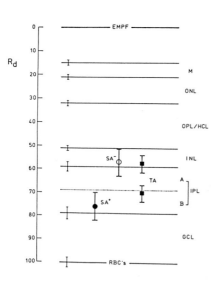

Fig. 8. An assessment of the stratification of amacrine cell dendrites within the inner plexiform layer (i.p.l.) by focal plane measurement. Rd, retinal depth (relative units; 0%, mid focal plane of the photoreceptor ellipsoids; 100%, layer of red blood cells within the inner limiting membrane, which are labelled by the diamino-benzidine reaction procedure used. The division of the retinal thickness (100%) into the various layers was achieved by making reference to histological sections of retinas prepared for electron microscopy. EMFP, ellipsoid mid-focal plane; M, myoids; ONL, outer nuclea layer; OPL, outer plexiform layer; HCL, horizonal cell layer; INL, inner nuclear layer; IPL, inner plexiform layer, sub-divided equally into sublaminae A and B; GCL, ganglion cell layer; RBC, layer of red blood cells. SA^+, SA^-, sustained depolarizing and hyperpolarizing units (closed and open circles), respectively; TA, transient amacrine cells (squares). The error bars associated with the different levels denote S.E.M.'s)

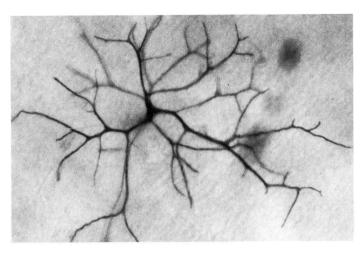

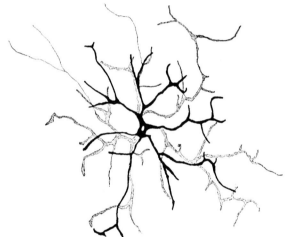

Fig. 9. Tangetial views of the p-type dendritic fields of a bi-stratified Type I amacrine cell (the light-evoked response of the cell was transient). Above, wholemount view photographed at the level of the proximal dendritic field. Below, camera lucida drawing showing the spatial relationship of the distal (black) and the proximal (dotted) dendritic fields. No relationship appears to exist between the two fields. Calibration bar 50 μm.

In the case of bi-stratified cells, we have questioned whether the two layers of dendritic field are in any way anatomically specialized with respect to each other in the plane of the retina. Fig. 9a shows a HRP stained Type I transient amacrine cell photographed at the level of the distal dendritic field. Fig. 9b is a composite camera lucida drawing of both dendritic fields. Clearly, there seems to be no special arrangement in the relative lay out of the two dendritic fields.

202

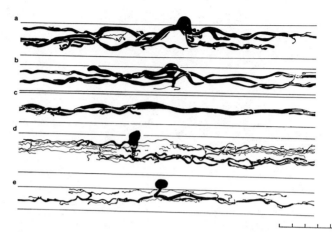

Fig. 10. Composite camera lucida drawings of transient amacrine cells from radial sections of retinas. In each case, the two horizontal lines denote the boundaries of the inner plexiform layer. x-c, Type I amacrine cells; d and e, Type II amacrine cells. Calibration bar 50 μm (5 x 10μm). Note that the full horizontal/tangetial extents of the cells are not shown.

We have recently been sectioning our collection of amacrine cells radially for further light microscopical analyses and eventual electron microscopical examination. Using the data that we have so far obtained, we would finally like to address the following question "Is the dendritic organization of a given functional type of amacrine cell within the i.p.l. the same for all such cells?" To elucidate this point for transient amacrine cells, we have examined the radial views of a number of cells. Camera lucida reconstructions of some of these are shown in Fig. 10. Clearly, the dendrites of different TA's are confined to different combinations of the sub-laminae of the i.p.l., and even within the small sample of cells included here, the possible synaptic domain of these cells appears to encompass the entire i.p.l. At one extreme some TA's are diffuse (Fig. 10d), whilst at the other, they are monostratified (Fig. 10c). We have seen only a few of the latter, but they always seem to be confined to sub-lamina 3, for both Types I and II. Thus, the middle zone of the i.p.l. may be a specialized region where perhaps depolarizing and hyperpolarizing synaptic potentials meet, and some transient responses are generated (Toyoda et al 1973; Miller 1979). As already noted, the latter response type is well suited for control of sensitivity and adaptation in the retina. Interestingly, the dendrites of the amacrine cells that are immunoreactive to substance P, which we have also implicated in this role, ramify in this sub-lamina (Brecha et al 1982; Djamgoz and Osborne, unpublished observation in the roach).

Although the Famiglietti - Kolb rule seems to stand to preliminary testing, it is likely to represent an over-simplification of the functional sub-division of the i.p.l. As already noted, the light evoked responses of the amacrine cells (as well as the bipolars and ganglion cells) can be depolarizing or hyperpolarizing depending at least on the colour and/or the spatial configuration of the stimulus. This can be so even for monostratified units. It is also evident from Fig. 10 that although the transient units broadly correspond to bi-stratified or diffuse amacrine cells, the stratification of their dendrites within the i.p.l. vary from unit to unit. This question clearly requires further investigation using more elaborate stimuli.

References
Barlow, H.B., Hill, R.M. and Levick, W.R. J. Physiol (Lond). 173, 377-407 (1964).
Bauer, B. and Ehinger, B. Acta Physiol Scand. 108, 105-107 (1980).
Bloomfield, S. and Miller, R.F. J. Comp. Neurol. 208, 288-303 (1982).
Brecha, N., Sharma, S.C. and Karten, H.J. Neurosci. 6, 2737-2746 (1981).
Brecha, N. and Karten, H.J. in Molecular and Cellular Basis of Visual Activity. J. Sheffield and R. Hiller eds. (Berlin/Srpinger 1984) pp. 107-135.
Cajal, S.R. La retine des vertebres. La Cellule 9, 17-257 (1893).
Davis, G.W. and Naka, K.-I. J. Neurophysiol 43, 807-831 (1980).
Djamgoz, M.B.A. Ph.D. Thesis, University of London (1978).
Djamgoz, M.B.A. and Ruddock, K.H. Neurosci Lett. 7, 89-93 (1978a).
Djamgoz, M.B.A. and Ruddock, K.H. Neurosci Lett. 10, 23-28 (1978b).
Djamgoz, M.B.A., Stell, W.K., Chin, C.-A. and Lam, D.M.K. Nature 292, 620-623 (1981).
Djamgoz, M.B.A. and Ruddock, K.H. J. Physiol.(Lond) 339, 19P (1983).
Djamgoz, M.B.A.,Downing, J.E.G and Prince, D.J. Biochem. Soc. Trans. 11, 686-689 (1983).
Djamgoz, M.B.A., Downing, J.E.G and Wagner, H.J. J. Physiol (Lond) 349, 21P (1984).
Dowling, J.E. Proc. R. Soc. B. 170, 205-228 (1968).
Dowling, J.E. in The Neurosciences. F. O. Schmitt and F. G. Worden eds (MIT Press,Cambridge 1979) pp. 163-181.
Dowling J.E. and Werblin, F.S. J. Neurophysiol 32, 315-338 (1969).
Dowling J.E. and Ehinger, B. Science 188, 270-273 (1975).
Ellias, S.A. and Stevens, J.K. Brain Res. 196, 365-372 (1980).
Famiglietti, E.V. jr. Brain Res. 261, 138-144 (1983).
Famiglietti, E.V. Jr. and Kolb, H. Science 194, 193-195 (1976).
Famiglietti, E.V. Jr., Kaneko, A. and Tachibana, M. Science 198, 1267-1268 (1977).
Johns, P.R. Amer. Zool. 21, 447-459 (1982).
Kaneko, A. J. Physiol (Lond) 207, 623-633 (1970).
Kaneko, A. J. Physiol (Lond) 235, 133-153 (1973).
Kaneko, A. and Hashimoto, H. Vis. Res. 9, 37-55 (1969).
Kaneko, A. and Tachibana, M. Nature 293, 220-222 (1983).
Kato, S. Negishi, K. Teranishi, T. and Sugawara, K. Vis. Re. 23, 355-393 (1983).
Kolb, H. Phil. Trans. R. Soc. Lond. B. 298, 355-393 (1982).
Mariani, A. Nature 198, 654-655 (1982).
Marshak, D.W. and Dowling, J.E. Soc. Neurosci Abstr. 10, 21 (1984).
Miller, R.F. in The Neurosciences. F.O. Schmitt and F.G. Worden eds. (MIT press, Cambridge 1979) pp. 227-245.
Miller, R.F. and Dacheux, R.F. Brain Res. 104, 157-162 (1976).
Mitarai, G., Goto, T. and Takagi, S. Sensory Processes 2, 375-382 (1978).
Murakami, M. and Shimoda, Y. J. Physiol. (Lond) 265, 802-818 (1977).
Naka, K.-I. Invest. Ophthal 15, 926-935 (1976).
Naka, K.-I. Vis. Res. 20, 961-965 (1980).
Naka, K.-I. Vis. Res. 22, 653-660 (1982).
Naka, K.-I. and Ohtsuka, T. J. Neurophysiol. 38, 72-91 (1975).
Naka, K.-I., Marmarelis, P.Z. and Chan, R.Y. J. Neurophysiol. 38, 92-131 (1975).
Naka, K.-I., Davis, W. and Chan, R.Y. Sensory Processes 2, 366-374 (1978).
Naka, K.-I., and Christensen, B.N. Sciences 214, 462-464 (1981).
Neal, M.J. Biochem. Sco. Trans. 11, 684-686 (1983).
Stell, W.K. in Handbook of Sensory Physiology v. VII/II M.G.F. Fuortes ed. (Berlin, Springer 1972) pp. 111-214.

Stell, W.K. and Lightfoot, D.O. J. Comp. Neurol. 159, 473-502 (1975).
Toyoda, J.-L, Hashimoto, H. and Ohtsu, K. Vis. Res. 13, 283-294 (1973).
Werblin, F.S. J. Neurophysiol. 33, 342-350 (1970).
Werblin, F.S. J. Physiol Lond 264, 767-785 (1972).
Werblin, F.S. and Copenhagen, D.R. J. Gen. Physiol. 63, 88-110 (1974).
Witkovsky, P. and Dowling, J.E. Z. Zellforsch. 100, 60-82 (1969).

The Serotonin-Accumulating Cells in the Rabbit Retina

N. N. Osborne, D.W. Beaton, S. Patel
Nuffield Laboratory of Ophthalmology
University of Oxford
Oxford, England

A specific population of amacrine neurones in the mammalian retina accumulates exogenous serotonin (Ehinger, 1982; Osborne, 1984). There has also been a recent report that a set of horizontal cells in the squirrel monkey retina can take up extrinsic serotonin (Floren and Hendrickson, 1984). Furthermore, in one species of Long-Evans hooded rats it has been reported that elements in the outer plexiform layer which probably make contact with terminals of photoreceptor cells take up tritiated serotonin (Redburn and Mitchell 1984; Redburn, 1984).

The purpose of this report is to describe the characteristics of the serotonin-accumulating neurones in the rabbit retina. The studies are based purely on immunohistochemical results where neurones were first loaded with exogeous serotonin. Particular attention is paid to the developmental aspect of these neurones and to the uptake and release of the accumulated amine.

Methods

Cells were dissociated from 2 days postnatal Dutch rabbit retinas by a controlled trypsinisation procedure and resuspended in culture medium (for details see Beale and Osborne, 1983; Beale et al, 1982). The culture medium ($37^{\circ}C$) was changed after the third and sixth days. Normally on day 10 living cells were exposed to a culture medium containing $10^{7}M$ serotonin for 30 minutes, and subsequently fixed in 4% paraformaldehyde with 0.1M phosphate buffer (pH 7.4) for 20 minutes. Thereafter the coverslips containing the fixed cells were processed for immunohistochemistry according to Coon's (1958)indirect procedure as described below.

Pieces of fresh retina (Dutch rabbit) were loaded with serotonin by incubating them in Krebs bicarbonate medium containing $10^{-7}M$ of the amine for 30 minutes at $37^{\circ}C$ (Osborne and Patel 1984). The pieces of retina were recovered with forceps, rinsed in ice cold medium and fixed in 4% paraformaldehyde in 0.1 M phosphate buffer (pH 7.4) for 1-3 hours. Frozen sections 10 um thick were subsequently produced at $-20^{\circ}C$ and recovered on gelatine-coated glass slides.

Glass slides containing fixed frozen sections of retina, or coverslips containing fixed retinal cell cultures, were incubated overnight at $4^{\circ}C$ with a rat x rat monoclonal serotonin antibody (Consolazion et al 1981) and then developed with rabbit anti-rat IgG conjugated either to rhodamine or to fluorescein. The monoclonal and development fluorescent antibodies were diluted 1:200 and 1:20 respectively in phosphate buffer saline (PBS) containing 0.2% Triton X-100. The glycerol/PBS mounted sections were viewed with a microscope equipped with epifluorescence optics and photographs were taken with Kodak Tri-X film (ASA 400).

Localisation of serotonin uptake in adult (2 months or more) retina:
As already discussed elsewhere (Osborne, 1982a, 1984), and mentioned before, negative results are obtained in rabbit and other mammalian retinal tissues subjected to immunofluorescence studies for the localisation of serotonin (Fig. 1b). However, tissue from adult animals first incubated in serotonin and then processed by immunofluorescence for serotonin localisation, shows that the amine is taken up into a population

Neurocircuitry of the Retina, A Cajal Memorial
A. Gallego and P. Gouras, Editors

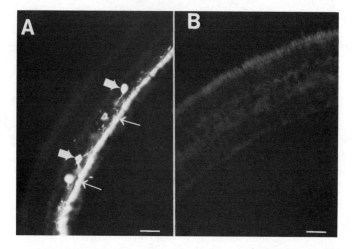

Fig. 1. Immunohistochemical localisation of serotonin in rabbit adult retina incubated in exogenous serotonin (A). The amine is localised in amacrine cell bodies (large arrows) as well as processes in the inner plexiform layer (small arrows). Retinas processed for the localisation of serotonin without previous incubation in exogenous serotinin exhibited no specific fluorescence (B). Scale bar = 50 µm.

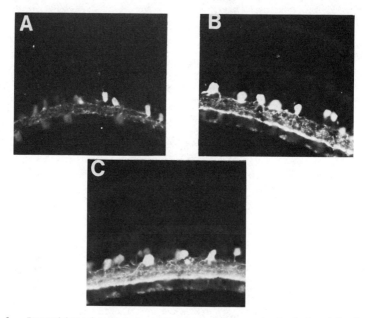

Fig. 2. Immunohistochemical localisation of serotonin in 2-day (A), 6-day (B) and 10-day (C) rabbit retinas following incubation with exogenous serotonin. In these sections the indoleamine is localised in specific amacrine cells. Scale bar = 50 µm.

of large amacrine cell bodies and terminal processes in the inner plexifrom layer (Fig. 1a). Positive staining is never seen in the outer plexiform layer, outer nuclear layer or photoreceptor layer. On very rare occasions a positive cell may be seen in the ganglion cell layer; these are thought to be displaced amacrine cells. Generally, though, one can conclude that a single population of amacrine cells in the adult (2 months or more) retina takes up exogenous serotonin.

Localisation of serotonin uptake in developing retina

The capacity of specific neurones in the rabbit retina to take up exogenous serotonin is not restricted to the adult retinal Figure 2a shows specific neurones from a two-day-old rabbit retina which have accumulated exogenous serotonin. At this stage there is a distinct inner plexiform layer, although the retina is morphologically and physiologically immature (Kong et al 1977; McArdle et al 1977). The outer plexiform layer cannot be clearly discerned. At 6 to 10 days (Fig. 2b,c), after birth, the retina is still quite immature, but the serotonin-accumulating cells are less elongated and there is a clearly defined outer plexiform layer. The actual intensity of fluorescent processes in the inner plexiform layer is more abundant and distinct as development progresses. In fig. 2a,b,c, all the results are consistent with what we observe in the adult retina. One may, therefore, conclude that a distinct population of amacrine neurones takes up exogenous serotonin and that these cells can be observed in 2-day postnatal retinas. However, a close examination of retinal sections reveals discrepancies which make it difficult to draw such a straightforward conclusion. On some occasions processes situated in the outer plexiform layer were also found to take up exogenous serotonin (Fig. 3). Figure 3 shows examples from 2,8,10,15 and 30 day-old retinas. It can be seen that in addition to the amacrine cells which take up exogenous serotonin, other neurones which appear morphologically similar to interplexiform, bipolar and/or horizontal cells take up extrinsic serotonin. These observations were particularly clear in 6-15 day postnatal retinas and were evident in some sections from all retinas (of these ages) analysed. Positive staining for serotonin in neurones other than amacrine is rarer in retinas from more advanced animals. In a one month old animal a few positive processes in the outer plexiform layer have been observed (Fig. 3), but this is unusual. We have never observed any processes in the outer plexiform layer in retinas from animals of two months or more which have taken up exogenous serotonin.

Localisation of serotonin uptake in retinal cultures

Specific neurones in rabbit retinal cultures take up exogenous serotonin (Fig. 4). Specific neurones derived from 2 day old retinas show positive staining after 24 hours in culture (Fig. 4a). At this state the neurones have no obvious processes, yet have the ability to take up exogenous serotonin. After six days in culture, neurones, as exemplified by those which take up serotonin, are more mature with long processes (Fig. 4b). As the neurones grow in culture (Fig. 4c) the processes increase in length. Details concerning the development of neurones in rabbit retinal cultures are described elsewhere (Osborne and Beaton, in preparation).

Specificity of serotonin uptake by intact or cultured neurones

The effect of 10^{-5}M of chlorimipramine and benztropine on the uptake of exogenous serotonin by intact rabbit retinas and cultures of retinal neurones are shown in Figs. 5 and 6. It can be seen that in each instance chlorimipramine blocks the uptake of endogenous serotonin while the effect of benztropine is negligible. It is known that chlorimipramine is a

208

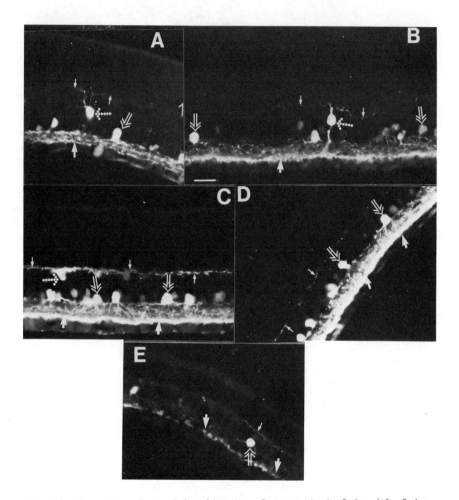

Fig. 3. Immunohistochemical localisation of serotonin in 2-day (A), 8-day
(B), 10-day (C), 15-day (D) 30-day (E) rabbit retinas following incubation
with exogenous serotonin. These sections show various examples where the
indoleamine is associated not only with amacrine perikarya (double arrows)
and terminals (single arrow) but also with other cell-types (dotted
arrows) and the outer plexiform layer (very small arrows). Scale bar = 50
μm.

specific blocker for the transport of serotonin while benztropine plays
the same role in the uptake of dopamine. These results show, therefore,
that the transport of serotonin into specific neurones in the intact
retina or cultures of cells is fundamentally the same.

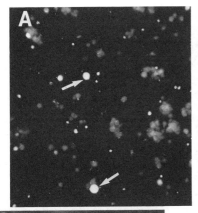
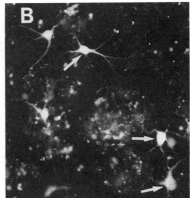
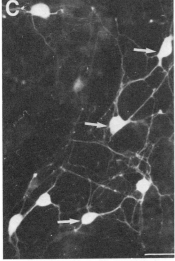

Fig. 4. Immunohistochemical localisation
of serotonin in retinal cultures of 2-day
old animals following incubation with
exogenous serotonin. A = a culture of 24
hours, b = a culture of 6 days; C = a
culture of 12 days. The neurones which
take up exogenous serotonin are shown by
the arrows. Scale bar = 50 μm.

Potassium-stimulated release of accumulated serotonin

Constant with biochemical findings from rabbit and other retinas
(Ehinger and Floren 1978; Osborn 1980; 1982b), Fig. 7 demonstrates that
25mM KCl causes a release of the accumulated serotonin. Exosure of
retinas to normal physiological saline for the same period doesnot result
in a significant release of the accumulated amine. Furthermore, the
effect of 25mM KCl is encounteracted by the inclusion of 15mM KCl is
encounteracted by the inclusion of 14mM $CoCl_2$.

Experiments on cell cultures carried out in an identical way to that
described for intact retinas failed to demonstrate a potassium-induced
release of accumulated serotonin (Fig. 8). Even when higher
concentrations of potassium were used (30mM)no effect was observed.

210

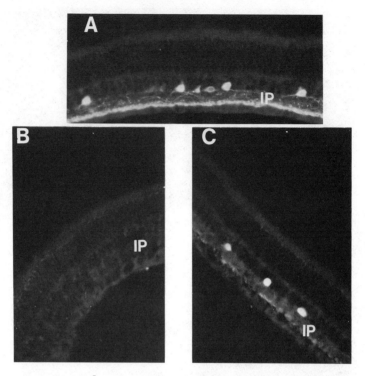

Fig. 5. Effect of 10^{-5}M chlorimipramine (B) and benztropine (C) on the uptake of serotonin by adult retina. The control is hown in (A). It can be seen that chlorimipramine blocks the uptake of serotonin with the amacrine neurones which specifically take up the amine. Benztropine does not block the uptake of serotonin though it does have a mild effect. IP - inner plexiform layer. Scale bar = 50 μm.

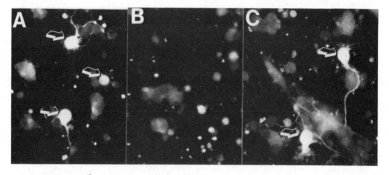

Fig. 6. Effect of 10^5M chlorimipramine (B) and benztropine (C) on tne uptake of serotonin by 6-day old rabbit retinal cultures. The cultures were derived from 2-day old retinas. A= control. The arrows show neurones which have taken up serotonin. It can be seen that positive cells were not observed in the chlorimipramine treated cultures (B) while benztropine (C) had little effect. Scale bar - 50 μm.

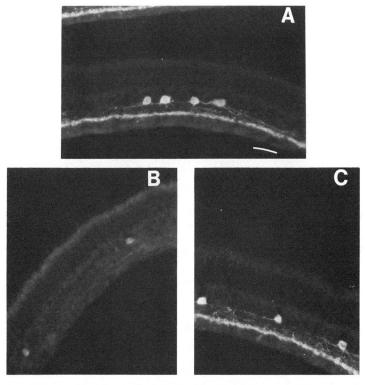

Fig. 7. Effect of either physiological saline (A) or saline containing 25mM KCl (B) or saline containing 25mM KCl plus 15 mM $CoCl_2$ (C) following an incubation in exogenous serotonin (for details see Osborne and Patel, 1984). It can be seen that KCl has the effect of stimulating the release of previously accumulated serotinin. The inclusion of $CoCl_2$ counteracts the effect of KCl. Scale bar - 50 µm.

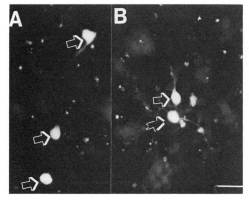

Fig. 8. Effect of physiological saline (A) or saline containing 25mM KCl (B) following an incubation of rabbit retinal cells in exogenous serotonin. Conditions of experiments were identical to those for the intact retina. It can be seen that KCl does not stimulate the release of previously accumulated serotonin by specific cells (arrows). Scale bar - 50 µm.

Discussion

The presented data show that serotonin-accumulating neurones in the adult retina are restricted to a specific population of amacrine neurones. These neurones appear immediately after birth at a stage when the eyes are unopened and synaptic connections of the individual neurones have not yet been established. However, the serotonin-accumulating neurones in young rabbits (1-30 days) are not restricted to a population of typical amacrine neurones but are also associated with spasmodic cells which appear morphologically to resemble interplexiform, bipolar and horizontal cells. The neurones other than amacrine neurones which accumulate exogenous serotonin are more pronounced in the 1-15 day old retinas and only signs of their existence are apparent in retinas up to 30 days old.

The finding that processes in the outer plexiform layer and possible horizontal cells of a vertebrate retina accumulate serotonin is surprising but not unique. Floren and Hendrickson (1984) have shown that a population of horizontal cells in the squirrel retina take up radioactive serotonin. A system of neuronal processes in the outer plexiform layer of Long-Evans hooded rats has also been shown to take up exogenous serotonin (Redburn and Mitchell 1984; Redburn 1984). The results presented in this article describe a thire mammalian species where the uptake of serotonin is not restricted to a population of amacrine cells. This report is, however, unusual in its demonstration that the occurrence of this phenomenon in the rabbit retina is restricted to young animals and is most pronounced at the very early stages (1-15 days).

The finding that neurones other than amacrine neurones take up exogenous serotonin, but only in very young retinas, suggest that these neurones might play a specific part during the development of the rabbit retina. Could it be that a specific class of serotonergic neurones has a role to play in synaptogenesis? Once the neurones have fulfilled their role they may differentiate into other types of neurones with a different biochemistry? It is known that cultured sympathetic neurones, for example, may become coded to produce the appropriate neurotransmitter at a critical stage in their development and simultaneously lose their ability to respond to previous instructions (Chun and Patterson 1977; Patterson et al 1976, 1978). An alternative explanation is that these neurones are misplaced amacrine neurones with no specific function and as development proceeds they degenerate. This would explain their absence from the process of synaptogenesis (Hume et al 1984), but this does not apparently occur in the fully developed retina.

The neurones which take up exogenous serotonin in the intact adult retina show characteristics associated with serotonin-containing neurones. The uptake of serotonin is dependent upon sodium (Osborne, 1980, 1984), and as shown here, chlorimipramine inhibits the uptake of the amine while benztropine has only a minor effect. It is well known that chlorimipramine is a potent blocker of serotonin uptake in serotonergic neurones while benztropine has its effect on the uptake of dopamine in dopaminergic cells. Furthermore, the accumulated serotonin is released by potassium depolarisation. This release is calcium-dependent as it is inhibited by the presence of cobalt ions in the medium. It is thought that cobalt ions interfere with the entry of calcium into synaptic endings resulting in a reduction in, or abolition of, transmitter release (Weakly 1973). Whether the serotonin-accumulation neurones in the adult rabbit retina utilise serotonin as a transmitter still remains to be proven, however. Serotonergic amacrine neurones have only been demonstrated in non-mammalina retinas (Osborne, 1982a,b, 1984; Osborne et al 1981, 1982) and all attempts to localise such neurones in mammalian retinas have

213

failed (Ehinger and Floren 1980; Ehinger, 1982; Osborne 1984). It has, therefore, been suggested by certain authors that the true transmitter of serotonin-accumulating neurones in mammalian retinas is a substance closely related to the amine (Ehinger 1982; Ehinger et al 1981; Floren and Hendrickson 1984). The other view is that the inability to localise endogenous serotonin in neurones of mammalian retinas may simply be due to a lower level of amine in these neurones when compared with the same cells in non-mammalian retinas (Osborne, 1982a, 1984).

The findings that serotonin-accumulating neurones occur in the retina immediately after birth meant that it was possible to study them in a culture system. These neurones, like the serotonin-accumulating neurones in the intact retina, do not take up other putative transmitters like GABA, dopamine, aspartate and noradrenaline (Osborne and Beaton in preparation). As demonstrated in this report, the uptake of serotonin into a population of cultured neurones is blocked by chlorimipramine but not by benztropine. However, potassium depolarisation did not cause a release of the accumulated serotonin. Thus, while the characteristics of neurones which take up serotonin in rabbit cultures and intact retinas are very similar, they appear to respond differently to an impulse of potassium. This may be due to the fact that the neurones in culture are immature and/or lack appropriate cell contacts. The finding is of some interest and clearly warrants further study.

In summary, the data in this paper show that a subpopulation of amacrine cells in the adult mammalian retina has the ability to take up, store and release serotonin following potassium depolarisation. The release of serotonin is calcium-dependent. The subpopulation of neurones appears to be determined prenatally. However, during the initial stages of the retina's development some serotonin-accumulating neurones are associated with the outer plexiform layer in the form of interplexiform and/or bipolar and/or horizontal cells. These neurones could have an additional function of their own or simply be misplaced amacrine serotonin-accumulating neurones destined to degenerate in the process of synaptogenesis. The serotonin-accumulating neurones can be cultured from 2-day old retinas. They behave differently from the same neurones in intact adult retinas in response to an elevated level of potassium chloride, but in other respects are the same.

Acknowledgement

This work was supported by the Wellcome Trust to whom we are grateful.

References

Beale, R. and Osborne, N.N. Brain Res. 7, 107-120 (1983).
Beale, R., Nicholas D., Neuhoff, V. and Osborne, N.N. Brain Res. 248, 141-149 (1982).
Chun, L.L.Y., and Patterson, P.H. J. Cell Biol 75, 694-704 (1977).
Consolazione, A., Milstein, C., Wright, B. and Cuello, A.C. J. Histochem. Cytochem. 29, 1425-1431 (1981).
Coons, A.H. in General cytochemical methods. J.F. Danielli ed., Academic Press New York 1958) pp 399-422.
Ehinger, B. Retina 2, 305-321 (1982).
Ehinger, B., Floren, I. Exp. Eye Res. 26, 1-11 (1978).
Ehinger, B., Floren, I. Neurochem. Internatl. 1, 209-229 (1980).
Ehinger, B., Hansson, Ch., Tornquist, K. Exp. Eye Res. 33, 663-672 (1981).
Floren, I. and Hendrickson, A. Invest. Ophthal. 25, 997-1006 (1984).
Hume, D.A., Perry. H. and Gordon, S. J. Cell Biol. 97, 253-257 (1983).

Kong, Y.C., Fung, S.C. and Lam, D.M.K. J. Comp. Neuorl. 193, 1127-1135 (1980).

McArdle, C.B., Dowling, J.E. and Masland, R.H. J. Comp. Neurol. 175, 253-274 (1977).

Osborne, N.N. Brain Res. 184, 283-297 (1982).

Osborne, N.N. in Biology of Serotonergic Transmission. N.N. Osborne ed. (John Wiley and Sons, Chichester, U.K. 1982a) pp. 401-430.

Osborne, N.N. J. Physiol (Lond) 331, 469-479 (1982b).

Osborne, N.N. in Progress in Retinal Research v. 3. N.N. Osborn and G. Chader eds. (Pergamon Press 1984) pp. 61-103.

Osborne, N.N. and Patel, S. Exp. Eye Res. 38, 611-620 (1984).

Osborne, N.N., Nesselhut, T., Nicholas, D.A. and Cuello, A.C. Neurochem. Internat. 3, 171-176 (1981).

Osborne, N.N., Nesselhut, T., Nicholas, D.A., Patel, S. and Cuello, A.C. J. Neurochem. 39, 1519-1528 (1982).

Patterson, P.H., Potter, D.D. and Furshpan, E.J. Scientific American 38-47 (1978).

Redburn, D.A. Fed. Proc. 43, 2699-2703 (1984).

Redburn, D.A., Mitchell, C.K. Invest. Ophthal. Vis. Sci. Suppl. 25, 85 (1984).

Weakley, J.N. J. Physiol. 234, 597-612 (1973).

Functional Neurocircuitry of Amacrine Cells in the Cat Retina

H. Kolb, R. Nelson[*]
Physiology Department, University of Utah
Salt Lake City, Utah

Laboratory of Neurophysiology[*]
National Institutes of Health
Bethesda, Maryland

Amacrine cells are a diverse group of third order neurons found in the vertebrate retina. First described in bird retina by Cajal in 1888 as spongioblasts he later renamed them amacrine cells because he could find no axon on them: however, as an advocate of the "Neuron doctrine" he could never quite reconcile himself with the lack of an axon on this nerve cell type. Later electron microscopic examination has shown that many neurons, chief amongst them amacrine cells of the retina engage in demdrodendritic synapses, and so Cajal, had he lived to know this, might have been more satisfied with the axonless morphology of retinal amacrine cells.

Although Cajal (1892) classified amacrine cells into several morphological types and advocated that they formed important architectural elements of the five-tiered stratification of the inner plexiform layer, later research stressed a simpler organization of the neural networks in the retina, eschewing stratification as a morphological distinction between amacrines, or other retinal cell types (Boycott and Dowling 1969). Retinal amacrines were given a single function with stereotypical ON-OFF response patterns and were thought to be responsible for AC or temporal image processing alone (Werblin and Dowling 1969; Werblin 1972). Although these were important simplifying concepts with immense functional significance, they led to a period of disregarding Cajal's original important morphological descriptions and more importantly his concept of morphology underlying functional pathways.

A renewed look at the morphology of retinal neurons became feasible with the development of whole-mount Golgi staining techniques (Ogden et al 1974; Stell and Witkovsky 1973; Ogden 1974; Kolb 1974; Boycott 1974; Gallego 1975; Mariani and Leure-Dupree 1977). Stained retinal neurons now had their complete dendritic trees visible for scrutiny, and could be more readily distinguished on morphological criteria such as dendritic field size and dendritic branching patterns (Kolb et al 1981; Vallerga and Deplano 1984) as compared with vertical section techniques. Furthermore, after Nelson and coworkers (1978) demonstrated that the dendrties of OFF centre ganglion cells in cat branched in a different neuropil than those of ON centre ganglion cells, an organization now known to be typical of vertebrate retinas, the potential importance of stratification of amacrine cells as relating to ganglion cell receptive field organization became apparent. A diverse amacrine population was also emerging from studies of retinal microcircuitry (Kolb and Famiglietti 1974; Nelson et al 1976; Sterling 1983) intracellular recordings and pharmacology (Kaneko 1973; Naka 1976; Murakami and Shimoda 1977; Miller 1980; Frumkes et al 1981; Kolb and Nelson 1981; Nelson 1982 Belgum et al 1984).

Moreover, research using induced fluorescence (Ehinger and Falk 1969; Tork and Stone 1979; Mariani et al 1984), autoradiographic (Ehinger 1983 review; Freed et al 1983; Frederick et al 1984; Pourcho 1981, 1982; Pourcho and Goebel 1983, 1984) and immunocytochemical staining techniques (Karten and Brecha 1983; Brecha et al 1984 for review) suggested a

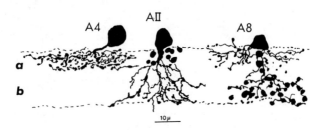

Fig. 1. Camera lucida drawings of three small-field amacrine cells as seen in vertical section. A4 has a small field of tufted varicose dendrites which branch in sublamina a close to the amacrine cell bodies. AII is the bistratified amacrine cell with lobular appendages branching in sublamina a and finer dendrites ramifying through sublamina b. A8 is a small field cell with spidery dendrites branching in sublamina a and varicosities in sublamina b. Scale bar 10 μm.

multitude of amacrine subtypes, most of which could be independently confirmed in Golgi staining descriptions.

In the cat retina a significant advance in our understanding of amacrine cell function has come from intracellular recordings and stainings with horseradish peroxidase (HRP). Physiological evaluation allows us to determine whether amacrine cell activity is sustained, transient or ON/OFF, what its centre response sign might be, the organization of its receptive field and whether it is involved in the rod or cone systems or both. The HRP staining of the amacrine cell allows us to perform both light and electron microscopy on the sectioned cell so that we can confirm the system (rod or cone) that the cells are involved in, provide explanations for specific synaptic inputs that might be responsible for receptive field characteristics, and yield dimensional data to use for modelling spread of electrical signals and weighting of synapses (Miller and Bloomfield 1983; Stevens and Jacobs 1983). Thus using these combined physiological and anatomical techniques we have been able to gain some understanding of several amacrine cell types in the cat retina (Kolb and Nelson 1981, 1982, 1984; Nelson 1982). These are amacrine cell types on which, in most cases, we have intracellular recordings, morphology and neurocircuitry and furthermore by correlating our findings with those of Pourcho and group (Pourcho 1982; Pourcho and Goebel 1983; 1984) we have some idea as to the neurotransmitter these amacrine cells might use.

Amacrine cells primarily of the cone pathway in cat retina

Intracellular recordings and stainings with Procion or horseradish peroxidase have revealed three amacrine cell types that appear to be primarily involved in the cone driven pathways of the cat retina. By comparison with our morphological classification (Kolb et al 1981) these cells are identified as A4, A8 and A19. Amacrines A4 and A 8 are illustrated in the camera lucida drawings of vertically sectioned retina in Figure 1.

As can be seen A4 is a small-field amacrine with a 50 μm dendritic field size. The dendrites are varicose, densely branched and intertwined and, moreover, restricted to branching in an area of neuropil of the IPL below the amacrine cell bodies i.e. in sublamina a. Electron microscopy of such an amacrine cell (Kolb 1979) indicated that it is postsynaptic to cone bipolar cells cb2 ending in sublamina a and presynatpic to a type ganglion cells of the OFF centre variety ramifying in sublamina a. In

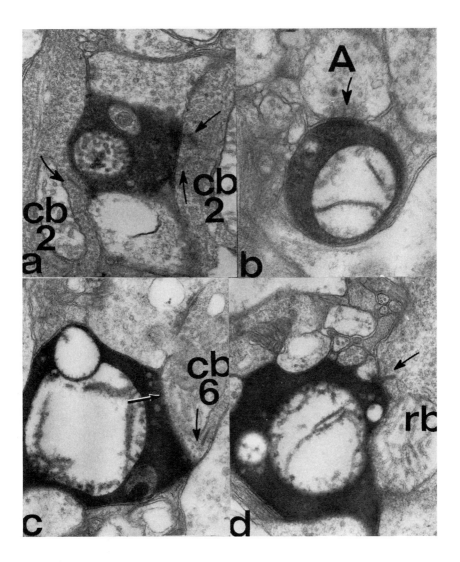

Fig. 2. a) Electron micrograph of HRP stained dendrites of A8 in synaptic contact with cone bipolars (cb2, arrows) in sublamina a_. b) Stained A8 profile postsynaptic to an amacrine dendrite in sublamina a_. Note dense-cored vesicle in unidentified amacrine. c) stained profile of A8 postsynaptic to a cone bipolar axon terminal (cb6, arrow) in sublamina b_. The A8 dendrite makes a reciprocal synapse to the cone bipolar (black and white arrow). d) stained A8 profile postsynaptic to a rod bipolar axon terminal (rb, arrow). All x 25,000.

addition A4 receives input from other unidentified amacrine cells and makes reciprocal feed back synapses upon the cone bipolars providing synaptic input. The A4 appears to function as an intermediary between OFF centre bipolars and OFF centre ganglion cells. The physiological response of A4 is a sustained hyperpolarization to light (Fig. 9) and its receptive field as measured by displacing slits of light from the centre of the receptive field (Nelson 1977) is three times larger than its dendritic field (approximately 150 μm compared 50 μm) (Kolb and Nelson 1984). Stimulation of A4 with rod matched red and blue lights indicates that at higher intensities A4 is driven primarily by cone signals (Fig. 9).

A8 has a different branching pattern from A4 (Fig. 1). It is a small-field, bi-stratified cell with a curious dichotomy of dendritic morphology in sublamina a and sublamina b of the IPL. Fine spidery dendrites emerge from the cell body region and branch only in sublamina a whereas globular dendrites with large varicosities spread down into the neuropil of sublamina b to end running along the top of the ganglion cell bodies. It was possible to examine this HRP stained A8 amacrine cell in the electron microscope to determine its synaptic circuitry. The finer dendrites confined to sublamina a were postsynaptic to ribbon synapses of cb2 type cone bipolar terminals (Fig. 2a), presynaptic to OFF centre ganglion cell dendrites and postsynaptic to amacrine cell profiles (Fig. 2b). Interestingly the presynaptic amacrine process illustrated in Fig. 2b contains a dense-cored vesicle which may indicate that it is a dopamine containing amacrine cell type. As will be seen later in our description of rod/cone amacrine cells, the dopaminergic amacrine cell of the cat retina, A8, is strongly involved with the AII amacrine cell. A8 and AII have many features in common i.e. their small-field, bi-stratified morphology, dichotomy of inputs in sublaminas a and b and common occurrence of gap junctions with similar profiles, but one is involved in cone system A8, while the other is more strongly involved in the rod system, AII. It is possible, that both A8 and AII are influenced by the dopaminergic amacrine. Dopamine may be involved in a functional reorganization of retinal circuits during light adaptation (Mariani et al., 1984).

The electron microscopic examination of A8 further shows that the globular dendrites in sublamina b are postsynaptic to both rod and cone bipolar cell axon terminals (Figs. 2c,d). Because the A8 amacrine gives a strongly hyperpolarizing response to cone pathway stimulation we suspect that the cone bipolar cell with which it is postsynaptic in sublamina b is the hyperpolarizing cone bipolar cb6 (Nelson and Kolb 1983). Small gap junctions are seen between HRP stained A8 dendrites in sublamina b and similar appearing dendrites, which we presume are other A8 dendrites.

Intracellular recording from the A8 amacrine cell show that it has a hyperpolarizing response to full field illumination with a pronounced spike at stimulus off (Fig. 3). Furthermore, stimulation with rod matched red light produces a response that grows beyond the rod saturation level indicative of cone driven sensitivity. The intracellular responses of the A8 to displacing a slit of light from the centre of the receptive field are shown in Fig. 3. As can be seen, the receptive field centre as measured by the hyperpolarizing response, stretches across 300-400 μm of slit displacement. However, when the slit of light illuminates an area 700 μm to either side of the central point (0), an ON depolarization is seen and there is a reduction of the OFF spike. In other words the receptive field organization of A8 is clearly concentric: it has an OFF centre and an ON surround.

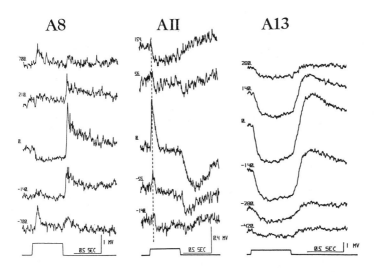

Fig. 3. Receptive field plots of A8, AII and A13 amacrine cells. The maximum intracellular response occurs at the centre of the receptive field (0 point). 200 μm wide slits are flashed at distances from the centre (indicated in μm to the left of each trace) to map the extent of the receptive field. A8 and AII show a concentric organization with a hyperpolarizing (A8) or depolarizing (AII) central response and the surround of opposite polarity. A13 shows a simple hyperpolarizing response throughout its receptive field. Note spikey depolarization at ON for AII and at OFF for A8. Stimulus conditions: A8, 200 μm slit, 647 nm log quanta μm^{-2}s^{-1}; AII, 25 μm slit, 441 nm, 3.1 log quanta μm^{-2}s^{-1}.

In contrast to A4 and A8, A19 is large-field, unistratified cell with completely different morphological characteristics. Figure 4 shows camera lucida drawings of the large-field cells we will discuss in this paper. The drawings are of cells as seen in a whole-mount of retina, viewing them from the ganglion cell side of the retina. All but A13 (see later section) have dendritic fields stretching across 750 to 1000 μm. It can be appreciated that such cells could not be well characterized in vertical sections where only a small fraction of the dendritic tree or even only one dendrite might be visualized. In any event, A19 is the large-field amacrine cell of the cone system that we have studied by intracellular recordings and electron microscopy, and found to be involved most heavily in cone driven pathways. It has rather thick, linear dendrites with a sparse branching pattern. Only few small appendages occur on the dendrites. In addition, A19 is monostratified with branches running purely in s2 (Cajal's nomenclature, 1892) or just above the sublamina a and sublamina b border in the IPL.

Electron microsocpy of an A19 amacrine cell indicates that this cell receives synaptic input from cone bipolar cells that terminate in sublamina a. By cytological appearance the cone bipolar terminals are of two sorts. One (Fig. 5a) has globular, rounded axonal branches, typical of cb1 (Kolb 1979): the other has thinner more horizontally oriented axon terminals running parallel to the surface of the A19 dendrites (Fig. 5c), more typical of cb2 terminals. Thus we are proposing that A19 receives input from both cone bipolar types that end in sublamina a, cb1 and cb2.

220

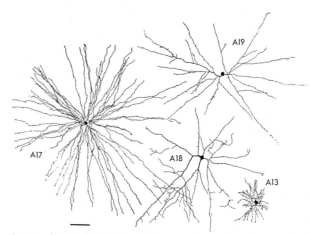

Fig. 4. Camera lucida drawings of large field amacrine cells in the cat
as seen in whole mount views. A17 is a diffusely branched cell with a
1000 um dendritic spread of very fine dendrites bearing synaptic beads
every 10 µm; HRP stained. A19 is a monostratitied cell with radiate
linear dendrites running in sublamina a just above the a/b border; HRP
stained. A18 is a Golgi stained dopaminergic amacrine cell. It has a
large cell body and thick major dendrites but cob-web wike fine dendrites
that fill in the space between large dendrites (example is understained
except for lower left region). A18 dendrites stratify under the amacrine
cell bodies in sublamina a. A13 is smaller field than the other amacrines
here but has a diffuse dendritic tree covering 150 µm. The many fine
dendrites swell into beads intermittently; Golgi stained. Scale bar 100
µm.

A19 cell dendrites also make reciprocal synapses upon both these cone
bipolar types (not shown). Considerable amacrine input also occurs to
both large and smaller diameter dendrites of A19 (Fig. 5b). A19 dendrites
contain conspicuous numbers of neurotubules (Fig. 5b and c, nt). Such
neurotubule-filled, thick linear profiles have been noted to engage in gap
junctions as shown in Fig. 5d (arrows). The two large neurotubule filled
profiles in this micrograph are from material being analysed for another
amacrine cell type A17 (see later section), and one of the profiles
involved in the gap junction turned out to be presynaptic to the HRP
stained A17 cell. Indirect evidence, thus, suggests that A19 amacrine
cells are joined in gap junctions with other A19 cells, forming a kind of
laterally running syncytium in the IPL. In addition, during the analysis
of the A8 cell we noted large diameter, neurotubule filled amacrine
profiles to be postsynaptic to the A8 dendrites in sublamina a. The EM
analysis of the A19 provided little evidence of this cell being
presynatpic to alpha or beta type ganglion cells (Boycott and Wässle 1974)
although we did note the A19 to be pre-synaptic to a ganglion cell with
small diameter dendrites, either the dendritic tips of an alpha type
ganglion cell, or the dendrites of another, unidentified small class of
ganglion cell.

Intracellular recordings of A19 show that this cell gives an ON/OFF
response to light stimulation (Fig. 6). The cell is driven strongly by
cone pathway stimulation as judged by its OFF response to red light. Its
receptive field is indicated in Fig. 6. The receptive field as mapped
with 200 µm wide slits of red light (647 nm) is over 1000 µm, a

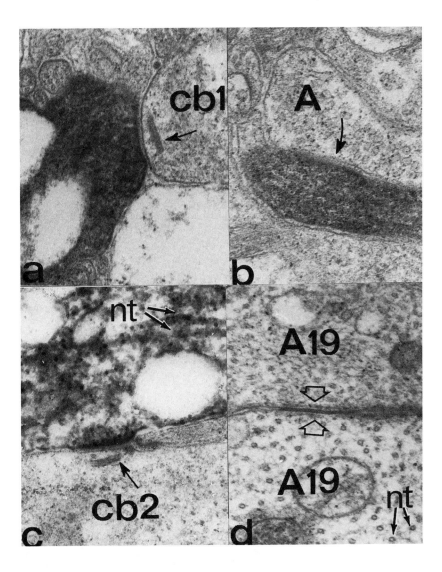

Fig. 5. a) Electron micrograph of an HRP stained A19 amacrine cell dendritic appendage which is postsynaptic to cone bipolar cb1 (arrow) in sublamina a of the IPL. b) The A19 dendrite is postsynaptic to an amacrine cell (A arrow). C) A major dendrite of the stained A19 cell receives synaptic input (arrow) from a cb2 type of cone bipolar cell. Note the prominent neurotubular content (nt, black and white arrows) of the major dendrites of A19. d) in other material two neurotubular filled large dendrites (nt black and white arrows), presumed to be A19 cells, engage in a gap junction (open arrows). All X 75,000.

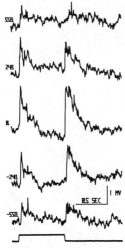

Fig. 6. Intracellular responses and receptive field map of an A19 amacrine cell. The response is a depolarizing transient at both onset and at offset of the light. This ON/OFF amacrine has a receptive field of about 1100 microns edge to edge, as measured by a 200 um wide slit presented at different distances from the centre of the receptive field (given in μm to the left of each trace). Stimulus 647 nm, 5.6 log quanta μm^{-2}s^{-1}.

measurement larger than its dendritic field and consistent with such cells being coupled at gap junctions to neighboring similar cell types. The ON/OFF response of A19 suggests that it is allied with the "local edge detector" seen in extracellular ganglion cell recordings (Cleland and Levick 1974).

Amacrine cells interconnecting rod and cone pathways

The small-field bistratified AII amacrine cell (Fig. 1) is by now well known to be an amacrine cell of the rod pathways serving as an interneuron between rod bipolar cell axon terminals and OFF centre ganglion cells (Kolb and Famiglietti 1974; Famiglietti and Kolb 1975; Nelson et al 1976; Kolb 1979; Nelson 1982; Kolb and Nelson 1983; Sterling 1983; Famiglietti 1983). The small dendritic tree has a bistratified morphology and functional separation of the dendritic tree. As shown in Fig. 7a the lobular appendage-like dendrites of sublamina a are presynaptic at punctate synapses to a type ganglion cells which are known to be OFF centre types. The lobular appendages are also pre- and postsynaptic to cb1 bipolar cells and postsyanptic to amacrine cells one type of which is known to be the dopaminergic amacrine cell (see below). AII dendrites in the lower neuropil of the IPL, sublamina b, are postsynaptic to rod bipolar axon terminals and additionally make gap junctions with other AII dendrites (Fig. 7b). The AII amacrine cell fits into the cone system by making both chemical syanpses upon cb1 cone bipolar terminals in sublamina a, making electrical synapses with cone bipolar type cb5, branching in sublamina b of the IPL (Fig. 7b). In fact we consider the gap junctions with cb5 as being one of the major routes whereby rod signals reach ON centre ganglion cells in sublamina b (Nelson and Kolb, 1983), as rod bipolar cells make very few synapses directly with ganglion cell dendrites (Freed and Sterling, 1983).

A13 is a small to medium field amacrine cell of the cat retina. Its dendritic tree spans 75 to 150 um, dependent on its location relative to the area centralis. A typical A13 cell from 2 mm eccentricity is shown in Figure 4 and as can be seen, in comparison to the large-field cells it looks diminutive. It is an amacrine with a diffuse branching pattern where the beaded dendrites ramify through all parts of the IPL. Electron microscopy of an HRP stained A13 is shown on Figs. 7c and d. The

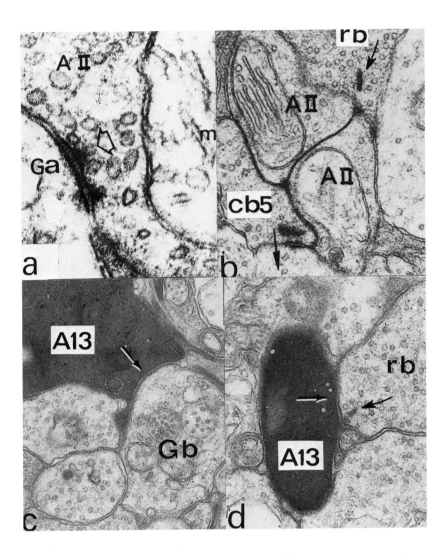

Fig. 7. a) Electron micrograph showing a small punctate synapse (open arrow) between an AII amacrine lobular appendage and an OFF centre ganglion cell dendrite (Ga) .in sublamina a of the IPL. m, mitochondrion in AII profile. X 150,000. b) Two AII amacrine dendrites are postsynaptic to a rod bipolar terminal (rb, arrow) in sublamina b. The two AII dendrites form a gap junction between each other and cone bipolar type cb5. The latter cone bipolar is presynaptic to another amacrine cell dendrite (arrow). c) HRP stained A13 amacrine dendrite is presynaptic (black and white arrow) to an ON centre ganglion cell (Gb) dendrite. d) A13 amacrine cell postsynaptic to a rod bipolar terminal in sublamina b of the IPL, and makes a reciprocal synapse (black and white arrow). b,c and d X 60,000.

dendrites are postsynaptic to both rod bipolar and cone bipolar axons in sublamina a making, in each case, a reciprocal synapse with the bipolar terminal (Fig. 7d). It makes most sense to interpret the cone bipolar input to be from a cb6 cone bipolar cell, because, as will be seen later, the A13 is a hyperpolarizing unit like the cb6 cone bipolar cell type. The A13 dendrites are also seen to be presynaptic to ganglion cell dendrites ramifying in the lower portion of the IPL i.e. in sublamina b (Fig. 7c).

Intracellular responses of A13 are markedly different from those of AII amacrines: the former are hyperpolarizing and the latter, depolarizing. Both units, however, show domination by rod driven input but with higher light intensities and particularly with red stimuli a small portion of the response of each can be attributed to the cone system. Figure 3 shows the typical receptive field properties of an AII and A13 amacrine cell. AII has a rather small receptive field region of less than 100 μm where the response is a transient ON-depolarization, but an antagonistic surround in the form of an ON-hyperpolarization occurs when the stimulus falls beyond the 100 μm centre (Fig. 3, AIII). A detailed study of the physiology of the AII cell has been given elsewhere (Nelson, 1982). In contrast to AII, A13 gives a slow hyperpolarizing response to light across its whole receptive field of 700 μm and there is no indication of an antagonistic surround response (Fig. 3, A13).

In Fig. 4 is illustrated a large field amacrine named A18. In our previous Golgi study (Kolb et al 1981) we suggested that this cell might be the equivalent of a rare cell type that fluorescesces brightly with with the formaldehyde vapor techniques that display retinal dopaminergic cells (Tork and Stone 1979). A18 has the same large cell body and very highly stratified dendritic tree. With fluorescent techniques very fine dendrites from one or more such cells can be seen wrapping around other cell bodies to form rings. The example stained by the Golgi technique (Fig. 4) is surely understained in this regard. Recent immunocytochemical localization of tyrosine hydroxylase in whole-mount of cat retina reveals dopamine-containing amacrine cells in far greater detail (Oyster et al 1984) than possible with the formaldehyde induced fluorescence techniques. The immunocytochemically marked cells appear identical with the A18 of the Golgi studies. These cells have cobweb-like dendritic tree with dendrites wrapping around other cell bodies or around clear spaces the sizes of cell bodies or thick amacrine dendrites. Electron microscopy by Pourcho (1982) of (H^3)-dopamine labeled cells in the cat retina indicates that this amacrine cell type is postsynaptic to unidentified amacrines and other labeled dopaminergic profiles, but is presynaptic to AII amacrine cell bodies, AII apical dendrites and AII lobular appendages in sublamina a of the IPL. In our analysis of the A17 cell (see below) we have noted that high branching amacrine dendrites, running close beneath the amacrine cell bodies and containing dense-cored vesicles, synapse upon similar dendrites and upon the A17 dendrites. Thus we interpret the dopaminergic amacrine in the cat retina as being very involved with two amacrine cells of the rod pathways, AII and A17, but because dopamine is known to be released from light adapted cat retinas by intermittent light stimulation (Kramer 1971) we suppose that A18 must be driven in some way by the cone bipolar and cone amacrine pathways prior to releasing transmitter upon the two aforementioned rod amacrine cells.

Pure rod amacrine cells of the cat retina

We have only found one amacrine cell in cat retina that appears purely to be driven by rod signals. This is the A17 amacrine cell, a whole-mount view of which is illustrated in Fig. 4. The cell has a 10 μm cell body

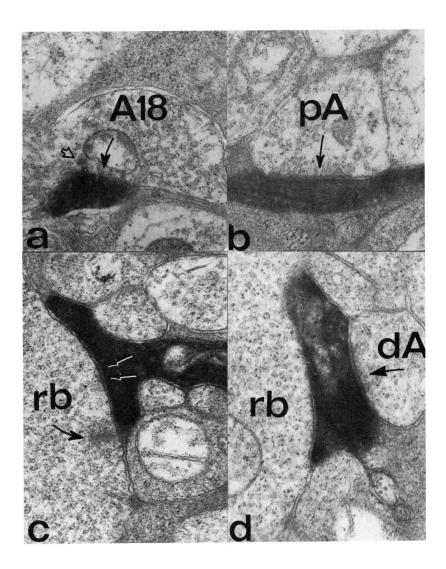

Fig. 8.   a)   Fine dendrite of an HRP stained A17 amacrine cell is
postsynaptic to a large pale amacrine cell profile (A18, arrow) lying
under the amacrine cell bodies in sublamina a.   The A18 profile contains a
dense-cored vesicle (open arrow). b) Stained A17 dendrite is postsynaptic
to a pale amacrine (pA, arrow) of unknown type in sublamina a of the IPL.
c) A17 amacrine process is postsynaptic to a rod bipolar axon terminal
(rb, arrow) in sublamina b of the IPL.   The stained A17 makes a
reciprocal synapse (black and white arrows). d) Stained A17 profile is
postsynaptic to a dark amacrine profile (dA, arrow) of unknown origin just
above the sublamina a/b border of the IPL. All X55,000.

and wide dendritic tree (800-1000 μm) of extremely fine dendrites bearing varicosities or beads at regular intervals. The dendrites spread through all the strata of the IPL and come eventually to run in the lower portion of sublamina b.

Electron microscopy of such A17 cells proves to be a difficult task because of the fine diameters of the dendrites and the relatively widely spaced beads (approximately every 10 μm) which are the primary synaptic loci. Figures 8a-c show sample electron micrographs through profiles of an HRP-stained A17 amacrine cell. Fine dendrites and small beads typical of the dendrites of sublamina a are frequently postsynaptic to amacrine dendrites. One type of amacrine profile running in neuropil just below the amacrine cell bodies contains dense-cored vesicles (Fig. 8a) and is a candidate for being the dopaminergic amacrine cell type (A18). Other amacrine profiles either labeled as pA, pale amacrines, or dA, dark amacrines, are also presynaptic to fine dendrites of A17 cells in the neuropil of sublamina a, either or both of which could be candidates for A19 and A4 synaptic input. In sublamina b, on the other hand, A17 dendrites proved only to have synaptic exchange at the large beads. These beads cluster up against rod bipolar axon terminals, one rod bipolar terminal per synaptic bead usually, and here also make a clear reciprocal synapse upon the rod bipolar terminal (Fig. 8c).

Intracellular recordings of the A17 cells indicate that they have a sustained depolarizing response to light, a large receptive field little bigger than their dendritic field, and no evidence of a surround (Nelson and Kolb 1985). Figure 9 shows responses of the A17 cell to rod-matched red and blue stimuli and as can be seen the responses are essentially superimposable through the entire intensity range: thus our conclusion that A17 cells are purely driven by rod mechanisms, presumably the rod bipolar input that we have observed in electron microscopy. The rod matched responses of A17 contrast nicely with the small field A4 amacrine cell of the cone system (Fig. 9, A4). Not only is the cone amacrine of a different response sign, i.e. hyperpolarizing compared to depolarizing, but because of the strong cone (560 nm) driven component of the response, responses to red stimulation surpass those to blue at every intensity used in these rod-matched stimulus pairs. A17 is clearly a rod driven amacrine while the A4 is in the cone pathways.

We have discussed seven different amacrine cell types of the cat retina in this paper. These are amacrines that have been studied by combined anatomical and physiological techniques so that we now have some idea as to their neurocircuitry, their function within the rod and cone systems and their interchange with other amacrines cells. Furthermore, we have some clues as to which ganglion cell system, ON centre or OFF centre, these amacrine cells might be driving. From some very ingenious experiments by Pourcho and Goebel (1983, 1984) where Golgi stained cells can be labeled with the different tritiated neurotransmitter substances, we can also identify a neurotransmitter candidate for each of these seven amacrine cells. Table 1 summarizes all the combined data, and Figure 10, 11 and 12 provide summary diagrams of the connectivity of these cells.

A4 is a small field, sustained OFF centre unit with a small receptive field and no surround. It is mostly cone driven and appears to intercede between OFF centre bipolars cells, unknown amacrine cells and OFF centre ganglion cells (Fig. 10). Its neurotransmitter is thought to be glycine (Pourcho and Goebel 1983). We speculate that A4 may be involved in post-excitatory inhibition of OFF centre ganglion cells as suggested by Miller and Frumkes and coworkers in mudpuppy (1981, 1982). Although in cat Ikeda and Sheardown (1983) have discovered glycine to be responsible for ON inhibition of OFF centre ganglion cells.

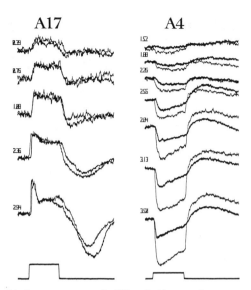

Fig. 9. Intracellular response of A17 and A4 amacrines to rod matched red and blue stimuli. The depolarizing responses of the A17 are essentially the same to these pairs of stimuli throughout the intensity range. The hyperpolarizing responses of the A4 show a size variation dependent on the wavelength of the stimulating light. In each pair the response of greater amplitude was elicited by the red stimulus. This is indicative of a large amplitude input from the long wavelength (560 nm peak absorbing) cones of the cat, which respond much more strongly to red than to blue rod-matched stimuli. Stimulus conditions: red, 647 nm, 4.6 log quanta $\mu m^{-2} s^{-1}$; blue, 441 nm, 3.1 log quanta $\mu m^{-2} s^{-1}$; Broad field flash.

A19 is a large field amacrine with a transient ON/OFF response to light. In fact, this is the only amacrine type we have seen so far in cat retina, with a response type corresponding to the stereotypical phasic amacrine cells of cold blooded vertebrates (Werblin and Dowling, 1969; Werblin 1972). A19 cells in cat appear to be driven by two types of cone bipolar and by several amacrine types, one of which is A8 a phasic OFF centre unit. Gap junctions probably interconnect large numbers of A19 cells across the retina (Fig. 11). Its transmitter is thought to be GABA. We suggest that A19 cells may play some role in the formation of complex receptive fields recorded from certain ganglion cells. For example the "local edge detector" ganglion cells (Cleland and Levick, 1974b) have an ON/OFF response possibly driven by an ON/OFF amacrine cell type.

A8 is another small field bistratified amacrine cell mostly involved in the cone system. It receives input from rod and OFF centre cone bipolars and has output to A19 amacrines amongst others and to OFF centre ganglion cells (Fig. 10). Its physiology shows cone driven phasic OFF centre responses and its receptive field is concentrically organized with an antagonistic surround. Its neurotransmitter is probably glycine (Pourcho and Goebel, 1984). Like AII this cell type appears capable of transmitting a concentric receptive field directly to its ganglion cell of contact. Thus it is probably involved in the formation of the receptive field of OFF centre beta ganglion cells.

228

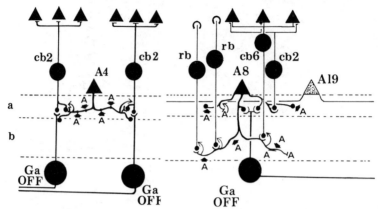

Fig. 10. Wiring diamgrams of two amacrine cells of the cone pathways in the cat retina. A 4 is a small field amacrine that receives input from cone bipolars (cb2), on which it makes reciprocal synapses. Many unidentified amacrines also have synaptic input to A4 and its output is to other amacrines and to OFF centre ganglion cells. A8 receives synaptic input in sublamina a from cone bipolar cb2 and amacrine cells, and in sublamina b from rod and cone bipolar terminals upon which it makes reciprocal synapses. Its dendrites are joined in gap junctions with other A8 cells in sublamina b. A8 has synaptic output to OFF centre ganglion cells and other amacrine cells amongst them A19.

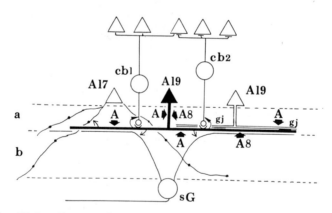

Fig. 11. Wiring diagram of the A 19 amacrine cell in the cat retina. A19 is a monostratified large field cell with dendrites in sublamina a at the a/b border. It receives synaptic input from two types of cone bipolar, cb1 and cb2 and other amacrine cells amongst them A8. It engages in reciprocal synapses with the cone bipolar axon terminals, and makes synapses upon small caliber ganglion cell dendrites (sG) (not yet identified as to ganglion cell type) and A17 amacrine cell dendrites in sublamina a. A19 amacrine cells appear to be joined by gap junctions (gj) to other A19 cells.

T A B L E 1

Summary of Functional Neurocircuitry of Seven Amacrine
Cells in the Cat Retina

AMACRINE	FIELD SIZE	CENTER TYPE	RESPONSE	SYSTEM	TRANSMITTER
A4	Small	OFF	Sustained	Cone	Glycine
A19	Large	ON/OFF	Transient	Cone	GABA
A8	Small	OFF	Transient	Cone	Glycine
A18	Large	?	?	Cone/Rod	Dopamine
AII	Small	ON	Trans/Sust	Rod/Cone	Glycine
A13	Medium	OFF	Sustained	Rod/Cone	GABA
A17	Large	ON	Sustained	Rod	GABA

A18 is the dopamine amacrine cell that Pourcho (1982) has shown to
have synapses upon the AII cell and we have some evidence for it having
synaptic interactions with another amacrine of the rod system, A17 (Fig.
12). It is a large field cell with as yet unknown physiology and as yet
unknown input, other than from unidentified amacrine cells. We suggest
that A18 should be indirectly cone bipolar driven through other cone
system amacrines because dopamine is known to be released under photopic
light conditions (Kramer 1971; Iuvone et al 1978). We think that cone
system driven dopamine cells are inhibiting AII and A17 cells.
Furthermore, because of dopamine's effect on electrical synapses
(Teranishi et al 1983) the A18 may be uncoupling AII amacrine cells from
each other and from cone bipolars, so that the AII pathway to ON centre
ganglion cells is severed during photopic conditions. In the dark
however, the A18 should not be releasing transmitter (Kramer 1971) thus
allowing A17 cells to function effectively and allowing the coupling of
AII signals both to other AIIs and through cone bipolar routes to ON
centre ganglion cells.

AII is by now rather well known to be glycinergic (Pourcho 1981;
Frederick et al 1984; Marc 1984). This largely rod driven amacrine with a
depolarizing response to light and a concentric receptive field
organization is known to have output upon OFF centre ganglion cells
directly, and ON centre ganglion cells indirectly through the ON centre
cone bipolar cell cb5 (Fig. 12). Nelson (1982) has suggested its function
is to quicken rod signals to ganglion cells in the mospic range. As it
has a centre surround organization and appropriate circuitry we presume it
transmits this organization directly to ganglion cells.

A13 is a medium field sustained OFF centre unit. Although mainly rod
driven it also has cone driven components. Its input is from rod bipolars
and cone bipolars of sublimina b and its synaptic output is to ON centre
ganglion cells (Fig. 12). A13 is probably GABAergic (Pourcho and Goebel
1983) and for this reason we suggest it is a good candidate for providing
OFF inhibition in ON centre ganglion cells, as described by Ikda and
Sheardown (1983) in cat retina.

230

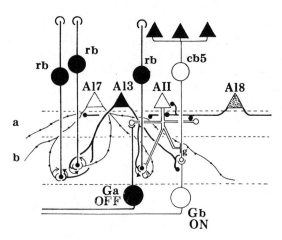

Fig. 12. Wiring diagram of four amacrine cell types involved primarily in the rod system in the cat retina. A17 is wide field and diffuse receiving synaptic input in sublamina b only from rod bipolar axon terminals upon which it makes reciprocal synapses. In sublamina a, A17 receives amacrine input primarily from A18, but also from probably A4 and A19. A13 is a medium field diffuse amacrine cell with synaptic input from rod and cone bipolar axons in sublamina b. It makes reciprocal synapses to the bipolars and has synaptic output upon ON centre ganglion cells. AII is the bistratified cell of the rod system. Receiving synaptic input from rod bipolars in sublamina b where it also makes gap junctions (g) with cb5 type cone bipolar cells, in sublamina a it receives input from cb1 and makes synapses upon cb1 and dendrites of OFF centre ganglion cells. In addition, in sublamina a, A18 cells make synapses upon the AII cell body, apical dendrite and lobular appendages. A18 is the dopaminergic amacrine of the cat retina. It is a wide-field cell with its dendrites restricted to the upper part of sublamina a where it has synaptic output upon AII and A17 amacrine cell dendrites. It probably has synaptic input (not shown) from other A18 cells and cone amacrine cells of as yet unknown type.

Lastly A17 is the most purely rod driven of the amacrine cells. Its only output so far discovered is reciprocal synapses back upon rod bipolar axons although it receives input from various amacrine cells amongst them A18 (Fig. 12). It has a wide-field sustained depolarizing response, but its receptive field is difficult to define because under some circumstances it appears to have a smaller receptive field than under others (Nelson and Kolb 1985). It receives amacrine input from probable A4 (pA), A19 (dA) and A18, the dopamine cell. As a GABAergic cell its presumed inhibitory function is still a puzzle to us. We can only suggest it has a local adapting effect on rod bipolars and a sensitivity to temporally changing large stimuli in mesopic light conditions. But it is not clear how such information might be passed to ganglion cells.

Acknowledgement
    Supported in part by grant EY 03323 from the National Institutes of Health.

References
Belgum, J.H., Dvorak, D.R. and McReynolds, J.S. J. Physiol. (London) 354, 273-286 (1984).
Boycott, B.B. in Essays on the nervous system: A Festschrift for Professor J.Z. Young, R.M. Bellairs and E.G. Gray eds. (Clarendon Press, Oxford 1974) pp. 223-257.
Boycott, B.B. and Dowling, J.E. Phil. Trans. Roy. Soc. B 225, 14-176 (1969).
Boycott, B.B. and Wassle, H. J. Physiol (Lond) 240, 397-419 (1974).
Brecha, N.C., Eldred, W., Kuljis, R.O. and Karten, H.J. in Progress in Retinal Research. N. Osborne and G. Chader, eds. (Pergamon Press 1984) pp. 185-226.
Cajal, R.S. Rev. trim. d. Histol. norm. etr. Numero 1 y 2 (1888).
Cajal, S.R. in The Structure of the Retina. S.A. Thorpe and M. Glickstein Trans. (Thomas, Springfield 1972).
Cleland, B.G. and Levick, W.R. J. Physiol. (Lond.) 240, 457-492 (1974).
Ehinger, B. Vis. Res. 23, 1280-1292 (1983).
Ehinger, B. and Falck, B. Albrech. v. Graefes Arch. klin. exp. Ophthal. 178, 295-305 (1969).
Famiglietti, E.V. Vis. Res. 23, 1265-1280 (1983).
Famiglietti, E.V. and Kolb, H. Brain Res. 84, 293-300 (1975).
Frederick, J.M., Rayborn, M.E. and Hollyfield, J.G. J. Comp. Neurol. 227, 159-172 (1984).
Freed, M.A., Yasuhisa, N. and Sterling, P. J. Comp. Neurol. 219, 295-304 (1983).
Freed, M.A. and Sterling, P. Ann. Meet. Soc. Neurosci. 9, 806 (1983).
Frumkes, T.E., Miller, R.F., Slaughter, M. and Dacheux, R.F. J. Neurophysiol 45, 783-803 (1981).
Gallego, A. in Neural Principles in Vision. F. Zettler and R. Weiler eds. (Springer Verlag 1975) pp. 26-62.
Ikeka, H and Sheardown, M. Vis. Res. 23, 1161-1174 (1983).
Iuvone, P.M. Galli, C.L, Garrison-Gund, C.K. and Neff, N.H. Science 202, 901-902 (1978).
Kaneko, A. J. Physiol (Lond) 235, 133-153 (1973).
Karten, H.J. and Brecha, N. Vis. Res. 23, 1197-1205 (1983).
Kolb, H. J. Comp. Neurol. 155, 1-14 (1974).
Kolb, H. J. Comp. Neurocytol. 8, 295-329 (1979).
Kolb, H. in Molecular and Cellular Basis of Visual Acuity. S.R. Hilfer and J.B. Sheffield eds. (Springer Verlag 1984) pp. 55-78.
Kolb, H. and Famiglietti, E.V. Science 186, 47-49 (1974).
Kolb, H. and Nelson, R. Vis. Res. 21, 1625-1633 (1981).
Kolb, H., Nelson, R. and Mariani, A. Vis. Res. 21, 1081-1114 (1981).
Kolb, H. and Nelson, R. Vis. Res. 23, 301-312 (1983).
Kolb, H.J. and Nelson, R. in Progress in Retinal Res. N. N. Osborne and G. J. Chader eds (Pergamon Press 1984) pp. 21-60.
Kramer, S.G. Invest. Ophthal. 10, 438-452 (1971).
Marc, R.E. and Liu, W.S. J. Comp. Neurol. (1984).
Mariani, A.P. and Leure-Dupree, A.E. J. Comp. Neurol. 175, 13-26 (1977).
Mariani, A.P., Kolb, H. and Nelson, R. Brain Res. 322, 1-7 (1984).
Miller, R.F. in Neuronal Interactions in the Vertebrate Retina. F.O. Schmitt and F.G. Worden eds. (MIT Press,Cambridge, MA London, England 1980).
Miller, R.F, Frumkes, T.E., Slaughter, M.M. and Dacheux, R.F. J. Neurophysiol. 45, 743-763 (1981).
Miller, R.F., Slaughter, M.M. and Dick, E. in Neurotransmitter interactions and Compartmentation. H.F. Bradford ed. (Plenum, New York 1982).
Miller, R.F. and Bloomfield, S.A. Proc. Natl. Acad. Sci. 80, 3069-3073 (1983).
Murakami, M. and Shimoda, Y. J. Physiol (Lond) 264, 801-818 (1977).

232

Naka, K-I. Invest. Ophthal. 15, 926-935 (1976).
Nelson, R. J. Comp. Neurol. 172, 109-135 (1977).
Nelson, R. J. Neurophysiol. 47, 928-947 (1982).
Nelson, R., Kolb, H., Famiglietti, E.V. and Gouras, P. Invest. Ophthal. 15, 935-946 (1976).
Nelson, R., Famiglietti, E.V. and Kolb, H. J. Neurophysiol 41, 472-483 (1978).
Nelson, R. and Kolb, H. Vis. Res. 23, 1183-1195 (1983).
Nelson, R. and Kolb, H. Ophthalmic Res. 16, 21-26 (1984).
Nelson, R. and Kolb, H. J. Neurophysiol. in press (1985).
Ogden, T.E. J. Comp. Neurol., 153, 399-428. (1974).
Ogden, T.E., Green, J.D. and Petesrson, R.G. Stain Technol. 49, 81 (1974).
Oyster, C.W., Takahashi, E.S., Brecha, N.C. and Cilluffo, M. Invest. Ophthal. Vis. Sci. Suppl 25, 87 (1984).
Pourcho, R.G. Brain Re. 215, 187-199 (1981).
Pourcho, R.G. Brain Res. 252, 101-109 (1982).
Pourcho, R.G. and Goebel, D.J. J. Comp. Neurol. 219, 25-35 (1983).
Pourcho, R.G. and Goebel, D.J. Invest. Ophthal. Vis. Sci. Suppl 25, 284 (1984).
Stell, W.K. and Witkovsky, P. J. Comp. Neurol. 148, 33-46 (1973).
Sterling, P. Ann. Rev. Neurosci. 6, 149-185 (1983).
Stevens, J.K. and Jacobs, J.R. Ann. Meet. Soc. Neur. 9, 686 (1983).
Teranishi, T., Negishi, K. and Kato, S. Nature 301, 243-245 (1983).
Tork, I. and Stone, J. Brain Res. 169, 261-273 (1979).
Vallerga, S. and Deplano, S. Proc. Roy. Soc. B, 221, 465-477 (1984).
Werblin, F.S. and Dowling, J.E. J. Neurophysiol. 33, 339-355 (1969).
Werblin, F.S. Science, 175, 1008-1010 (1972).

The Neurocircuitry of Primate Retina

Peter Gouras, Hans U. Evers
Columbia University
Department of Ophthalmology
630 W. 168 St.
New York, N. Y. 10032

We are gradually moving toward a better understanding of the synaptic circuitry of the primate retina by continued anatomical and physiological studies of single cells. Our own research has concentrated on interpreting the possible synaptic circuits that intervene between functionally identifiable photoreceptor mechanisms and different parallel systems of retinal ganglion cells subserving the same or similar populations of photoreceptors. In this paper we propose a hypothetical model of the synaptic circuitry of the primate retina emphasizing the influence of recent experiments done with a probe for the action of the shortwave (S) cone mechanism (Gouras and Eggers 1983) and others (Evers and Gouras 1985) in which APB (2-amino-4-phosphonobutyric acid) is used to block on-center bipolars and consequently specific components in the electroretinogram (ERG).

Physiology indicates that there is considerable autonomy in the way signals of each photoreceptor system are organized before they influence either the center or surround mechanism of primate retinal ganglion cells. For example, one cone mechanism can mediate the center and another the antagonistic surround of one ganglion cell and show the converse organization on a neighboring ganglion cell. In a third cell both of these cone mechanisms can act synergistically in the center and surround of the receptive field and all of these ganglion cells can share the same or a very similar population of photoreceptors.

Figure 1 shows schematically the major ganglion cells systems in primate retina which subserve in parallel a common pool of cone and rod photoreceptors. Figure 1 shows only cones and thereby emphasizes the foveal region where rods are sparse. One system is thought to subserve shortwave sensitive (S) cones (Fig. 1, right) which comprise about 5% of primate cones. The strong signal from S cones detectable in these cells is antagonized by an opponent signal from the middle (M) and/or long (L) wavelength sensitive cones. Usually, perhaps always, the S cone mechanism excites and another cone mechanism(s) inhibits these cells. Each ganglion cell has a relatively large receptive field within which the opposing cone systems appear to be organized more coextensively than concentrically (Gouras, 1984).

The other two major retinal ganglion cell systems subserve the L and M cone systems, perhaps exclusively. Most of these cells appear to have a concentrically organized receptive field structure (Fig. 1, middle and left). One of these ganglion cell systems (Fig. 1, middle) receives from both L and M cones in both the center and antagonistic surround of the receptive field. The other system is composed of ganglion cells in which either the L or M cone mechanism, alone, forms the center and the other forms a concentrically organized surround in the receptive field. Both of these ganglion cell systems can have either an on- or an off-center response, making six possible varieties of these type of ganglion cells. These together with the system of ganglion cells subserving S cones comprise at least seven to eight functional varieties. This does not encompass all the varieties encountered but they form a large part and can serve as a starting point for considering the neurocircuitry of the primate retina.

© 1985 by Elsevier Science Publishing Co., Inc.
Neurocircuitry of the Retina, A Cajal Memorial
A. Gallego and P. Gouras, Editors

234

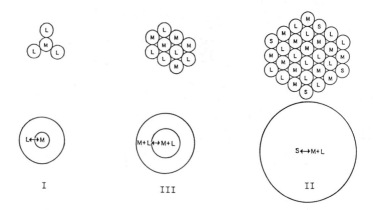

Fig. 1. A scheme of how parallel systems of retinal ganglion cells subserve the same cone photoreceptor mosaic. Each small circle in the mosaic signifies a single cone. There are equal numbers of M and L but fewer S cones. An S/M+L ratio of 0.18 is used but 0.1 is probably a better estimate (Gouras, 1984). Type I units have an input from only one type of cone in the center and another cone type in the surround. Type II units receive antagonistic (S versus M+L) signals from a quasi-coextensive population of cones; their receptive fields are relatively large. Type III cells have a concentrically organized receptive field organization but with both center and surround mechanisms receiving signals from M and L cones.

The Circuitry of the S cone Retina

Figure 2 illustrates a hypothetical synaptic circuit for the S cone mechanism. Light absorbed by S cones excites an on-center bipolar cell which only contacts S cones. An on-center bipolar is a logical choice since most or all of the S cone signals excite primate retinal ganglion cells. This arrangement requires a sign inverting synapse from the S cone to the on-center bipolar. Sign inverting synapses between cones and on-center bipolars are known to exist in the outer plexiform layer of retinas of other vertebrates (Tomita 1984). This syanptic arrangement requires a sign preserving excitatory synapse between the S cone bipolar and its corresponding ganglion cell. Such an hypothesis is in accord with Mariani's (1983) silver staining of a class of bipolars, the dendrites of which contact a select group of cones having the suspected spatial distribution of S cones. This S cone bipolar cell terminates in the on-center lamina of the inner plexiform layer.

The hypothesis that the S cones transmit their signals to specific ganglion cells via a system of on-center bipolars agrees with our recent results with the S cone ERG. The primate S cone ERG is an E-type ERG by Granit's terminology (1947). E-type ERGs have a small a-wave, a large, slow b-wave to the onset and a corneal negative wave to the offset of a light stimulus. The prototype E-type ERG is produced by rods and is illustrated in Fig. 3 (right side, blue stimulus). Notice the negative off-response which saturates with the brightest stimuli. Figure 3 (left side, red stimulus) illustrates an I-type ERG, which is characteristically produced by cones. These two ERGs are obtained from the cynomolgus monkey (M. fascicularis) in the dark-adapted state. Under these conditions the response to blue light is dominated by rods but the cone response can also be exposed with longwave (red) stimuli. The I-type ERG is characterized

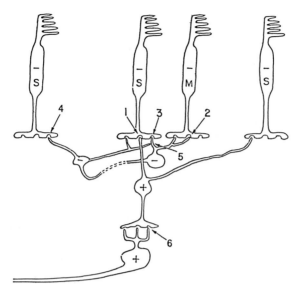

Fig. 2. Hypothetical neurocircuitry of the S cone system in primate retina. A large field on-center bipolar (+) cell is postsynaptic to several S cones at the sign inverting synapse (1) and presynaptic to a S cone subserving ganglion cell (+) at sign preserving synapse (6). A horizontal cell (-) is postsynaptic to M (and/or L) cones at sign preserving synapse (2) and presynaptic to S cones at sign inverting synapse (3). Another horizontal cell (-) is postsynaptic to S cones at sign preserving synapse (4) and presynaptic to the previous horizontal cell at sign inverting synapse (5).

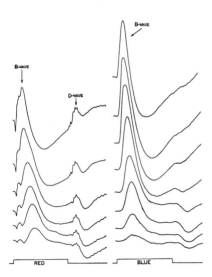

Fig. 3. The dark-adapted primate ERG elicited by a pulse (0.6 sec) of red (640 nm) and blue (460 nm) light. The red light elicits a large a-wave, two discrete b-waves, an early cone, and a later rod b-wave; with strong red light, oscillations can be seen on the rising phase of the combined rod and cone b-wave. At off, red light elicits a corneal positive d-wave, considered to reflect mainly the depolarizing responses of off-center midspectral cone bipolars. The blue light elicits a very small a-wave with the brightest stimuli and a single large rod b-wave without any oscillations. At off, blue light elicits a negative off-response thought to be due to the hyperpolarization of on-center rod bipolars and amacrines. With very bright stimuli, this negative rod off-response is lost as a result of saturation of the rods.

by a large a-wave, a quicker b-wave to the onset and a corneal positive
(d-) wave to the offset of a light stimulus. The I-type ERG seen on the
left of Fig. 3 is produced by the M and L cone mechanisms (Evers and
Gouras 1985). The S cones contribute a relatively small signal to the
primate ERG which is only detectable with wavelengths shorter than 500 nm.
In order to facilitate detecting this response, a steady yellow adapting
field is used to saturate the rods and desensitize the longer wavelength
sensitive (L and M) cones. This leaves the S cones in relative darkness.
Figure 4 illustrates the primate S cone ERG under these circumstances.
The response is best detectable with wavelengths from 400 to 500 nm. Not
only is the S cone ERG small with stimuli of longer wavelengths, but the
response of the M and L cone ERG becomes so large that it swamps the
smaller S cone response. The S cone ERG has its maximum sensitivity to
440-450 nm which distinguishes it from the rod ERG with a maximum at
500-510 nm. The S cone ERG, like that of the rods, is an E-type response.
We have suggested that the difference between an I and an E type ERG
depends on the presence or absence, respectively, of an off-center bipolar
system (Evers and Gouras 1985; Gouras et al 1985). On-center bipolars can
contribute to a corneal positive b-wave and a corneal negative
off-response; off-center bipolars can contribute to the corneal negative
a-wave and a corneal positive off-response. This presumes that the ERG
current depends on extracellular K^+ current. We have used this reasoning
to test the hypothesis that S cones have only on-center but M and L cones
have both on- and off-center bipolars by injecting small amounts of APB
into the vitreal chamber. This drug specifically blocks the synaptic
transmission between photoreceptors and on-center bipolars (Slaughter and
Miller 1981). Figure 5 illustrates how APB changes the S, L and M cone
ERG in primate retina. The b-waves of these ERGs are eliminated. The
corneal positive off-response (d-wave) of the L and M cone ERG becomes
supernormal whereas the negative off-response of the S cone ERG
disappears. These results are consistent with the hypothesis that all
three cone mechanisms have on-center but only L and M cones have
off-center bipolar systems. Other investigators have used APB to study
the primate (Knapp and Schiller 1985) and rabbit (Masey et al 1983) ERGs.
In their experiments no attempt was made to eliminate the relatively large
rod components in these ERGs; consequently their results reflect the rod
system almost entirely. APB, in this case, also eliminates the b-wave of
the ERG, which is consistent with the hypothesis that E-type ERG are
generated by receptor systems with on-center bipolars. This hypothesis
also agrees with Dacheaux and Raviola's finding (1984) that rod bipolars
in rabbit retina are on-center. For these reasons, the neurocircuitry in
Fig. 2 incorporates a sign inverting synapse (1) between S cones and S
cone bipolars and a sign-preserving (excitatory) synapse (6) between S
cone bipolars and S cone subserving ganglion cells.

We also know from physiology that all of these S cone subserving
ganglion cells receive a maintained antagonistic signal that originates in
L and/or M cones. The most logical interneuron to carry such a signal is
a horizontal cell that is postsynaptic to L and/or M cones and presynaptic
to S cones and/or S cone bipolars. Horizontal cells carrying maintained
antagonistic signals between cone mechanisms are well known in fish and
turtle retina (Tomita 1984) and are thought to release an inhibitory
synaptic transmitter, gamma-aminobutyric acid (Murakami et al 1982). Such
a horizontal cell system has been incorporated into the synaptic circuitry
of the S cone retina as synapses (2) and (3).

Synapses 1, 2, 3 and 6 in Fig. 2 are sufficient to explain a unique
phenomenon nicknamed "transient tritanopia" and exhibited by S cone
ganglion cells (Gouras 1968), the b-wave of the S cone ERG (Valeton and
van Norren 1979; Evers and Gouras 1985) and subjective threshold detection

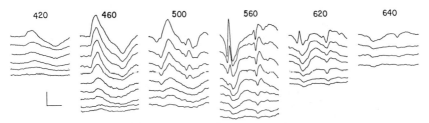

Fig. 4. Electroretinograms of cynomolgus monkey in the presence of a
yellow (Wratten 12) field of 500 ft.-lamberts. The stimulus is a light
pulse (0.1 sec) which produces an on- and an off-response, shown next to
each other. The wavelength (nanometers) of stimulation is shown above
each column of responses. The energy of stimulation is reduced
successively from above down. The calibration signifies 50 microvolts
vertically and 50 milliseconds horizontally.

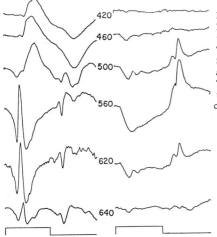

Fig. 5. The cynomolgus monkey's
ERG before (left) and after (right)
the intravitreal injection of APB.
The upper three recordings show the
S cone and the lower three, the L
and M cone ERG (as in Fig. 4).
The b-wave is lost after APB but
the positive off- effect (d-wave)
of the L+M cone ERG is increased.

mediated by the S cone mechanism (Mollon and Polden 1977). This
phenomenon characterized mainly by a transient elevation of
threshold of the S cone mechanism occurring whenever a long wave adapting
field, which has no direct effect on S cones, is turned off. In the
circuit of Fig. 2 this results in a depolarization of S cones by the
horizontal cell which receives an excitatory (depolarizing) transmitter
from L and/or M cones and releases an inhibitory (hyperpolarizing)
transmitter onto S cones. Light hyperpolarizes the L and/or M cones which
in turn stops the release of the excitatory transmitter at synapse (2)
which leads to hyperpolariz ation of this horizontal cell and the stopping
of the release of its inhibitory transmitter at synapse (3). This
depolarizes the S cone which consequently releases its sign inverting
transmitter, assumed to be a Na$^+$ conductance decreasing transmitter and
hyperpolarizes the on-center S cone bipolar. When the L and/or M cones
are put into darkness, the reverse occurs and the S cone on-center bipolar
is depolarized. We assume that this off-depolarization produced by
darkening the L and/or M cones saturates synapse (1) in the excitatory

direction so that any stoppage of transmitter release by light being absorbed by S cones (hyperpolarizing) remains ineffective. Such a saturation of synapse (1) in the excitatory direction would mean that sufficient transmitter has been released to block more than all the available Na^+ channels on the postsynaptic membrane of the S cone bipolar. This model can explain transient tritanopia (Gouras and Zrenner 1983).

An additional horizontal cell interneuron is present in the synaptic circuitry of the S cone retina depicted in Fig. 2. The purpose of this interneuron is to enable the S cone mechanism to disinhibit the S cones from the antagonism which is considered to reach them by the horizontal cell postsynaptic to the L and/or M cones. We require such a circuit because the S cone subserving ganglion cell is excited not only by blue but by white (blue + yellow) light (Gouras and Eggers 1983). This horizontal cell interneuron is postsynaptic to S cones and presynaptic to the horizontal cells described above. It is not presynaptic to L and/or M cones because this would interfere with the parallel action these cones perform in addition to antagonizing S cones. It is interesting that Kolb Mariani and Gallego (1980) have described a second type of horizontal cell in monkey retina which has two functionally distinct parts, one of which could subserve the role of this hypothetical horizontal cell postsynaptic to S cones.

The six synapses and the neuronal arrangements depicted in Fig. 2 are all that are required to explain the behavior of the S cone subserving ganglion cells. It assumes that all such ganglion cells are excited by S cones through a system of on-center bipolars and that there are no off-center S cone bipolars or ganglion cells. There is evidence for this both in the retina (Gouras and Zrenner 1979) and the lateral geniculate nucleus (Malpeli and Schiller 1978).

We have found no need to involve amacrine cell interactions in the S cone retina although undoubtedly such interactions exist. This is not so when considering the synaptic circuitry of the L and M cone retinas, where amacrine cell interactions seem essential to explain some of the physiology.

The L and M Cone Retinas

The M and L cones are more numerous than S cones in primate retina (Bowmaker et al 1980) and have many more ganglion cells subserving them (Gouras 1984). There are two major systems of retinal ganglion cells subserving L and M cones. One system resembles the S cone subserving ganglion cells in responding tonically to a maintained stimulus and usually showing opponent interactions between different cone mechanisms. The other system shows phasic responses to a maintained stimulus and no overt evidence of cone opponent interactions. The former system, together with the S cone subserving ganglion cells, appears to project mainly to the parvo- while the latter appears to project mainly to the magnocellular layers of the lateral geniculate nucleus (Gouras 1984).

Tonic System

Figure 6 shows a hypothetical neurocircuit of the tonic system of ganglion cells subserving the M and L cones. Each M and L cone is subserved by at least two bipolar cells, one sign preserving (off-center), the other sign reversing (on-center). We believe a double or "push-pull" set of on- and off-center bipolars is a characteristic feature of primate L and M cone retinas. This arrangement provides for fine resolution with separate cells detecting an increment versus a decrement of light on each cone. By this means there can be a large dynamic range in the depolariz-

ing direction for both increments and decrements of light.

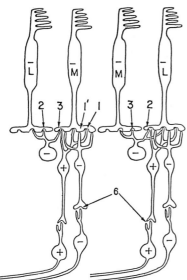

Fig. 6. Hypothetical neurocircuitry of the tonic L and M
cone ganglion cell systems. Two
small field bipolar cells, one on
(+), the other off (-) center,
are postsynaptic to each cone by
synapses(1) and (1') respectively
and presynaptic to ganglion cells
(6). Horizontal cells are post- ·
synaptic to L and presynaptic to
M (left) cones and the reverse
(right) by synapses (2) and (3)
respectively.

The on-center bipolar is considered to use the same synaptic
mechanisms as the S cone bipolar and terminates in the on-center lamina of
the inner plexiform layer with dendrites of small on-center ganglion
cells. There are at least four such on-center bipolars, one subserving M
and the other subserving L cones. The off-center bipolar uses a sign
preserving synapse and therefore an excitatory one designated 1' in Fig.
6. This synapse would logically use a Na^+ conductance increasing
transmitter between cone and bipolar cell. The transmitter released by
the cone is probably the same for both bipolars but the receptor protein
on the postsynaptic membrane is different (Bailey and Gouras 1985). This
off-center bipolar synapses in the off-center (outer) lamina of the inner
plexiform layer with the dendrites of an off-center ganglion cell. Again
the same sign preserving, excitatory syanpse (6) is used here as elsewhere
in our model of primate retina. Again there are at least two of these on-
and off-center channels, one pair for L and one for M cones.

Most of these L or M cone subserving ganglion cells are antagonized by
the cone mechanism that does not form the center mechanism in their
receptive field. This antagonistic signal like the center mechanism is
also maintained but integrates over a relatively larger retinal area than
the center; it is routinely referred to as a concentrically organized
antagonistic surround. An L cone center ganglion cell has an antagonistic
M cone surround and vice versa. We have chosen the horizontal cell to
mediate this maintained antagonism between cone mechanisms. We must
assume that these horizontal cells are cone specific with one set
transmitting an antagonistic signal from M to L and another set from L to
M cones. These synapses are referred to as (2) from cone to horizontal
cell and (3) from horizontal to cone. The synapses, themselves otherwise
resemble those in Fig. 2.

This synaptic circuitry explains why such ganglion cells shown cone
opponency and why this integrates over a relatively larger retinal area
since it is mediated by horizontal cells. It fails to explain why there
are strong differences in the strength of the cone opponency among
different ganglion cells subserving the same or very similar area of the
retina. To explain this without mixing different cone outputs on the same

bipolar cell, requires that some degree of cone opponency be exerted on the bipolar and/or ganglion cell at a point in the retina that is not common to all such ganglion cells. Therefore we have proposed that there is a subpopulation of bipolars and/or tonic ganglion cells to produce stronger cone opponent interactions in certain ganglion cells (Gouras and Zrenner 1981). An alternative explanation is that cone specific primate horizontal cells are presynaptic to certain bipolars; this has not been reported in primate or cat retina but has been in rabbit (Dowling et al 1966).

Phasic System

A parallel system of ganglion cells share the same L and M cones. Figure 7 shows the hypothetical neurocircuitry of these ganglion cells. We assume that there is a separate subsystem of on- and off-center bipolar cells, each of which is postsynaptic to both L and M cones. We reject the alternative model of using the tonic bipolar cell system to feed a separate class of phasic ganglion cells for the following reasons. We envisage tonic bipolrs to be small cells with slower conduction velocities and without any extensive contacts on more than one relatively small ganglion cell, with the midget system being the paragon among this class of cells. Having a larger bipolar cell system with each bipolar contacting several cones would provide the larger receptive field centers these ganglion cells have, would give this system a more rapid intraretinal conduction velocity which these cells have (Gouras 1968), and would allow for an extensive degree of antagonistic amacrine to bipolar cell interaction in order to produce the phasicity these cells exhibit. These ganglion cells would therefore have a two-tiered system of antagonistic interactions. The horizontal cells antagonistically interacting L and M cones would be one tier which the phasic would share with tonic ganglion cells; and the amacrine cells antagonistically interacting phasic on-center with on-center and phasic off-center with phasic off-center bipolars would be a tier which the phasic would not share with the tonic ganglion cells. The former system would confer L and M cone opponent interactions on phasic ganglion cells but this would not be overt since the phasic bipolars receive direct input from both L and M cone. Such an

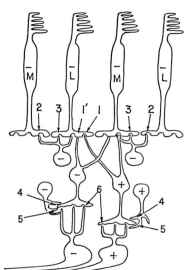

Fig. 7. Hypothetical neurociruitry of the phasic L and M cone ganglion cell systems. Two large field bipolar cells, one on (+), the other off (−) center, are postsynaptic to both L and M cones by synapses (1) and (1') respectively and presynaptic to ganglion cells. The horizontal cell circuitry is identical to that of the tonic cell system (Fig. 6). A separate system of on (+) and off (−) center amacrines are both pre- and postsynaptic to the corresponding bipolars by synapses (4) and (5) to produce phasicity.

arrangement would make these ganglion cells sensitive to color contrasts but would not allow them to code for color, per se. This is what has been found for such cells in the retina (Gouras and Eggers 1983) and the lateral geniculate nucleus (Colby and Schiller 1983).

The first tier of horizontal cell interactions would be identical to that facing the tonic cell system and therefore involve identical neurocircuitry. The second tier or amacrine cell interactions would be unique to the phasic cell system. There latter interactions would produce their phasic response. Dowling and West (1972) proposed that phasicity in ground squirrel retinal ganglion cells was due to an amacrine cell intervening between bipolars and phssic ganglion cells. We favor the circuit in which the amacrine system gates the bipolar which feeds the phasic ganglion cells directly because the latency of phasic ganglion cells to light stimulation of the photoreceptors is relatively short compared to tonic ganglion cells.

The Rod System

In mammalian retina, the rods are subserved by a separate system of rod bipolars which end deeply in the on-center lamina of the inner plexiform layer (Missotten 1965; Dowling and Boycott 1966; Raviola and Raviola 1967). The rod bipolars do not synapse directly with ganglion cells but use a amacrine cell interneurons which subsequently synapse on ganglion cells (Kolb and Nelson 1985). The horizontal cell system for rods is composed of the so called axon terminal end of a horizontal cell, the other end of which subserves cones. These two parts of the same cell are connected by a long, thin process that serves to electrically isolate the rod from the cone end of the cell (Nelson et al 1976). The rod oraxon terminal end sends numerous processes) into rod spherules(Boycott and Kolb 1973; Gallego and Sobrino 1975).

Figure 8 illustrates the hypothetical neurocircuitry of the primate rod retina. We assume that rod bipolars are on-center cells receiving a Na^+ conductance decreasing transmitter released by rods and designated synapse (1) as in the cone systems (Figs. 2, 6 and 7). This is consistent with the fact that APB eliminates the rod b-wave of the ERG in primates (Knapp and Schiller 1985) and rabbits (Massey et al 1983). It also agrees with Dacheaux and Raviola's finding (1984) that rod bipolars in rabbit retina are on-center cells.

The rod bipolar appears to excite the rod amacrine interneuron (Nelson et a 1976; Kolb and Nelson 1985) which in turn forms chemical synapses (5) on off-center ganglion cells and electrical synapses (7) on on-center cone bipolars. By this means the rod system appears to be able to excite the same on- and off-center ganglion cells as cones.

In primates, the rod receptive field center of a ganglion cell appears to be larger than the cone receptive field and the antagonistic surround tends to be weaker than it is for cones (Gouras 1967). This relative independence of rod and cone receptive fields is undoubtedly a result of the separate neurocircuits these systems use before they influence ganglion cells.

The horizontal cell system of rods is still inadequately explored in vertebrate retina. We assume that the rod horizontal cell system performs a similar role as cone horizontal cells, namely to provide an antagonistic surround to photoreceptors. By having separate horizontal cell systems for rods and cones, inappropriate antagonistic feedback is eliminated.

242

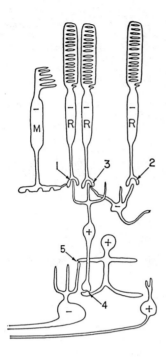

Fig. 8. Hypothetical neuro-circuitry of the rod system in primate retina. A large field on-center bipolar is postsynaptic to a number of rods by sign inverting type synapses (1) and presynaptic by sign preserving excitatory synapses (4) to a rod amacrine cell. The latter is presynaptic to off-center ganglion cells by a sign inverting inhibitory synapse (5) and electrically coupled to on-center ganglion cells.

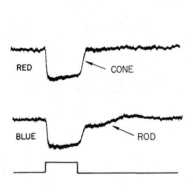

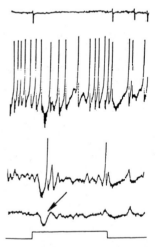

Fig. 9. Illustration (left) of maintained S potential in the outer part of the inner nuclear layer of primate retina, considered to be a horizontal cell response with a strong cone and a weak rod response.
Illustration (right) of an intracellular response of an off-center phasic ganglion cell. The upper record is the response before penetration; the lower three are intracellular responses; the lowermost shows the phasic hyperpolarization of this cell (arrow) to a maintained stimulus after spike generation has ceased. The duration of the light pulse (below) is 100 (left) and 200 (right) msec.

Figure 9 (left) illustrates that both cone and rod signals can be detected in an S potential of monkey retina. These responses resemble those in cat retina which are known to be produced by horizontal cells (Steinberg 1969; Niemeyer and Gouras 1973; Nelson 1977). These responses are maintained, which we believe to be characteristic of events in the outer retinal layers where horizontal cell interactions occur. Figure 9 (right) illustrates the intracellular response of a phasic off-center ganglion cell. This response is transient to a maintained stimulus and is considered to depend on strong amacrine cell interactions as depicted in Figure 7.

Discussion

We have attempted to describe the synaptic circuitry of the primate retina. Our strategy has been to decompose the retina into separate retinas according to each photoreceptor mechanism. Each receptor system is then considered in relationship to its own on- and off-center bipolar system. The M and L cone subretinas are additionally divided into two separate tonic and phasic systems. By this means we envision four separate retinal circuits (modules) processing each area of visual space by at least seven parallel channels of ganglion cells. Each ganglion cell isolates specific cone signals from others within its receptive field center. The tonic system, including the S cone subserving ganglion cells, provide the ultimate in cone specificity and consequently form the substrate for color vision (Gouras 1984). The rod system does not have any separate ganglion cell system but appears to influence all ganglion cells to some degree.

Acknowledgement

This work is supported by National Institutes of Health Grant #EY 02591, National Retinitis Pigmentosa Foundation, Alcon Laboratories and St. Giles the Cripple.

References

Bailey, C.H. and Gouras, P. in Principles of Neuroscience. E. Kandel and J. Schwartz eds. (Elsevier Holland 1985) Chapt. 27.
Bowmaker, J.K. Dartnall, H.J.A. and Mollon, J.D. J. Physiol. 298, 131-143 (1980).
Colby, C.L. and Schiller, P.H. Vis. Res. 23, 1631-1641 (1983).
Dacheux, R.F. and Raviola, E. Invest. Ophthal. Vis. Sci. Suppl. 25, 203 (1984).
Dowling, J.E. and Boycott, B.B. Proc. Roy. Soc. B. 166, 80-111 (1966).
Dowling, J.E., Brown, J.E. and Major, D. Science 153, 1639-1641 (1966).
Evers, H. and Gouras, P. Invest. Ophthal. Vis. Sci. Suppl. 26, 112, 1985.
Gouras, P. in Progress in Retinal Research. N. Osborne and G. Chader, eds. (Pergamon Press 1984) Chapter 8.
Gouras, P. J. Physiol. 192, 747-760 (1967).
Gouras, P. J. Physiol. 199, 533-547 (1968).
Gouras, P. J. Physiol. 204, 407-419 (1969).
Gouras, P. and Eggers, H.M. Vis. Res. 23, 1175-1182 (1983).
Gouras, P., MacKay, C., Evers, H.U. and Eggers, H.M. in Retinal Degeneration: Contemporary Experimental and Clinical Studies. G.Anderson, J. Hollyfield and M. LaVail eds. Alan R. Liss Inc. New York (1985).
Gouras, P. and Zrenner, E. Exerpta Medica Int. Cong. Ser. 450/1: 379-384 (1979).
Gouras, P. and Zrenner, E. Vis. Res. 21, 1591-1598 (1981).

244

Gouras, P. and Zrenner, E. in Colour Vision: Physiology and Psychophysics. J.D. Mollon and L.T. Sharpe eds. (Academic Press, London 1983) pp. 515-526.

Granit, R. Sensory mechanisms of the retina. Univ. Press Oxford (1947).

Knapp. A.G. and Schiller, P.H. Vis. Res. 24:, 1841-1846 (1984).

Kolb, H., Mariani, A.,Gallego, A. J. Comp. Neurol. 189, 31-44 (1980).

Kolb, H. and Nelson, R. Vis. Res. 23, 301-312 (1983).

Malpeli, J.G. and Schiller, P.H. Brain Res. 141, 385-389 (1978).

Massey, S.C. Redburn, D.A. and Crawford, M.L.J. Vis. Res. 23, 1607-1614 (1983).

Mariani, A.P. Nature 308, 184-186 (1984).

Missotten, L. Bull. Socl Belge d'Ophth. 136 (1) 1-203 (1964).

Mollon, J.D. and Polden, P.G. Philos. Trans. R. Soc. Lond. B 278, 207-240 (1977).

Murakami, M., Shimoda, Y., Nakatani, K., Miyachi, E. and Watanabe, S. Jpn. J. Physiol. 32, 911-926 (1982).

Nelson, R. J. Comp. Neurol. 172, 109-135 (1977).

Niemeyer, G. and Gouras, P. Vis. Res. 13, 1603-1612 (1973).

Slaughter, M.M. and Miller, R.F. Science 211, 182-185 (1981).

Steinberg, R.H. Vis. Res. 9, 1319-1329 (1969).

Tomita, T. in Foundations of Sensory Science. W.W. Dawson and J.M. Enoch eds. (Springer Berlin-Heidelberg 1984)

Valeton, J.M. and Van Norren, D. Vis. Res. 19, 689-693 (1979).

West, R.W. and Dowling, J.E. Science 178, 510-512 (1972).

Zrenner, E. and Gouras, P. Invest. Ophthal. Vis. Sci. 18, 1076-1081 (1979).

Afferent and Efferent Peptidergic Pathways in the Turtel Retina

Reto Weiler
Zoological Institute
University of Munich
Munich, West Germany

Most neuropeptides, previously identified in several regions of the brain and thought to act as neurotransmitters (Krieger 1983) have also been localized in retinal tissue (Stell et al 1980). This localization was mainly achieved with immunohistochemical methods, in some instances detection with radioimmunoassays or the demonstration of binding sites was also used. Some of the preceding articles in this volume are good illustrations of the results obtained with these techniques. The majority of immunohistochemical studies carried out on the retina have been able to correlate each neuropeptide recognized with a distinct morphological class of amacrine cells. Here they seemed to exist in a mutually exclusive manner and no coexistence with other putative neurotransmitters such as amino acids, catecholamines and indoleamines, which have all been demonstrated in amacrine cells, has been reported. The enormous variety of putative neurotransmitters in amacrine cells seemed to parallel the great morphological diversity of amacrine cells demonstrated with classical anatomical methods. The almost total restriction of neuropeptides to amacrine cells was somehow disappointing for the retinal physiologist since amacrine cells belong to the functionally most unexplored retinal neurons. There was hope, however, that a specific neuropeptide would exist in similar morphological subtypes of amacrine cells in retinas of different species, thus giving us a reliable functional-morphological criterion. This hope was only marginally fulfilled and the comparison of the immunohistochemical results from different species showed that different neuropeptides do exist in different species and no neuropeptide common to all retinas was discovered. Furthermore, one neuropeptide could exist in two or more different subclasses of amacrine cells in the same retina. All these findings imply that neuropeptides do not have a general, simple function in the retina but are rather involved in local circuits with very specific functional tasks in neuronal processing within the inner plexiform layer of the retina. This will make the exploration of their role a real challenge for the physiologist.

Compared to the vast data on the appearance of neuropeptide-like immunoreactivity in the retina, additional criteria supporting their role as retinal neurotransmitters, are rather scanty. Using radioimmunoassay techniques and high performance liquid chromatography, the peptides neurotensin and somatostatin (Brecha et al 1981), enkephalin (Watt et al 1983) and substance P (Osborne 1984) have been studying qualitatively and quantitatively. Elevation of the potassium concentration increased the released amount of substance P and enkephalin, a process found to be calcium dependent (Osborne 1984; Su and Lam 1983). The release of dopamine and GABA from the retina could be influenced by the exogenous administration of enkephalin (Djamgoz et al 1981; Dubocovich and Weiner 1983; Watt et al 1984).

Astonishingly there are very few reports presenting electrophysiological data, although the retina is a neural tissue electrophysiologically well explored. All the existing data have been obtained by extracellular recording of ganglion cell activity. The results showed that exogenously applied synthetic enkephalin suppressed ganglion cell firing in the mudpuppy retina (Dick and Miller 1981) but increased the firing in goldfish (Djamgoz et al 1981). Neurotensin and substance P both increased ganglion cell firing in the mudpuppy anc carp (Dick and Miller 1981; Glickman et al 1982) and LHRH also increased the firing in the goldfish retina (Stell et al 1984). The rather unspecific action of neuropeptides was in contrast to the above mentioned localization of immunoreactivity in distinct cell populations and the resulting idea of an involvement in local circuits. The unspecificity, however, could result simply from the limitation of extracellular recording technqiues to detect such specific action. We therefore decided to screen the retina for possible peptidergic action using intracellular recording techniques in combination with intracellular staining.

This approach demanded a much more detailed analysis of the peptidergic cell itself and I will report here some of the results obtained during this study. The analysis concentrated on the following questions: what is the physiological photoresponse of an amacrine cell containing a neuropeptide, how is this cell integrated into a local circuit, is there a coexistence with an other transmitter in the same cell, is there a specific release of the neuropeptide upon appropriate stimulation?

Since this approach involves the application of several techniques it was necessary to find a suitable retinal preparation where all these techniques can be applied. The retina of the turtle Pseudemys scripta elegans seemed appropriate, it contains only few neuropeptides in different subclasses of amacrine cells (Eldred and Karten 1983), has a well layered inner plexiform layer and intracellular recordings are possible from all neuronal elements contributing to it (Weiler and Marchiafava 1981).

Immunocytochemical demonstration of neuropeptide-like antigenicity was done either in frozen sections of the retina or in retina slices which were subsequently resin-embedded (Weiler, 1985; Weiler and Ball 1984). The putative transmitters; amino acid dopamine and taurine were localized revealing high affinity uptake systems by incubation with the tritiated substances and subsequent autoradiography (Weiler and Ball, 1984). Intracellular recordings were obtained using glass-microelectrodes filled with either horseradish peroxidase or Lucifer Yellow for subsequent cell identification. For signal amplification and storage, conventional techniques were used (Marchiafava and Weiler 1982).

The physiology of amacrine cells exhibiting neurotensin-like immunoreactivity

In a frozen section of the retina, neurotensin-like immunoreactivity (NTLI) is seen in two different amacrine cell populations (Fig. 1a), (Eldred and Karten 1983). Less frequently it can be observed in interstitial and displaced amacrine cells (Weiler and Ball 1984). The morphology of the two cell populations differs very markedly (Fig. 1b). One cell type (NT-A) has a large soma and sends one thick primary process into the inner plexiform layer (IPL) where it branches horizontally into few branches, which spread in different directions but remain in the middle layer of the IPL. In contrast, the other cell type (NT-B) has a small soma sending several fine processes into the IPL which run along the outer border of the IPL before dropping. The processes branch extensively at layers 3 and 4 and then reach the inner border of the IPL.

The localization of the same immunoreactivity in such morphological different cell types raises the question whether both types are also functionally different. This would imply that a neuropeptide is released with different time courses from different cells. We therefore paralleled the immunocytochemical studies with intracellular recordings to obtain

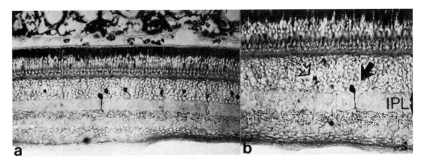

Fig. 1. Neurotensin-like immunoreactivity in the turtle retina. a) immunoreactivity was revealed in a frozen section using the peroxidase-antiperoxidase method and is visible in two amacrine cell populations. b) same section at higher magnification. NT-A cells (arrow) have one principal process which branches into few horizontally running branches at the middle of the inner plexiform layer (IPL). NT-B cells (open arrow) send several thin processes into the IPL which cross the entire IPL and branch predominantly at layers 3 and 4 of the IPL.

physiological data from amacrine cells and by subsequent dye-marking also morphological data. In Figs. 2 and 3 these data are summarized for the NT-A and NT-B cells, respectively.

An immunoctyochemically labelled NT-A cell is shown at high magnification in Fig. 2a. The thick principal process remained undivided up to the middle of the IPL and there it branched into three processes, two of them were partially in the plane of the section and run horizontally. Labelled profiles seen in the inner half of the IPL belong to processes of NT-B cells.

Intracellularly stained amacrine cells have been morphologically classified in the turtle retina into three main groups: monostratified, multistratified and diffuse cells (Weiler and Marchiafava, 1981). The data obtained during this study confirmed this basic classification. From 47 stained cells, 12 were monostratified and from these 5 cells had a principal process branching into three processes running along the middle of the IPL. One such cell, stained intracellularly with horseradish peroxidase is seen in a flat mounted retina in Fig. 2b. The transretinal distribution of its processes was analyzed by centering a set of concentric circles with an equidistance of 30 μm at retinal level over the soma of a camera lucida drawing (Marchiafava and Weiler, 1982). At each crossection of a circle with a process, the depth of this point within the IPL was measured. The IPL was divided into five equal layers and the number of points was plotted against the layer number (Fig. 2c). The histogram for the cell of Fig. 2b clearly reveals the monostratified character of the cell. After reembedding some of the cells were cut transversally and camera lucida drawing of subsequent sections (Fig. 2d) confirms the distribution of processes along the middle of the IPL. All the anatomical data from the 5 monostratified amacrine cells were identical with the data of NT-A cells, making it very likely that they are the same. All these cells responded to light stimulation with transient membrane depolarizations at the on- and offset of a light stimulus (Fig. 2e). Enlarging the stimulus area did not alter this basic property of the photoresponse although the transients were reduced in amplitude and decayed more slowly.

248

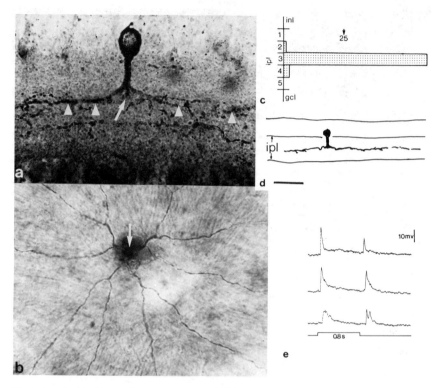

Fig. 2   Comparison of NT-A cells with intracellularly stained amacrine cells. a) NT-A cell in a thick section of resin-embedded material. Note the division of the principal process into three branches (arrow) which run horizontally (arrowheads). Labelled profiles in the inner half of the IPL belong to NT-B cells. b) Intracellularly horseradish peroxidase labelled amacrine cell in the flat mounted retina observed from the vitreous side. Three branches (arrow) leave the principal process. c) analysis of the radial distribution of the stained processes in b) see text for method. There is a prominent peak at the middle of the IPL (layer 3). inl = inner nuclear layer; glc = ganglion cell body layer. d) Camera lucida drawing of subsequent transverse sections from a retina containing a monostratified amacrine cell injected with Lucifer Yellow. Scale 50 um.   e) Photoresponses recorded from the cell of Fig. 2b. The stimulus was a white light spot (1.6 erg x s-1 x cm-2) of increasing size (500 um, 1000 um, 3500 um from top to bottom).

NT-B cells are characterized by their fine processes which run about 50 to 100 um along the outer border of the IPL before dropping into the IPL, where they branch extensively mainly in layers 3 and 4 (Fig. 3a). From the 47 injected cells 6 had a similar diffuse branching pattern, varying only in size of their receptive fields. In the falt mount view (Fig. 3b), the focus is at layers 3 and 4 revealing the dense network at this level. The soma and the fine processes leaving it are partially masked by spillage of horseradish peroxidase. The depth analysis demon-strates the diffuse branching pattern with a maximum at layers 3 and 4 (Fig. 3c), also confirmed in camera lucida drawings of subsequent trans-

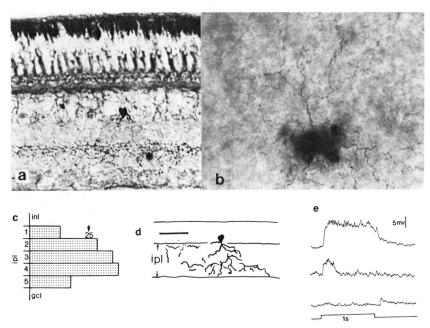

Fig. 3. Comparison of NT-B cells with intracellularly stained amacrine
cells. a) NT-B cell in a frozen section. Note the dense network of the
thin processes in layers 3 and 4. b) Intracellularly horseradish
peroxidase labelled amacrine cell in the flat mounted retina observed from
the vitreous side. Several branches protrude into the IPL, the dense
network in focus is at the inner half of the IPL. Dark reaction product
is located around the soma due to spillage during injection. c) See
Fig. 2c. The radial distribution of labelled processes in b) is diffuse
across the whole IPL with a maximum at layer 4. d) Camera lucida drawing
of subsequent sections containing profiles of a Lucifer Yellow injected
amacrine cell. Scale 50 μ. e) Photoresponses of the diffuse amacrine cell
of Fig. 3b. See Fig. 2e.

versal sections (Fig. 3d). The morphological data of these diffuse cells
are identical to the one of NT-B cells and again it is very likely that
they are the same. All these cells responded to light stimulation with a
graded, sustained membrane depolarization during light on (Fig. 3e). The
photoresponse was shaped with oscillations and increasing the stimulus
area inhibited the response suggesting an antagonistic surround.

It is remarkable that the different morphology of the two amacrine
cells with NTLI also reflects a different physiological behaviour.
Assuming the release of a neuropeptide upon membrane depolarization, a
neurotensin-like peptide is released in a time-space specific manner
within the IPL: at the on- and offset of a light stimulation, in the
middle of the IPL and through light stimulation in the inner half of the
IPL.

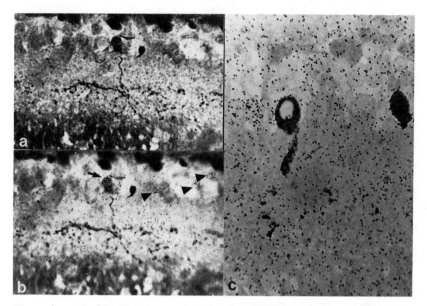

Fig. 4. Co-localization of neurotensin-like immunoreactivity and
(3H)-glycine high affinity uptake system in NT-B cells. a,b) Thick
sections of resin embedded retina. In a) NB soma and its processes
(arrows) are immunocytochemically labelled. In b) the focus is on the
autoradiographic film emulsion covering the section. Autoradiographic
label is present over several somas (arrow heads) among them also the NT-B
soma (arrow). The label within the IPL is diffuse with a higher density
in the inner half. c) Thin section of another double labelling
experiment. The somas of an NT-A (arrowhead) and a NT-B cell (arrow) are
visible. Autoradiographic label is present only over the NT-B soma; NT-A
cells do not have a high affinity uptake system for (3H)-glycine.

Co-existence of glycine uptake system with neurotensin-like immunoreactivity and peptide release

Amino acids, catecholamines, indoleamines and acetylcholine have all
been reported as putative neurotransmitters in amacrine cells and the
likelihood existed that one of these substances co-exists with a
neruopeptide in the same cell. Such co-localization has been established
in various regions of the CNS (Gilbert and Emson 1983) but in the retina
attempts to do so failed (Stell et al 1980). Only in recent studies was
it possible to localize a high affinity uptake system for glycine and NTLI
in the turtle retina (Weiler and Ball 1984) and a high affinity uptake
system for GABA and enkephalin-like immunoreactivity in the pigeon retina
(Watt etl 1984). We therefore made slices of retinas previously incubated
with (3H)-glycine and treated them immunocytochemically to reveal NTLI.
In a thick section (Fig. 4a) the soma and part of the arborization of a
stained NT-B cell are recognizable. Changing the focus onto the silver
grain in the autoradiographic film emulsion (Fig. 4b) clearly reveals
concentrated label over the soma of this cell. The small dark soma on the
right which is part of another NT-B cell is also labelled with silver
grains but the strong immunocytochemical label masks the autoradiographic

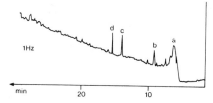

Fig. 5. HPLC elution profile of 100 μl Ringer solution which was kept for 40 min within an eyecup. The eye was stimulated with a flickering white light at hz (1.6 erg x sec-1 x cm-2) and kept in an oxygenated chamber. Elution was performed in a gradient system (acetonitril/TFA) over 45min using a Vydac column. See text.

label in the photograph. Concentrations of silver grains are visible over several soma without NTLI and although each NT-B cell contains both labels, these cells comprise only 7% of the cells labeled for glycine high affinity uptake system. A thin section of another double labelling experiment containing stained profiles of NT-A and NT-B cells shows autoradiographic label exclusively over the NT-B soma; NT-A somas were never double labelled. The demonstration of the two labels in NT-B cells makes it likely that these cells use glycine and a neurotensin-like peptide in their neuronal processing. From Fig. 3 we can determine that NT-B cells are sustained amacrine cells and consequently both substances would be co-released during light stimulation. In the mudpuppy retina the effects of both these exogenously applied substances have been investigated. Neurotensin had an excitatory and glycine an inhibitory influence on the spike activity of extracellularly recorded ganglion cells (Dick and Miller 1981; Miller et al 1981). Certainly much more information is needed to explain the functional significance of the co-existence of an inhibitory amino acid transmitter and an excitatory neuropeptide in the same amacrine cell in the retina. In this regard an important step is to analyze whether both substances are released from the retina under appropriate stimulus conditions and whether such a release is mutually influenced. We have already initiated such a study using high performance liquid chromatography. Eyecups or isolated retinas were placed into an oxygenated chamber and covered with 100 μl of Ringer solution. After a fixed stimulus programme the Ringer solution was analyzed in a Vydac column using a gradient system. Figure 5 shows the elution profile of such a run. The peak height of peaks a-d was influenced by different light stimulations and all peaks were drastically reduced in a Ringer solution containing cobalt. The elution profiles from the experiments with the isolated retina were identical to the ones with eyecup preparations. Peak a corresponds to serotonin which is present in amacrine and bipolar cells (Witkovsky et al 1984; Weiler and Schutte 1985); peak c to the neuropeptide glucagon which is present in amacrine cells (Eldred and Karten 1983) and peaks b and d are not yet analyzed but do not correspond to the neurotensin peak. We are currently analyzing the amino acid sequence of these peaks and are trying to enhance some of the small peaks. The results, however, indicate a release of peptides influenced by stimulus parameters. One goal of these experiments is the collection of enough material from these endogenously released peptides to use them in subsequent electrophysiological experiments.

Met-enkephalin-like immunoreactivity in amacrine cells and in a mesencephalic efferent pathway to the retina

Antisera against several opiate peptides have been tested in the turtle retina (Weiler unpublished) and Met-enkephalin-like immunoreactivity (ELI) was revealed in a distinct population of amacrine cells (Eldred and Karten 1983). These amacrine cells are bistratified

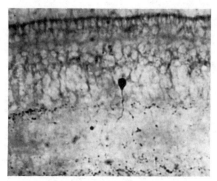

Fig. 6. Frozen section of the retina in which immunoreactivity against Met-enkephalin antiserum was revealed using the peroxidase-antiperoxidase method. An amacrine cell with two dense networks of processes at layers 1 and 5, respectively, is stained.

(Fig. 6); one thin process leaves the small soma and develops a very dense network of fine processes in layer 1 of the IPL before dividing into several fine processes which drop to the inner border of the IPL where they form another dense network in layer 5. Sometimes a few small processes arise in layer 3 giving the cell a tristratified appearance. Although the great majority of the intracellularly stained cells in the parallel electrophysiological study were multistratified, among these were also bistratified cells, I never recorded from a cell with a morpholog y identical to that of an amacrine cell with ELI. Therefore the physiological behaviour of this cell type is still unknown. The antiserum against Met-enkephalin did not only stain the described amacrine cells but also some fibres within the ganglion cell axon layer (Fig. 7a). Ganglion cell, however, never exhibited ELI and it could therefore be concluded that these fibres were not ganglion cell axons.Infortunate sections it was possible to follow collaterals of these fibres through the ganglion cell body layer up to their terminal arborization within the IPL at layers 3 and 4 (Fig. 7b). This confirmed that these fibres do not belong to ganglion cells. The fibres can also be recognized in the optic nerve (Fig. 7c) and the total number ranged between 3 and 6 fibres per optic nerve. They were beaded, had a diameter of 1½ μm and were unmyelinated (Weiler 1985).

The data obtained from the retina and the optic nerve demonstrate the existence of an efferent system in the turtle retina consisting of a small number of fibres containing an enkephalin-like neuropeptide. So far, only the neuropeptides, luteinizing releasing hormone and molluscan cardioexcitatory peptide have been demonstrated in efferent fibres in the goldfish retina, arising in the nervus terminalis (Stell et al 1984).

In order to reveal the origin of the fibres with ELI in the CNS, the fluorescent dye Nuclear Yellow (NY; Bentivoglio et al 1980) was injected into one eye. After a survival time of 1-5 days the brain was removed, fixed and frozen and sections were cut on a cryostat in a frontal plane from the rostral telencephalon to the medulla. A small number of labelled cell nuclei was detected in sections of the mesencephalon. 4 to 12 cell nuclei were stained on the contralateral and 1 to 3 on the ipsilateral side in a mesencephalic region between the second visceral nucleus and the locus coeruleus, basal to the isthmus opticus (Fig. 8a,b). The labelled cells were located within a field of many similar shaped cells with a slight yellowish autofluorescence at 390 nm (Weiler 1985). In animals with a shell size of about 20 cm, the rostral-caudal extension where labelled cell nuclei were detected was about 700 μm. Injection of NY into the orbital cavity during control experiments did not stain any cell nuclei in this sesencephalic region. The relatively small number of retrogradally labelled cell nuclei was in good agreement with the number

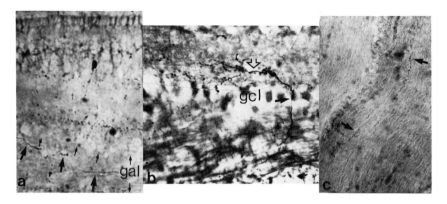

Fig. 7. Efferent fibres to the retina which exhibit Met-enkephalin-like immunoreactivity. a) Frozen section of the retina at the level of the optic disc. In addition to a labelled soma and profiles at layers 1 and 5 of the IPL, fibres with Met-enkephalin-like immunoreactivity (arrows) are present in the ganglion cell axon layer (gal). b) A collateral of such a fibre passes through the ganglion cell body layer (gcl: arrow) and enters the IPL where the terminal arborization terminates within layers 3 and 4 (open arrow). Stained profiles at layers 1 and 5 belong to amacrine cells (Fig. 6). c) Frozen section of the optic nerve. Immunoreactivity is visible in two beaded fibres (arrows).

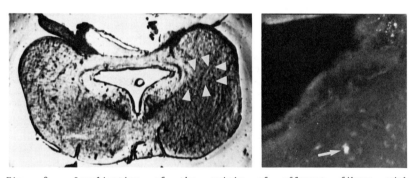

Fig. 8. Localization of the origin of efferent fibres with Met-enkephalin-like immunoreactivity using retrograde transport of Nuclear Yellow and subsequent immunohistochemistry. a) Frozen section of the turtle brain at the level of the caudal mesencephalon where the trochlear nerve enters the brain. The region with labelled cell nuclei is indicated with triangles. It is located between the lateral lumniscus and the locus coeruleus, basal to the isthmus opticus and belongs to the second visceral nucleus. b) Nuclear Yellow was incorporated into a cell nucleus of a cell located in the mesencephalon. In this frozen section of the brain only one cell nucleus (arrow) was stained within a field of cells of comparable size and shape. A total of 4 (n=12) to 12 labelled nuclei were found on the contralateral side and 1 to 3 on the ipsilateral side in the caudal mesencephalon.

of cells back labelled with (3H)wheat germ agglutinin (Schnyder and Kunzle 1983). The small number, however, exceeded the number of fibres with ELI within the optic nerve and it was therefore essential to show which NY labelled cell nuclei belonged to cell somas exhibiting ELI. To answer this question, double labelling experiments with NY and subsequent immunohistochemical treatment were performed. In these experiments about 25-50% of the NY labelled cells reacted with the antiserum against Met-enkephalin. This cell number is almost identical to the number of fibres with ELI in the optic nerve. This implies tht there is at least one additional efferent system in the turtle retina also consisting of only few fibres.

Localization of efferent input to multistratified amacrine cells

Although the number of efferent fibres with ELI is rather small, they could have a substantial influence on retinal processing. The fibres have several collaterals within the retina and they may project onto retinal neurons with a large receptive field.

Influences of efferent fibres on the photoresponses of ganglion cells have been described in the turtle and pigeon (Cervetto et al, 1976; Miledi 1972). This influence was thought to act through amacrine cells which responded, in the turtle, to optic nerve stimulation with a graded membrane depolarization (Marchiafava 1976). No attempt was made to further characterize the type of amacrine cell that was the target of such efferent input. To clarify this question, I used optic nerve stimulation during most of the intracellular recordings from amacrine cells. I distinguished three functional classes of amacrine cells, based on the already described morphological classes and previous work (Weiler and Marchiafava 1981). Electrical stimulation of the optic nerve results in antidromic spikes in ganglion cells and this was used to distinguish successful optic nerve stimulation, and efferent input onto amacrine cells was only investigated in such preparations (Fig. 8, top).

The results demonstrated clearly that only slow transient amacrine cells received efferent input. These cells were multistratified in different layers of the IPL and comprised the largest group of recorded cells. However, only 4 of 21 such cells responded with very complex membrane depolarizations to efferent stimulation. The response was graded with the intensity of the stimulation current and had a threshold (Fig. 9, bottom). None of the monostratified, fast on-off transient cells nor of the diffuse, sustained cells reacted to optic nerve stimulation and it is therefore unlikely that they are target neurons of efferent fibres (Fig. 9).

The experimental set up did not allow a pharmacological investigation of the synaptic events leading to the complex membrane depolarization. It is therefore not yet possible to assign these events to the efferent system described above. The intracellular recordings, however, have been made in the region of the retina where these fibres project and the peripheral location of these fibres in the optic nerve facilitated their electrical stimulation. In addition, the morphology of the affected amacrine cells would allow a direct synaptic input by these fibres in layers 3 and 4. The localization of an enkephalin-like neuropeptide in fibres within the optic nerve certainly offers a new chance to study the role of this neuropeptide in retinal processing: stimulation of the otpic nerve - in contrast to light stimulation -will cause localized endogenous release without activating the entire retina and will also circumnavigate the problems linked with the exogenous application of the synthetic peptide.

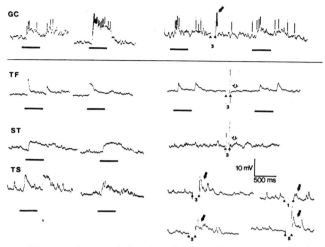

Fig. 9. Efferent input induced with optic nerve stimulation to intracellularly recorded amacrine cells. The traces on the left are the photoresponses of the cells following white light stimulation (black bars) with a spot (500 μm; C) and an annulus (o:3500 μm, i:1200μm;P). The irradiance was 10 (-4) erg x sec(-1) x cm(-2). According to their photoresponses the amacrine cells belong to the group of fast transient cells (TF), sustained cells (ST) and slow transient cells (TS). The traces on the right show responses to optic nerve stimulation (ONS; triangles) with current pulses applied through two chlorided silver hood-electrodes. The stimulator (WPI 305) was hand triggered and the stimulus artefact in the recording trace gives a measurement of the pulse duration. Cells TF and ST do not respond to ONS with a 3 mA pulse (open arrow), a current which produces antidromic spikes in ganglion cells (GC; arrow). In contrast, cell TS shows a complex depolarization following ONS (arrows). The membrane depolarization is related to the current strength with a threshold around 2 mA.

Conclusions

The data from the turtle retina, which I have reviewed briefly here, strongly suggest that neuropeptides are involved in neuronal processing within the retina. They have also shown that these peptides are most likely not involved in straight feedforward mechanism between amacrine and ganglion cells but rather - considering their co-existence with other putative neurotransmitters and their existence in efferent fibres - in neuronal communication between amacrine cells. Consequently, further functional studies should concentrate on this intrinsic neuron which possibly plays as many functional roles as it displays morphological varieties.

I wish to thank my colleagues Drs. Stell, Ball, Schneider and Marchiafava for the fruitful collaborations I enjoyed with them and which were the basis for many of the data reviewed and presented in this article. Drs. Wagner and Douglas gave valuable comments on the manuscript and I. Rambold helped with the illustrations. The research projects were supported by grants from the Alberta Heritage Foundation for Medical Research, the Swiss Academy for Medicine and the Deutsche Forschungsgeme inschaft SFB 220.

References

Bentivoglio, M., H.G.J.M. Kuypers, C.E. Catsman-Berrevoets, H. Lowew and O. Dann Neurosci. Lett. 18, 25-30 (1980).

Brecha, N., H.J. Karten and C. Schenker J. Neurosci. 6, 1329-1348 (1981).

Cervetto, L., P.L. Marchiafava and E. Pasino Nature, 160, 56-57 (1976).

Dick, E. and R.F. Miller Neurosci. Lett. 26,

Djamgoz, M.B.A., W.K. Stell, Chen-An Chin and D.M.K. Lam Nature 292, 620-623 (1981).

Dubocovich, M.L. and N. Weiner J. Pharmacol. & Exp. Therepeutics 22, 634-639 (1983).

Eldred, W.D. and H.J. Karten J. Comp. Neurol. 221, 371-381 (1983).

Gilbert, R.F.T. and P.C. Emson in Handbook of Psychopharmacology L. Iversen, S.D. Iversen and S.H. Synder eds. (Plenum Press Corp. V. 16 (1983)pp. 519-556.

Glickman, R.D., A.R. Adolph and J.E. Dowling Brain Res. 124, 81-99 (1982).

Krieger, D.T. Science 222, 975-985 (1983).

Marchiafava, P.L. J. Physiol 255, 137-155 (1976).

Marchiafava, P.L. and R. Weiler Proc. Roy. Soc. Lond 214, 403-415 (1982).

Miles, F.A. Brain Res. 48, 115-129 (1972).

Miller, R.F., T.E. Frumkes, M. Slaughter and R.F. Dacheux J. Neurophysiol 45, 764-782 (1981).

Osborne, N.N. J. Physiol. 349, 89-93 (1984).

Schnyder, H. and H. Kunzle Cell Tiss. Res. 234, 219-224 (1983).

Su, Y.Y.T. and D.M.K. Lam Soc. Neurosci. Abstr. 9, 282 (1983).

Stell, W.K., D. Marshak, T. Yamada, N. Brecha and H. Karten TINS 3, 292-295 (1980).

Stell, W.K., S.E. Walker, K.S. Chohan and A.K. Ball Proc. Natl. Acad. Sci. 81, 948-944 (1984).

Watt, C., D. Tavella, Y.Y.T. Su, Y.W. Peng and D.M.K. Lam Soc. Neurosci. Abstr. 9, 282 (1983).

Watt, C., Y.Y.T. Su, and D.M.K. Lam Nature 311, 761-763 (1984).

Weiler, R. Neurosci. Lett in press (1985).

Weiler, R. and P.L. Marchiafava Vis. Res. 21, 1635-1638 (1981).

Weiler, R. and A.K. Ball Nature, 311, 759-761 (1984).

Weiler, R. and M. Schutte Tiss. Res. in press (1958).

Witkovsky, P., W. Eldred and H.J. Karten J. Comp. Neurol 228, 217-225 (1984).

Postnatal development of GABA and glycine actions on the surround
inhibition of cat retinal ganglion cells in the area centralis

Hisako Ikeda and Jonathan Robbins
Vision Research Unit of Sherrington School
The Rayne Institute, St. Thomas' Hospital
London, England

The detection of contrast and the provision of spatial resolution are
the two major functional roles of the retinal ganglion cells, closely
packed in the area centralis where the density of cones is also highest.
On-centre cells which respond to a spot brighter than background and
off-centre cells which respond to a spot darker than background when
presented at the receptive field centre mutually enhance visual contrast.

In the area centralis of the cat, both on- and off-centre cells, which
give sustained firing to a stationary spot (classed as X or sustained
cells), are more frequently found than those which give transient firing
(classed as Y or transient cells). Under photopic conditions the
receptive field of a sustained cell in the area centralis of adult cats
consists of a sharply-defined, small excitatory centre and a strong,
sharply-defined inhibitory surround (surround inhibition).

The microionophoretic studies of the retinal ganglion cells in the
area centralis of adult cats (Ikeda and Sheardown, 1983a,b) under
predominantly cone mediated conditions, suggested that the surround
inhibition of on-cells is mediated by γ-aminobutyric acid (GABA), whereas
that of off-cells is mediated by glycine. Since on-cells are inhibited by
visual stimuli (black spot or white annulus) which excite off-cells, and
off-cells, separate inhibitory transmitters for on- and off-cells result
in the following condition: when on-cells are excited by a suitable
stimulus presented at a given point in the visual space, off-cells are
inhibited by one transmitter, glycine; conversely when off-cells are
excited, on-cells are inhibited by another transmitter, GABA. Therefore
the presence of specifically coding inhibitory transmitters used by on-
and off-cells in the adult area centralis may provide a mechanism to
enhance contrast detection in the vicinity of the visual axis.

Physiologically, the surround inhibition of sustained (X) on- and
off-cells in the area centralis of kittens at 7-9 weeks of age are still
weak and the inhibitory zone is widespread and ill-defined (Ikeda 1980).
Our question, then, is, has this physiological observation on the weak
inhibitory surround of kitten cells any pharmacological basis?

To answer this question we performed microionophoresis of GABA,
glycine and their selective antagonists, bicuculline and strychnine
respectively, and specifically evaluated their effects upon surround
response and inhibition of sustained cells in the adult and kitten area
centralis.

Methods
    Ten 18-22 week old cats and twelve 7-9 week old kittens were used.
The procedure of anesthesia and surgical preparation for intraretinal
ionophoresis using multi-barrelled electrodes has already been described
in detail elsewhere (Ikeda and Sheardown 1982). The eye was refracted by
retinoscopy and a correction lens placed in front of the eye to make the
retina conjugate with the stimulation plane. Methods of selection and
classification of retinal ganglion cells have been described previously
(Ikeda and Sheardown 1983).

ⓒ 1985 by Elsevier Science Publishing Co., Inc.
Neurocircuitry of the Retina, A Cajal Memorial
A. Gallego and P. Gouras, Editors

Cells were classified as on-centre or off-centre and sustained or transient using an optimal spot (a spot which produced optimal firing from the cell) generated on a TV screen (luminance 100 cd/m^2). Drug effects on on-cells were studied on the responses of cells to spots and annuli brighter (150-192 cd/m^2) than background, whereas those darker (20-30 cd/m^2) than background were used to study off-cell. Thus, the stimulating conditions were in the photopic range in order to study cone inputs to the ganglion cells. In this paper, the surround responses of sustained cells in the area centralis were exclusively studied using an annulus brighter or darker than background which produced optimal inhibition of these cells.

An electrode consisting of six-barrelled micropipettes was used throughout. The central barrel filled with 0.5 M sodium acetate (pH 7.7) recorded spikes generated by single ganglion cells and when positioned close to a soma picked up large biphasic isolated spikes with notched positive peaks (Fuortes, Frank and Becker 1957). A second barrel filled with sodium chloride (BDH 500 mM in water, pH 7.0) provided a balance current at the tip of the electrodes using the facility of a Neurophore BH-2 Unit (Medical Systems Corp). The four remaining barrels contained four drugs: GABA (Sigma, 500 mM in water, pH 3.0), Bicuculline Methobromide (Cambridge Res. Biochemicals, 5mM in water, pH 3.0), Glycine (Sigma, 500 mM in water, pH 3.0) and Strychnine Hydrochloride (Sigma, 5mM in 165 mM NaCl, pH 3.0). To prevent the drugs leaking out from the pipettes, a retaining current (35-45 nA) of polarity opposite to that of the ejection current was always applied except during the ejection period. The passage of the electrode was observed with an ophthalmoscope and the contact of the electode tip with the area centralis zone (a vessel-free zone, approximately 15° temporal and 5° superior, with respect to the optic nerve head which subtended to 5°) was closely guided using the pivot adjustments of the electrode advancing system (Ikeda and Osborne 1983).

Determination of the effective current

In order to compare the effects of drugs on adult and kitten cells, an effective current was determined for each drug in each cell. The effective current for bicuculline and strychnine was defined as that current which completely abolished the inhibition of the cell to optimal annulus at the receptive field surround. The effective current for GABA and glycine was defined as the strength of the current which extinguished at least 95% of the firing of a given cell to the optimal annulus "off".

In order to determine the effective current, after obtaining control responses, drug application was commenced at the 5 nA level. This was raised in 5 nA - 10 nA steps until the effective current was reached. Each ionophoretic current was maintained for exactly one minute and a further minute was allowed for recovery before an increased dose was given. For strychnine, a 2-4 minute recovery period was allowed for each dose. The negative effect of a drug was defined as less than 5% change in cell firing during 1 min application of the same current which is measured as the effective current of another drug (glycine in the case of GABA and vice versa: strychnine in the case of bicuculline and vice versa). All cells which showed no recovery from drug effects or revealed a change in spike height or waveform during drug application were rejected.

Results

The surround inhibition of ganglion cells could most clearly be demonstrated using an annulus brighter than background (white annulus)in on-centre cells, and an annulus darker than background (black annulus) in off-centre cells. The cells in the area centralis we studied showed strong inhibition when the annulus was present but fired when it was removed from the receptive field surround. Since the receptive field centre was small and the antagonistic surround is sharply defined in adult cells, small annulus (commonly the inner diameter was 2.5^{o} and the outer diameter, 4.5^{o}) produced optimal inhibition. On the other hand, in kitten cells, the receptive field centre was large and the antagonistic surround was widespread and ill-defined, a larger annulus (commonly the inner diameter was 3.3^{o} and the outer diameter, 9.9^{o}) was needed to evoke optimal inhibition.

Figure 1 illustrates responses of an adult on-, kitten on-, adult off- and kitten off-sustained cells in the area centralis stimulated by the optimal annulus at the receptive field surround, obtained before, during and after an application of bicuculline. The on-cells were stimulated by a white annulus, whereas the off-cells were stimulated by a black annulus. The sizes of the annuli were much larger for the kitten cells. All cells gave an inhibition of firing during the annulus "on" (3 sec period) and gave excitatory firing when the annulus was switched off. The strength of bicuculline current used is shown above therecords obtained during the drug application (middle column).

Whereas bicuculline 30 nA was required to block the inhibition of the adult on-cell, that of the kitten on-cell was blocked by as low a current level as 5 nA.

A 4-6 fold difference in the effective current of bicuculline required to block the surround inhibition between adult and kitten on-cells was a common finding. The mean effective bicuculline current which blocked the inhibition to annulus for adult on-cells was 26.0 nA (S.E. = 3.5 nA, n=13), whereas that for the kitten cells was 8.9 nA (S.E. = 1.4 nA, n=9). The difference was statistically significant (p- 0.0005).

However, as illustrated by the response of the off-cells in Fig. 1,

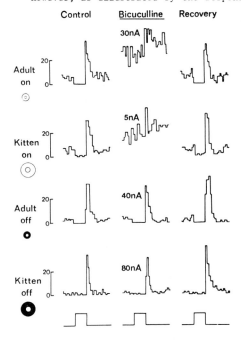

Fig. 1. Peristimulus histograms of responses of an adult on-, kitten on-, adult off- and kitten off-sustained cell in the area centralis to an optimal annulus which causes an inhibition of firing in the cells, obtained before, during and after ionophoretic aplication of bicuculline. The bottom line in each column indicates the timing of stimulus: the upward deflection being the period of the annulus "on" (3 seconds). The strength of current used is shown at the top left of each corresponding trace.

neither the inhibitions of adult off-cells nor those of kitten off-cells
were blocked by bicuculline.

Figure 2 illustrates the response of adult on-,kitten on-, adult off-
and kitten off-sustained cells in the area centralis obtained before,
during and after the effective current of strychnine. The inhibitions of
both the adult and kitten on-cells were unaffected by a relatively high
current of strychnine, whereas those of the adult and kitten on-cells were
completely blocked by strychnine. As for the bicuculline effect upon
on-cells, a much higher current of strychnine was required to block the
adult off-cell inhibition than that needed for the kitten cells'
inhibition. The effective current for the adult off-cell was 30 nA and
that for the kitten off-cell was 5 nA as shown in Fig. 2.

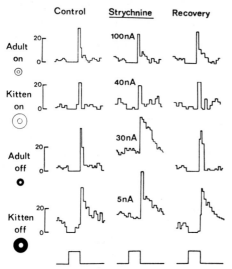

Fig. 2. Peristimulus histograms of responses of an adult
on-, kitten on-, adult off- and
kitten off-sustained cell in
the area centralis to an
optimal annulus which causes an
inhibition of firing in the
cells, obtained before, during
and after ionophoretic application of strychnine. The bottom
line in each column indicates
the timing of stimulus: the
upward deflection being the
period of the annulus "on" (3
seconds). The strength of
current used is shown at the
top left of each corresponding
trace.

The mean effective current of strychnine for blocking the surround
inhibition of adult off-cells was 31.2 nA (S.E. - 2.3 nA, n=25), while
that for the kitten off-cells, 10 nA (S.E. = 2.5 nA, n=9) (p= 0.0005).

Thus, in the kitten area centralis, a lower quantity of transmitter
antagonist was required to block endogenous GABA-mediated inhibition in
on-cells and endogenous glycine-mediated inhibition in off-cells compared
with that required to block the adult cell's visually induced surround
inhibition.

Figure 3 shows pen recorder tracings of the responses of adult on-,
kitten on-, adult off- and kitten off-sustained cells to the otpimal
annulus obtained before, during and after an ionophoretic application of
GABA. GABA virtually abolished the firing of cells to the annulus "off"
and spotaneous activity of both the adult and the kitten on-cells.
Contrary to the results of the antagonists, the kitten cell required a
much higher current (80 nA) than that required by the adult cell (30 nA)
and this observation was applicable to other kitten on-cells. The mean
effective current of GABA for the surround response of adult on-cells was
16.4 nA (S.E. = 2.0 nA, n=11), whereas that for kitten on-cells was 69.4
nA (S.E. = 13.4 nA, n=9) (p = 0.001).

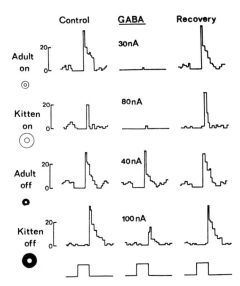

Fig. 3. Peristimulus histograms of responses of an adult on-, kitten on-, adult off- and kitten off-sustained cell in the area centralis to an optimal annulus which causes an inhibition of firing in the cells, obtained before, during and after ionophoretic application of GABA. The bottom line in each column indicates the timing of stimulus: the upward deflection being the period of the annulus "on" (3 seconds). The strength of current used is shown at the top left of each corresponding trace.

Furthermore, although kitten off-cells' visually induced surround inhibition could not be blocked by bicuculline, they were slightly inhibited by the exogenous GABA as illustrated by the kitten off-cell in Fig. 3. On the other hand, no such GABA-induced inhibition was observed in adult off-cells in the area centralis as shown by the adult off-cell in Fig. 3. The current level of GABA by which off-cells were examined was that equal to the effective current of glycine on off-cells as illstrated in Fig. 4. The current levels (40-100nA) of GABA which completely abolished the kitten on-cell firing, usually reduced the firing of kitten off-cells by 20-80%. Thus GABA receptors seem to be present not only upon on-cells but also upon off-cells in the kitten area centralis.

In Figure 4, the responses of adult on-, kitten on-, adult-off, and kitten off-sustained cells to optimal annulus, obtained before, during and after the effective current of glycine are shown. Glycine virtually abolished both the adult and kitten off-cells'firing and the effective current was higher (60 nA) for the kitten cell than the adult cell (25 nA). The mean effective current of glycine for kitten off-cells was 63.1 nA (S.E. - 18.8 nA, n=8), whereas that for adult off-cells, 19.3 nA (S.E. = 2.2 nA, n=14) (p = 0.025).

Furthermore, whilst glycine had no effect on adult on-cells, it inhibited kitten on-cells as Fig. 4 illustrates. When each of the on-cells were tested with the glycine current equal to the effective current of GABA, which completely inhibited these on-cells' firing, a partial inhibition resulting in a 20-80% reduction in cell firing was observed regularly. Thus, although the visually-induced surround inhibition of kitten on-cells was GABA mediated and strychnine failed to block that inhibition, externally-applied glycine could inhibit these cells' firing. This suggested that glycine receptors were indeed present on kitten on-cells but not on adult on-cells.

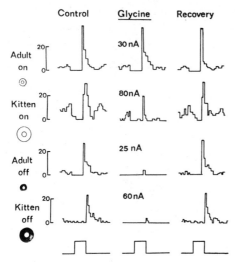

Fig. 4. Peristimulus histograms of responses of an adult
on-, kitten on-, adult off- and
kitten off-sustained cell in
the area centralis to an
optimal annulus which causes an
inhibition of firing in the
cells, obtained before, during
and after ionophoretic application of glycine. The bottom
line in each column indicates
the timing of stimulus: the
upward deflection being the
period of the annulus "on" (3
seconds). The strength of
current used is shown at the
top left of each corresponding
trace.

Discussion

We began this study by asking whether the neurophysiological
observation that the receptive field of 7-9 week old kittens' area
centralis had a weaker inhibitory surround and poorer spatial resolution
than that of adult cells in the area centralis had any pharmacological
basis. The main findings and conclusions were: 1) As in the adult, in
kitten area centralis the surround inhibition of on-cells is mediated by
GABA and that of off-cells is mediated by glycine. However, much higher
ionophoretic currents of GABA and glycine were required to inhibit the
kitten on- and off-cells than the adult on- and off-cells respectively,
i.e. kitten cells have low sensitivity to transmitter agonist . 2)
Whilst GABA had no effect on adult off-cells and glycine had no effect on
adult on-cells, GABA also inhibited the responses of kitten off-cells and
glycine, those of kitten on-cells in the area centralis (i.e. kitten on-
and off-cells have reduced selectivity to inhibitory transmitters). 3)
In spite of the non-selectivity of kitten cells to GABA and glycine, the
specificity of cells to inhibitory transmitter blocking agents was already
adult-like in that bicuculline blocked the visually induced surround
inhibitions purely in on-cells, whereas strychnine blocked the inhibition
purely in off-cells. 4) Nevertheless, much lower ionophoretic currents
of bicuculline and strychnine were enough to block the surround
inhibitions of kitten on- and off-cells than the adult on- and off-cells
respectively (i.e. kitten cells have high sensitivity to transmitter
antagonists).

These differences in GABA, glycine, bicuculline and strychnine actions
found between kitten and adult cells were very subtle. In the absence of
any developmental studies on the synaptic organisation of the cat retina,
the discussions remain speculative. However, we consider that the
observed differences between the kitten and adult cat in transmitter
actions on retinal ganglion cells may be analogous to those found in the
postnatal development of functional synapses at the neuromuscular junction
and sympathetic ganglia for the following reasons.

Firstly, the high sensitivity of kitten cells' inhibition to blocking agents (bicuculline and strychnine) may simply be due to the fact that lower quantities of endogenous GABA and glycine are released by immature presynaptic cells (amacrine). Physiologically this is reflected in the fact that visually-induced inhibitions of kitten cells are weak. A lesser amount of antagonist would be sufficient to block this weak inhibition of kitten cells mediated by a smaller quantity of transmitter than is required to block the strong inhibition mediated by a larger quantity of released transmitter. An analogous situation occurs in the postnatal development of the cholinergic synaptic terminals in the sympathetic ganglia (Bennett and Pettigrew 1974; O'Brien 1983; Hirst and McLachlan 1984). That is, presynaptic terminals which survive grow larger and release progressively larger quantities of transmitter during postnatal development.

Secondly, the low sensitivity of kitten on-cells to exogenous GABA and kitten off-cells to glycine may be explained by another analogy drawn with the developing sympathetic ganglia. Hirst and McLachlan (1984) found that the amplitude of synaptic current was much higher and their response to one quantum of transmitter was more variable in the immature synapse were greater than those in the mature synapse, thus the efficient receptor saturation for a quantum of released transmitter which occurs in the adult might not be present in the immature synapse. If this is so, the quantity of exogenous transmitter (GABA or glycine) required to occupy immature receptors and open ionic channels is larger than that required for mature receptors and this was what we found.

Thirdly, the reduced selectivity of on-cells and off-cells in the kitten to inhibitory transmitters suggests that in the kitten area centralis, GABA receptors are present upon off-cells and glycine receptors, upon on-cells, and that such inappropriate receptors are subsequently eliminated and are no longer present or become non-functional in the adult area centralis. Again examples from developing muscle fibres or Purkinje cells in the cerebellum and cortical cells suggest such mechanism (e.g. Crepel, Mariani, Delhaye-Bouchaud 1976; Rakic 1977; Johnson and Purves 1981; O'Brien 1983).

Kittens begin to have visual experience about 3 weeks after birth when they can climb up their mothers and explore the external visual field: then the development of functional capability of visual cells in the retina and subsequent pathways occurs. Since the postnatal development of chemical neuronal communication in the central nervous system is closely linked to the functional maturation of the specialised neuronal circuitry of the brain (Johnston and Coyle 1981), is it possible that similar developmental changes to those found elsewhere in the nervous system also occur in the maturation of ganglion cell synapses in the highly specialised area (area centralis)of the retina?

Acknowledgement

This work is supported by the Medical Research Council and the Special Trustees of St. Thomas' Hospital. We thank Drs. Gerta Vrbova, Norman Bowery, Jonathan Fry and Keith Ruddock for useful discussions.

264

References

Bennett, M.R. and Pettigrew, A.G. J. Physiol 241, 547-573 (1974).

Crepel, F., Mariani, S. and Delhaye-Bouchaud, N. J. Neurobiol. 7, 567-578 (1976).

Fuortes, MN.G.F., Frank, K. and Becker, M.C. J. Gen. Physiol. 40, 735-752 (1957).

Hirst, G.D.S. and McLachlan, E.M. J. Physiol. 349, 119-134 (1984).

Ikeda, H. J. Roy. Scc. Med. 73, 546-555 (1980).

Ikeda, H. and Osborne, A.E. J. Physiol 339, 4-5P (1983).

Ikeda, H. and Sheardown, M.J. Neurosci. 7, 25-36 (1982).

Ikeda, H. and Sheardown, M.J. Neurosci. 8, 837-853 (1983).

Johnson, D.A. and Purves, D. J. Physiol 318, 143-159 (1981).

Johnson, M.V. and Coyle, J.T. in The Fetus and Independent Life. Ciba Foundation Symposium 86. (London: Pitman 1981 pp. 251-270.

O'Brien, R.A.D. in Somatic and Autonomic Nerve-Muscle Interactions, G. Burnstock, R.A.D. O'Brien and G. Vrbova eds. (Amsterdam: Elsevier Science 1983) pp. 153-184.

Rakic, P. J. Comp Neurol 176, 23-52 (1977).

Are Dendritic Beads Related to Synaptic Loci

S. Vallerga, G. M. Ratto
Instituto di Cibernetica e Biofisica del CNR
Camogli, Italy

The response of retinal neurons depends both on diffusion properties, dictated by the fine morphology, and on the location of synapses over dendrites (Rall 1977; Butz and Cowan 1974; Koch et al 1982). It is therefore interesting to have a global view of all the morphological features contributing to the response, diameter and length of single branches, organization of bifurcations, and synaptic loci. Dendritic spines are light microscopy markers of synapses (Gray 1959), but in the retina they are sparse and barely visible. We studied dendritic beads, a dominant feature of amacrine cells in the fish retina (Vallerga and Deplano 1984; Ratto et al 1984) as alternative synaptic markers at the light microscopy level.

Methods

Retinae of adult specimens of the marine fish bogue (Boops boops) were stained according to a modified rapid Golgi technique (Vallerga and Deplano 1984). We did not measure any shrinkage possibly because the retinae were tightly sandwiched between filter papers throughout impreganation procedure. Camera lucida drawings (1250x, Reichert Polyvar) of well impreganated amacrine cells, viewed in tangential sections of the retina, were examined with a Leitz Mop image analyzer (provided by L. Agnati, Inst. di Fisiologia Umana e Endocrinologia, Univ. di Modena). The data were processed on a PDP11/40 computer with software developed by one of us (GMR).

Results

We measured the geometrical and topological properties of the dendritic beads evaluating their size, shape, total amount of their membrane surface, location over dendrites and their coexistence with cellular structures involved in information processing. The analysis was performed on amacrine cells shown in Figs. 1, 2 and 3; their typology and nomenclature have been described elsewhere (Vallerga and Deplano 1984).

Size
The distributions of the maximum diameters of the dendritic beads are given in Fig. 4. Neuron A and neuron B have similar distributions (Da=2+0.1 μm, Db=2.5+0.1 μm), neuron C has larger beads (Dc=3.1+0.1 μm). Apparently only these two populations of beads are present in the bogue retina.

Shape
To evaluate the bead shape we measured the form factor $F = 4*A/P**2$ which gives a measure of the eccentricity. The mean values of the distributions are: Fa=0.7+4.0.01. Fb=0.71+0.01, Fc=0.73+0.01 (Fig. 5) showing that the shape of dendritic beads is the same and does not depend on their size.

Membrane surface
We evaluated the total membrane surface of the bead population as the number of beads times the surface of the ellipsoid having as diameters the mean values of the major and minor axes of the beads.

266

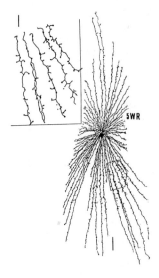

Fig. 1. Neuron A: wide field radiate amacrine cell of the bogue retina, narrowly stratified in the 5th sublayer of the inner plexiform layer (IPL). Upper left an enlargement of the marked area. Bars: bottom 50 μm, in the indent 10 μm.

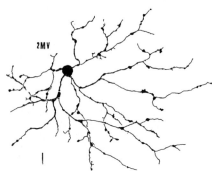

Fig. 2. Neuron B: medium field varicose amacrine cell of the 2nd sublayer of the IPL. Bar: 10 μm.

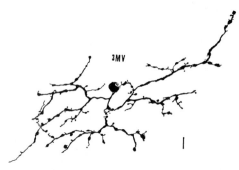

Fig. 3. Neuron C: medium field varicose amacrine cell of the 3rd sublayer of the IPL. Bar: 10 μm.

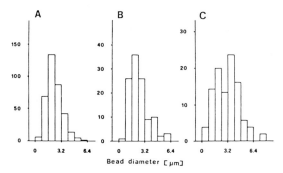

Fig. 4. Distribution of the maximum diameter of dendritic beads for neurons A, B and C. The mean values and standard errors are respectively: Da=2.4+0.1 um, Db=2.5+0.1 um, and Dc=3.1+0.1 um.

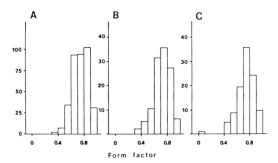

Fig. 5. Shape distribution of dendritic beads. Plots of the form factors (F=4*A/P**2) for neuron A, Fa=0.74+0.01, B, Fb=71+0.01, and C, Fc=0.73+0.01.

The occupancy of beads on dendrites has been calculated considering that the major axes of beads are oriented along dendrites:

Neuron	Total length	Bead length	Free portion
A	2983	871	29%
B	1923	282	15%
C	1146	335	29%

The value of lengths are in microns.

The dendritic membrane surface free from beads is the lateral surface of the cylinder with height equal to the free portion of dendrites and with diameter equal to the mean value of dendritic diameter.

The comparison of the amount membrane surfaces for soma, dendrites and beads gives:

Neuron	Soma	Dendrites	Beads
A	600	7050	5565
B	314	4653	1892
C	314	3639	2777

The values are in square microns.

Spatial Distribution

The maximum density of beads for neurons B and C, whose longest dendrites are within 200 um, occurs at about 100 um. The neuron A has the peak of bead density at 200 um.

Coexistence

a) Spines

In neuron C we counted 58 spines (a dozen of dubious cases were not considered); we investigated the correlation between bead population and spines. If we make the hypothesis of spines randomly located over dendrites, the probability for a spine to fall over a bead is:

$$Pc=BL/TL$$

Where BL is the linear occupancy of beads and TL the total length of dendrites. If we throw a spine over dendrites the possible events are:
1) the spine falls over a bead, with a probability P=0.29
2) the spine does not fall over a bead, with a probability P=0.71

We can test the hypothesis of correlation between beads and spines comparing the expected with the measure frequencies. From the binominal distribution the probability P(k) to have k events with n trials is:

$$P(k)=n! \ (**k) \ (q**(n-k)0/k!(n-k)!$$

In our case we have 58 spines, and 38 spines over beads

$$P(38) \qquad 1$$

Therefore the hypothesis of spines occurring independently of bead location must be disregarded.

In neuron A we have Pc=0.29, 65 spines and 49 coincidences between spines and beads. The probability that spine location does not depend on bead location is:

$$P(49) \qquad 1$$

Therefore also in this case the hypothesis of spines independent from beads does not hold.

b) Bifurcations

The unfolding of ramifications is determined by the number and position of bifurcations, that can be site particularly favorable for inhibitory synapses (Koch et al 1982). The neuron B has 31 bifurcations, of which 18 are occupied by beads, since the linear occupancy of beads over the dendrites is 0.15 a dependence of beads from bifurcations is suggested. We tested such hypothesis through computer simulation with a Monte Carlo-like method.

The simulated cell is defined by:
1) the observed statistics of morphological parameters
2) the observed distance distribution
3) every portion of dendrite has the same probability to receive a head.

The statement 3 derives from the observation that, statistically, the distance distribution for the beads follows the distribution of dendritic density. The distance is calculated along the direct pathway to the soma.

The test is therefore quite simple: we count the coincidences in the simulated cell, if such number is significantly smaller than the observed one, we should admit that bifurcations are privileged sites for beads. If there is no correlation between beads and bifurcations, the probability of coincidence in the simulated cell must be comparable with the same probability in the real cell.

The cell has 5 primary dendrites:

Primary dendrite	Number of bifurc.	Number of beads		Coincidence bead-bifur.		Coincidence bead-tip	
		Real	Simul	Real	Simul	Real	Simul
1	5	22	19	2	0	1	1
2	8	40	43	5	4	4	1
3	3	7	6	2	0	1	1
4	10	28	35	5	1	4	1
5	5	16	10	4	1	2	1

The number of dendritic tips is the number of principal dendrites plus the number of bifurcations. The observed frequency of coexistence of beads with bifurcations is:

$$Pc=0.58 \quad and \quad Pcs=0.14$$

Discussion

We observe in the amacrine cells of the bogue retina two populations of dendritic beads differing in size, but not in shape. They are not randomly distributed over the dendritic field, but preferentiate sites where are located cellular structures important for communication properties of the neuron as dendritic spines and bifurcation points. The total amount of membrane of dendritic beads is comparable with the dendritic membrane free from beads, and is an order of magnitude larger than the membrane surface of the soma.

If dendritic beads subserved a metabolic function one should expect larger size and higher density close to the soma, while their size is constant over the whole dendritic field and their maximum density correspond to the maximum density of dendrites. Furthermore the regression coefficient for bead diameter versus distance from the soma is $4=0.2$, indicating that there is no correlation between the size of a bead and its location over the dendritic field.

We suggest that the spatial relation of beads with cellular features dictating electrotonic properties such as bifurcations, dendritic tips and spines (Koch et al 1982) strongly argue in favour of their participation in neural transmission. A further support to this view is the observation of synapses on beads in amacrine cells of the cat retina (Kolb and Nelson 1983).

References

Butz, E.G. and Cowan, J.D. Biophys. J. 1, 661-689 (1974).
Gray, E.G. J. Anat. 93. (1959).
Koch, C. Poggio, T. and Torre, V. Philos. Trans. R. Soc. London B 298, 227-267 (1982).
Kolb, H. and Nelson, R. Invest. Ophthal. Vis. Sci. 20, 184 (1981).
Rall, W. in Handbook of Physiology. S.E. Geiger, ed. Am. Physiol. Soc. 39-97 (1977).
Ratto, G.M., Vallerga, S. and Cervetto, L. Invest. Ophthal. Vis. Sci. 20, 184 (1984).
Vallerga, S. and Deplano, S. Porc. R. Soc. London B 221, 465-477 (1984).

S U B J E C T   I N D E X

A

Acetylcholine, 171-187

Acidic amino acids (see Glutamate, Aspartate) 171-187

Amacrines

    cat, 215-232

    fish, 141-151, 188-204, 264-268

    primate, 233-244

    rod amacrine 215-232, 233-244

Ammonia (NH$_3$) 77-88

2-amino 4-phosphonobutyrate (APB) 45, 51-65, 236-237

Aspartate 34-50, 99-108

B

Benztropine 205-214

Bicuculline 66-76, 77-88, 256-262

Bipolars

    cat 215-232

    fish 34-50

    primate 233-244

    rods 34-50

Bombesin 152-160

C

Calcium effects 99-108

Carbon dioxide 77-88

Centrifugal fibers 171-187, 252-254

Chlorimipramine 205-214

Color vision 19-33, 194, 109-131, 233-244

Cones

    cat   109-121, 215-232

    double cones 89-98

    oil droplets 89-98

    primate 233-244

    turtle 19-33, 89-98

Corticotropin releasing factor 179

Chromatic adaptation 19-33

Cysteate 99-108

   D

Dendritic beads 265

Dopamine 171-187

    amacrine cells 226

    gap junctions 66-76, 77-88

    horizontal cells 1-18, 66-76

    interplexiform cells 77-88, 152-160

   E

Efferent fibers (see Centrifugal fibers)

Electrical synapses 1-18 (see gap junctions)

Electroretinogram (ERG) 233-244

Enkephalin 171-187

   F

Folic acid 99-108

Fish retina

    bogue (Boops boops) 264-268

    cat fish (Ictalurus punctatus) 141-151

    cyprinid (roach, Rutilis rutilis) 99-108, 188-204

elasmobranch (dogfish shark) 34-50

goldfish (Carrasius auratus) 161-170

mullet (Mugil cephalus) 77-88

white perch (Roccus americana) 1-18

G

Gamma amino butyric acid (GABA) 66-76, 89-98, 152-160, 161-170, 171-187, 215-232, 256-262

Ganglion cells 181

cat 215-232, 257-264

primate 233-244

Gap junctions 66-76, 77-88, 109-121, 215-232

Glutamate 1-18, 34-50, 51-65, 171-187

Glutamic acid decarboxylase (GAD) 161-170

Glucagon 155-156

Glycine 152-160, 171-182, 256-262

H

Horizontal cells 122-140

cat 109-121

fish 1-18, 34-50, 77-88, 99-108

primate 233-244

turtle 19-33, 66-76, 89-98

Horseradish peroxidase (HRP) staining 109-121, 188-204, 215-232

5-hydroxytryptamine (see Serotonin)

I

Indoleamine (see Serotonin) 175-176

Interplexiform cells (see Dopamine) 47-88, 152-160, 171-187

K

Kainate 99-108

Kynurenic acid 99-108

M

Monoclonal antibodies (horizontal cells) 1-18

Motion detection 195

N

Neuropeptides 177

Neuropeptide Y 155, 180

Neurostensin 156, 177-178

O

Oil droplets (in cones) 19-33, 89-98

P

Pancreatic polypeptide (see Neuropeptide Y) 180

Parallel processing 233-244, 257-264

Patch clamping 1-18

Q

Quisqualate 99-108

R

Rods

    amacrines 215-232

    bipolars 29-33

    circuits 109-121, 215-232, 241-242

    horizontal cells 122-140, 109-121

    transmission to bipolars and horizontals 19-33

274

S

Serotonin (5-hydroxytryptamine) 152-160, 171-187, 205-214

Somatostatin 152-160, 161-170, 178

Strychnine 256-262

Substance P 152-160, 177

T

Thyrotropin releasing hormone (TRH) 179-180

Tissue culture

    horizontal cells 1-16

    rabbit retina 205-214

U

Univariance for cones 19-33

V

Vasoactive intestinal peptide (VIP) 179, 156-159